Mind Maps
in
Surgery

Mind Maps
in
Surgery

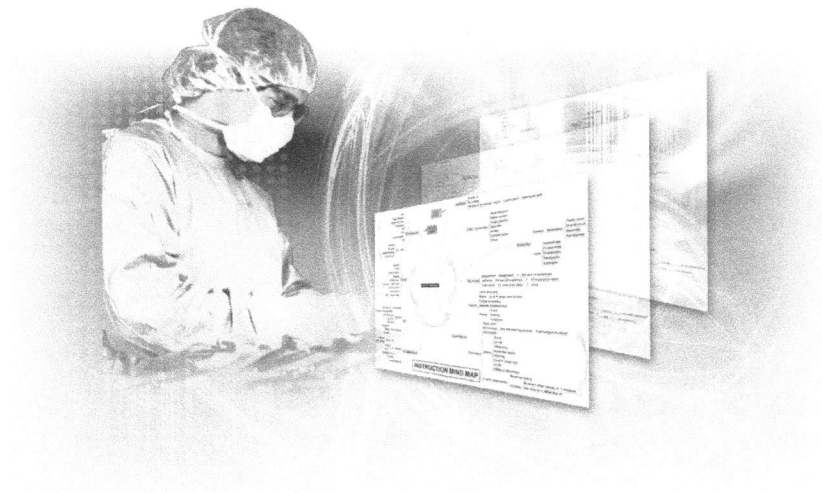

Pouya Youssefi
Pooneh Youssefi
Irving Taylor
University College London, UK

World Scientific

NEW JERSEY · LONDON · SINGAPORE · BEIJING · SHANGHAI · HONG KONG · TAIPEI · CHENNAI

Published by

World Scientific Publishing Co. Pte. Ltd.

5 Toh Tuck Link, Singapore 596224

USA office: 27 Warren Street, Suite 401-402, Hackensack, NJ 07601

UK office: 57 Shelton Street, Covent Garden, London WC2H 9HE

Library of Congress Cataloging-in-Publication Data
Youssefi, Pouya.
    Mind maps in surgery / Pouya Youssefi, Pooneh Youssefi & Irving Taylor.
        p. ; cm.
    Includes index.
    ISBN-13: 978-981-283-436-2 (hardcover : alk. paper)
    ISBN-10: 981-283-436-2 (hardcover : alk. paper)
    ISBN-13: 978-981-283-437-9 (softcover : alk. paper)
    ISBN-10: 981-283-437-0 (softcover : alk. paper)
  1. Surgery--Outlines, syllabi, etc. I. Youssefi, Pooneh. II. Taylor, Irving. III. Title.
    [DNLM: 1. Surgical Procedures, Operative--methods--Outlines. WO 18.2 Y83m 2008]

    RD37.3.Y68 2008
    617--dc22
                                                        2008033970

British Library Cataloguing-in-Publication Data
A catalogue record for this book is available from the British Library.

Typeset by Stallion Press
Email: enquiries@stallionpress.com

CONTENTS

ABBREVIATIONS

#	Fracture
Δ	Change
ΔΔ	Differential Diagnosis
AAA	Abdominal Aortic Aneurysm
ABC	Airway Breathing Circulation
ABPI	Ankle Brachial Pressure Index
Abx	Antibiotics
AF	Atrial Fibrillation
AFB	Acid-Fast Bacilli
AKA	Also Known As
ALP	Alkaline Phosphatase
ALT	Alanine Aminotransferase
AST	Aspartate Transaminase
ATN	Acute Tubular Necrosis
AV	Arteriovenous
AXR	Abdominal X-ray
B12	Vitamin B12
Ba	Barium
BM	Blood Glucose
BP	Blood Pressure
BPH	Benign Prostatic Hyperplasia
BS	Bowel Sounds
Ca	Cancer
Ca^{2+}	Calcium
CCF	Congestive Cardiac Failure
C. Diff	*Clostridium difficile*
CLL	Chronic Lymphocytic Leukaemia
CML	Chronic Myeloid Leukaemia
COC	Combined Oral Contraceptive
COPD	Chronic Obstructive Pulmonary Disease
CSF	Cerebrospinal Fluid
CVA	Cerebrovascular Accident
CVP	Central Venous Pressure
CXR	Chest X-ray

DM	Diabetes Mellitus
DVT	Deep Venous Thrombosis
ECF	Extracellular Fluid
ESWL	Extracorporeal Shock Wave Lithotripsy
ER	Oestrogen Receptor
ERCP	Endoscopic Retrograde Cholangiopancreatogram
FAST	Focused Abdominal Sonography in Trauma
FBC	Full Blood Count
Fe	Iron
GIT	Gastrointestinal Tract
Gynae	Gynaecology
Hb	Haemoglobin
HCl	Hydrochloric acid
HR	Heart Rate
Hrs	Hours
Hx	History
I&D	Incision & Drainage
ICF	Intracellular Fluid
ICP	Intracranial Pressure
IV	Intravenous
IVU	Intravenous Urogram
Ix	Investigation
JVP	Jugular Venous Pressure
K^+	Potassium
KUB	Kidneys Ureters Bladder
LFTs	Liver Function Tests
LIF	Left Iliac Fossa
LLQ	Left Lower Quadrant
LN	Lymph Node
LOC	Loss of Consciousness
LUQ	Left Upper Quadrant
LVF	Left Ventricular Failure
MAO	Monoamine Oxidase
MC + S	Microscopy, Culture + Sensitivity
Mets	Metastases
Mg^{2+}	Magnesium
MILS	Manual In-Line Stabilization
MOVU	Minimal Obligatory Volume of Urine
MRCP	Magnetic Resonance Cholangiopancreatogram
MRSA	Methicillin Resistant *Staphylococcus aureus*
MSU	Mid-stream Urine
Mx	Management
Na^+	Sodium
NBM	Nil By Mouth
NG	Nasogastric
NSAIDs	Non-Steroidal Anti-Inflammatory Drugs
O/E	On Examination
PE	Pulmonary Embolus
Pec	Pectoralis
PP	Pulse Pressure
PPI	Proton Pump Inhibitors
PR	Per Rectum

PR	Progesterone Receptor
PT	Prothrombin Time
PTC	Percutaneous Trans-Hepatic Cholangiography
PUO	Pyrexia of Unknown Origin
PV	Per Vaginum
Rh	Rhesus
RIF	Right Iliac Fossa
RLQ	Right Lower Quadrant
RUQ	Right Upper Quadrant
Rx	Treatment
SIADH	Syndrome of Inappropriate Anti-Diuretic Hormone
SBP	Systolic Blood Pressure
SOB	Shortness of Breath
Sx	Symptoms
TB	Tuberculosis
TED	Thrombo-Embolic Deterrant
TIA	Transient Ischaemic Attack
TIBC	Total Iron Binding Capacity
TNM	Tumour Node Metastases
U&Es	Urea & Electrolytes
USS	Ultrasound Scan
WCC	White Cell Count
X-Match	Cross-Match
Yrs	Years

ACKNOWLEDGMENTS

Medical Knowledge Acknowledgment

Whilst every effort has been made to ensure the information in this book is accurate and true at the time of going to press, neither the authors nor the publisher can accept any legal liability or responsibility for any omissions or errors that may have been made. Readers are strongly advised to confirm that the information is in keeping with current standards of practice, especially with regard to drug usage.

Buzan Acknowledgment

Mind Map is the Registered Trademark of the Buzan Organization, used with permission. Mind Mapping, originated by Tony Buzan in the late 1960s, is a powerful graphical technique which uses different cortical skills to aid information learning and memory acquisition.

Pouya Youssefi BSc (Hons) MBBS

Specialty Registrar in Cardiothoracic Surgery, The John Radcliffe Hospital. Core Surgery Trainee, Oxford Deanery. Anatomy Demonstrator, University of Oxford. Previous Foundation Doctor in Academic Surgery at University College London Hospital.

Pooneh Youssefi BSc MBBS

Specialist Registrar in General Practice. Previous surgical trainee and anatomy demonstrator at University College London Hospital and Royal Free Hospital.

Irving Taylor

Professor of Surgery, Vice-Dean and Director of Clinical Studies at University College London. Main surgical interests are surgical oncology and particularly colorectal cancer and liver metastases. Published over 600 publications in peer review journals, approximately half related to aspects of GI malignancy, and the author or editor of 24 books. Currently the President of the European Society of Surgical Oncology, Chair of the Royal College of Surgeons of England Professional Standards Committee and a member of the Chief Medical Officer's Medical Revalidation and Education Working Group.

MIND MAPS IN SURGERY

Introduction (*Pouya Youssefi, Pooneh Youssefi*)

Mind Maps® in Surgery uses a concise and visually-stimulating method to teach the reader the main topics in surgery. It is aimed at undergraduate medical students doing their surgical rotations, as well as revising for finals exams. It should also be useful for surgical trainees working towards their membership exams, as well as nurses in the surgical profession.

Each *Mind Map®* covers a particular topic, disease, or condition. All the information that can be found in multiple pages of a surgical text is summarized in one *Mind Map®*. It takes away the endless unimportant words which make up multiple paragraphs in a text, and presents the information in carefully structured pathways containing only the very important necessary keywords, without losing the details. What is produced is one *Mind Map®* covering a surgical disorder, which discusses pathophysiology; aetiology; symptoms and signs; investigation; differential diagnosis, and management. The branches are structured and wired in a very logical way — the same way that most people store information in their memory. The various shapes of the branches provide a visual stimulus for memory creation. Almost all the *Mind Maps®* follow the same structure, having main branches for aetiology, symptoms and signs, investigations, and treatment. This, again, provides a simple framework for learning and the revision of core topics. The reader will also be able to write notes to add information onto the *Mind Maps®* as they wish.

There are also *Mind Maps®* which are very exam oriented, e.g. Examining a Lump. These give the reader a very structured plan of method and are extremely useful for practical exams. This is one of the strengths of the book: it covers all the information needed for taking both written and practical exams. As well as covering all the major types of surgery, there is also a chapter on the Acutely Ill Patient. This topic covers the management of trauma, shock, head injuries, and burns. The chapter on The Surgical Patient provides information regarding pre-op management, post-op complications, as well as fluid and nutrition balance. These are topics that are vitally important for the student to have a good grasp of knowledge and understanding before their exams.

Pouya Youssefi
Pooneh Youssefi

Introduction (*Irving Taylor*)

Many years of bedside teaching to both medical students and postgraduates in surgery has convinced me of the imperative for trainees to develop logical ways of thinking about clinical problems so that information acquired by this experience can be retained and usefully developed both for primary learning as well as for passing examinations.

Medical students and junior trainees in surgery tend to learn in a similar fashion. They see and develop experience on clinical cases and management problems, and subsequently read available relevant literature so that they will remember the clinical condition. This technique allows reflection and defines the acquisition of experience and clinical wisdom.

When revising for summative examinations, these clinical scenarios act as a foundation and provide an infrastructure for retaining relevant information, supplemented by textbooks. Unfortunately, most texts are cluttered with flamboyant language which can camouflage the important necessary information for revision.

Mind Maps® in Surgery is an attempt to provide and connect all these necessary pathways in a manner which replicates the way in which we acquire and retain important information. Each *Mind Map®* deals with a single condition or topic in a structured and focussed manner. It follows the pattern by which we learn and provides in a logical manner relevant information as well as a visual stimulus and vehicle for memorising, creation and storage.

By following the clockwise nature of the *Mind Maps®*, students would be able to acquire the appropriate information and understand about the clinical conditions which otherwise would necessitate many pages of intense concentration and memorisation from surgical textbooks.

Needless to say, *Mind Maps®* should be used in collaboration with other techniques of learning and thus cannot displace the crucial bedside clinical experience. It is the hope of the authors that *Mind Maps® in Surgery* will provide a unique learning and revision technique such that it provides individuals with a simple, logical, and effective method of acquiring and retaining crucial and relevant information.

Irving Taylor

How to Use the Mind Maps

Mind Maps® use the technique of pathways to connect important relevant information, with only the important pertinent words being used. There will be one *Mind Map®* for each topic, for e.g. the acute abdomen. Visualize the *Mind Map®* as a clock. The reader has to start at the 12 o'clock position, and work their way in a clockwise direction around the *Mind Map®*. Each branch and sub-branch should in turn be read in a clockwise direction. Thus, for branches on the right hand side of the page, the sub-branches should be read starting from the top one, and working downwards. For branches on the left hand side of the page, the sub-branches should be read starting from the bottom one, and working upwards.

INSTRUCTION MIND MAP

ACUTE ABDOMEN

START HERE

FINISH HERE

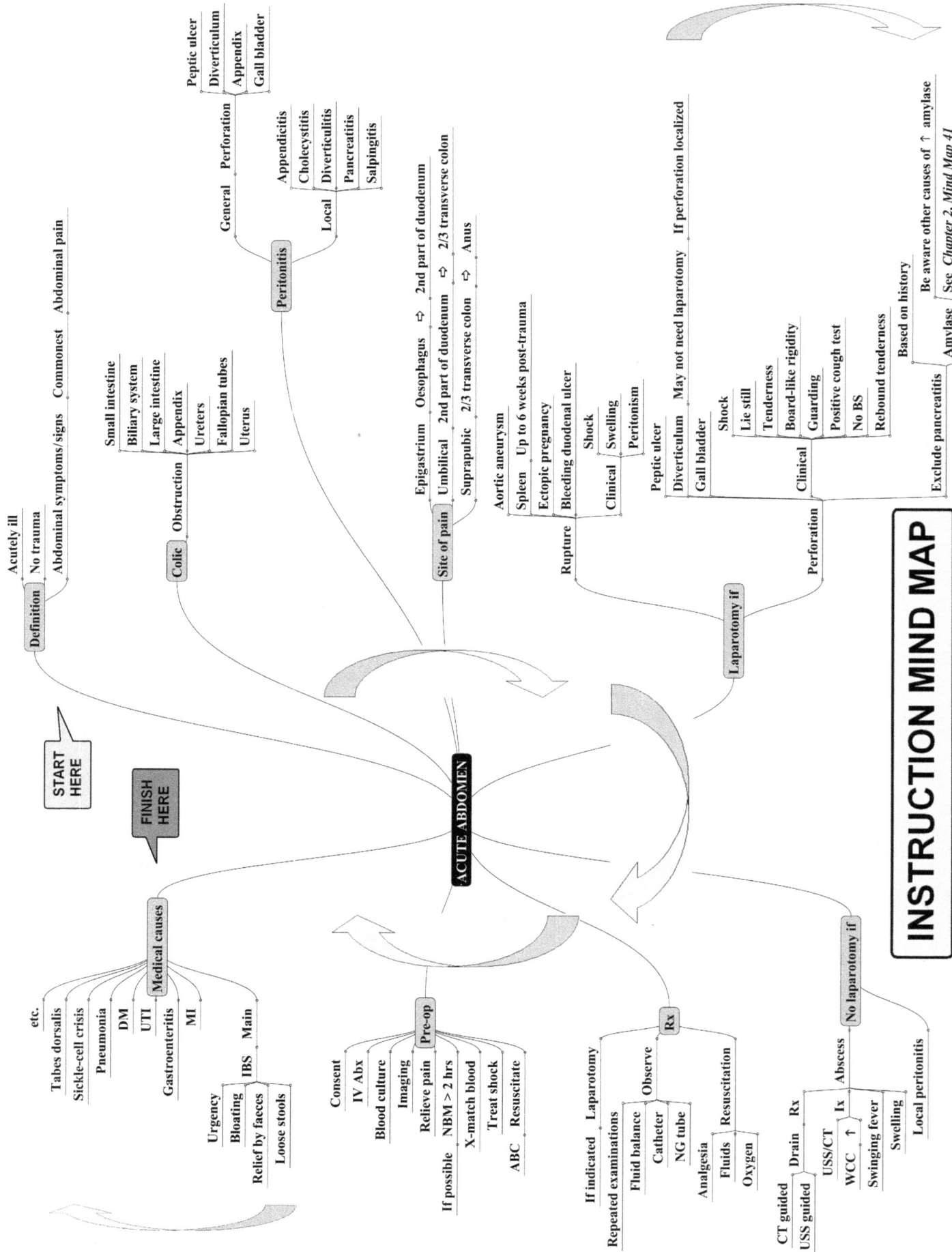

INSTRUCTION MIND MAP

Definition
- Acutely ill
- No trauma
- Abdominal symptoms/signs — Commonest — Abdominal pain

Colic — Obstruction
- Small intestine
- Biliary system
- Large intestine
- Appendix
- Ureters
- Fallopian tubes
- Uterus

Peritonitis
- General — Perforation
  - Peptic ulcer
  - Diverticulum
  - Appendix
  - Gall bladder
- Local
  - Appendicitis
  - Cholecystitis
  - Diverticulitis
  - Pancreatitis
  - Salpingitis

Site of pain
- Epigastrium — Oesophagus ⇔ 2nd part of duodenum
- Umbilical — 2nd part of duodenum ⇔ 2/3 transverse colon
- Suprapubic — 2/3 transverse colon ⇔ Anus

Rupture
- Aortic aneurysm
- Spleen — Up to 6 weeks post-trauma
- Ectopic pregnancy
- Bleeding duodenal ulcer
- Clinical — Shock / Swelling / Peritonism

Perforation
- Peptic ulcer
- Diverticulum — May not need laparotomy — If perforation localized
- Gall bladder
- Clinical
  - Shock
  - Lie still
  - Tenderness
  - Board-like rigidity
  - Guarding
  - Positive cough test
  - No BS
  - Rebound tenderness
- Exclude pancreatitis — Amylase — Based on history / Be aware other causes of ↑ amylase — See *Chapter 2, Mind Map 41*

Laparotomy if

No laparotomy if
- Abscess
  - Rx — Drain — CT guided / USS guided
  - Ix — USS/CT / WCC ↑ / Swinging fever / Swelling
- Local peritonitis

Rx
- If indicated — Laparotomy
- Repeated examinations
- Fluid balance
- Observe — Catheter / NG tube
- Resuscitation — Analgesia / Fluids / Oxygen

Pre-op
- Consent
- IV Abx
- Blood culture
- Imaging
- Relieve pain — If possible / NBM > 2 hrs
- X-match blood
- Treat shock
- Resuscitate — ABC

Medical causes
- etc.
- Tabes dorsalis
- Sickle-cell crisis
- Pneumonia
- DM
- UTI
- Gastroenteritis
- MI
- IBS — Main
  - Urgency
  - Bloating
  - Relief by faeces
  - Loose stools

Chapter 1

GASTROINTESTINAL

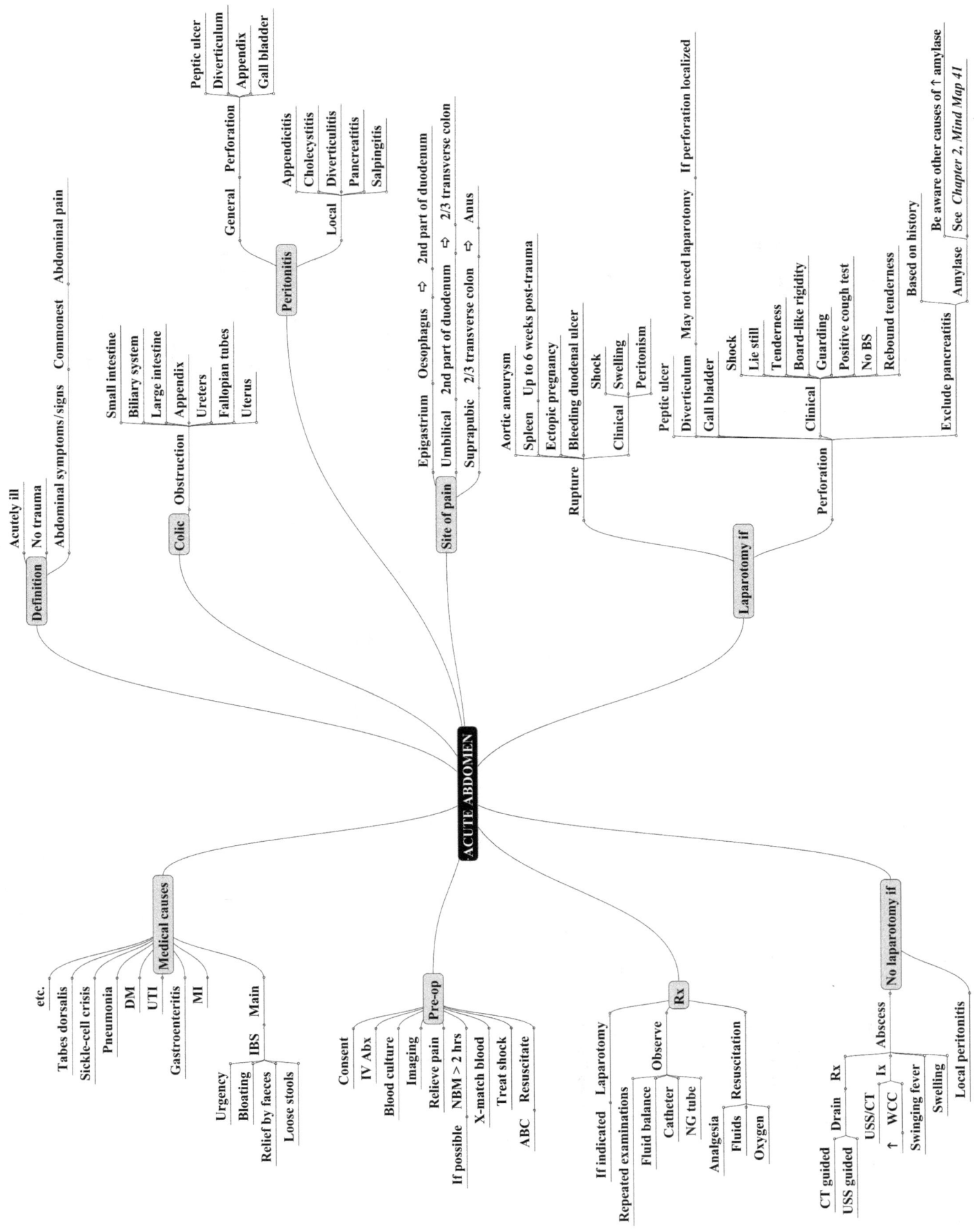

ACUTE ABDOMEN

Definition
- Acutely ill
- No trauma
- Abdominal symptoms/signs
- Commonest — Abdominal pain

Colic — Obstruction
- Small intestine
- Biliary system
- Large intestine
- Appendix
- Ureters
- Fallopian tubes
- Uterus

Peritonitis
- General — Perforation
  - Peptic ulcer
  - Diverticulum
  - Appendix
  - Gall bladder
- Local
  - Appendicitis
  - Cholecystitis
  - Diverticulitis
  - Pancreatitis
  - Salpingitis

Site of pain
- Epigastrium — Oesophagus ⇧ 2nd part of duodenum
- Umbilical — 2nd part of duodenum ⇧ 2/3 transverse colon
- Suprapubic — 2/3 transverse colon ⇧ Anus

Laparotomy if
- Rupture
  - Aortic aneurysm
  - Spleen — Up to 6 weeks post-trauma
  - Ectopic pregnancy
  - Bleeding duodenal ulcer
  - Clinical
    - Shock
    - Swelling
    - Peritonism
- Perforation
  - Peptic ulcer
  - Diverticulum — May not need laparotomy — If perforation localized
  - Gall bladder
  - Clinical
    - Shock
    - Lie still
    - Tenderness
    - Board-like rigidity
    - Guarding
    - Positive cough test
    - No BS
    - Rebound tenderness
  - Exclude pancreatitis — Amylase
    - Based on history
    - Be aware other causes of ↑ amylase
    - See *Chapter 2, Mind Map 41*

Medical causes
- etc.
- Tabes dorsalis
- Sickle-cell crisis
- Pneumonia
- DM
- UTI
- Gastroenteritis
- MI
- IBS — Main
  - Urgency
  - Bloating
  - Relief by faeces
  - Loose stools

Pre-op
- Consent
- IV Abx
- Blood culture
- Imaging
- Relieve pain — If possible — NBM > 2 hrs
- X-match blood
- Treat shock
- Resuscitate — ABC

Rx
- If indicated — Laparotomy
- Repeated examinations
- Fluid balance
- Catheter
- NG tube
- Observe
- Analgesia
- Fluids — Resuscitation
- Oxygen

No laparotomy if
- Abscess
  - Drain — Rx
    - CT guided
    - USS guided
  - Ix
    - USS/CT
    - ↑ WCC
    - Swinging fever
  - Swelling
- Local peritonitis

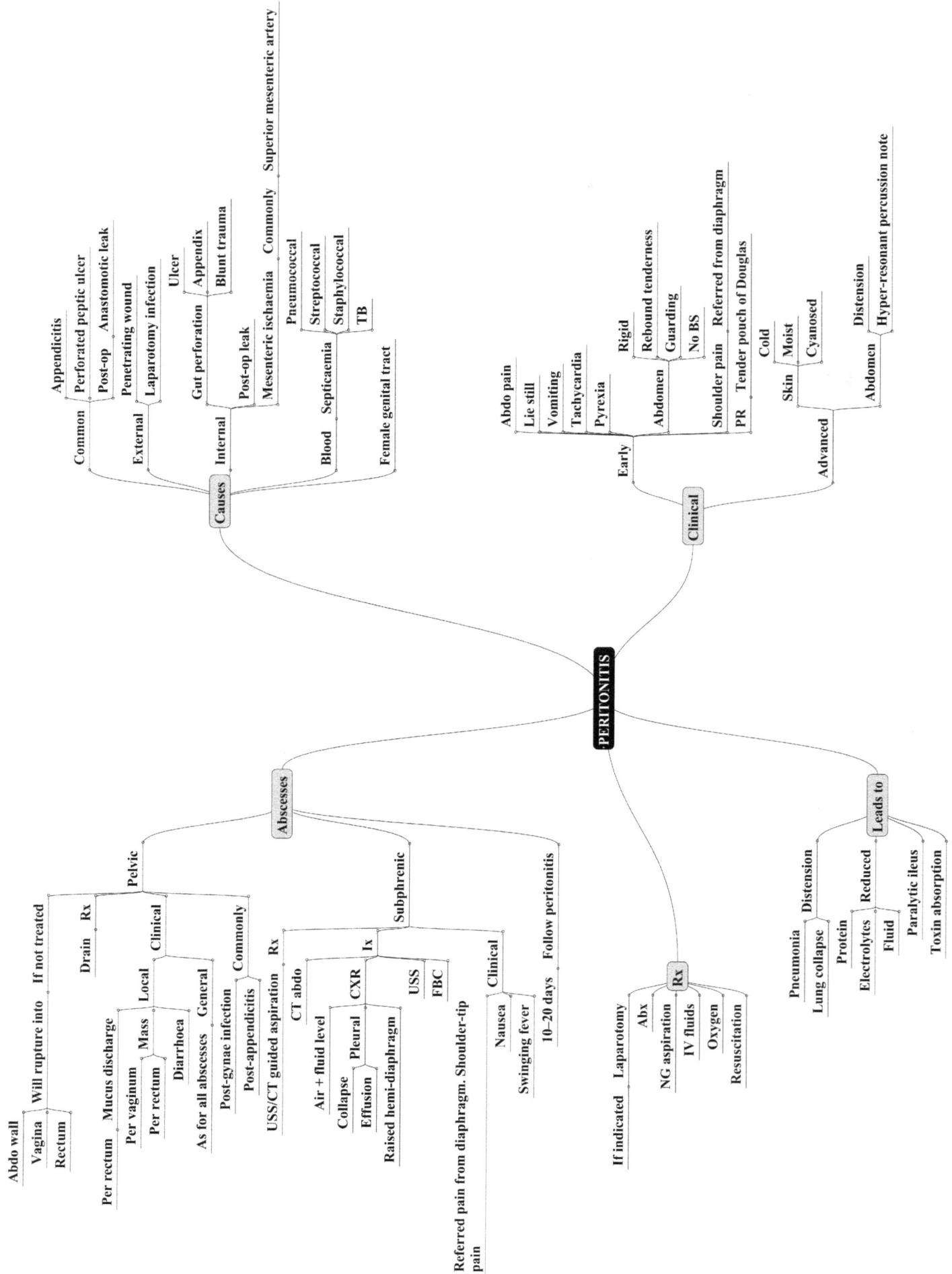

PERITONITIS

Causes

Common
- Appendicitis
- Perforated peptic ulcer
- Post-op — Anastomotic leak

External
- Penetrating wound
- Laparotomy infection

Internal
- Gut perforation
  - Ulcer
  - Appendix
  - Blunt trauma
- Post-op leak
- Mesenteric ischaemia — Commonly — Superior mesenteric artery
- Pneumococcal

Blood — Septicaemia
- Streptococcal
- Staphylococcal
- TB

Female genital tract

Clinical

Early
- Abdo pain
- Lie still
- Vomiting
- Tachycardia
- Pyrexia
- Abdomen
  - Rigid
  - Rebound tenderness
  - Guarding
  - No BS
- Shoulder pain — Referred from diaphragm
- PR — Tender pouch of Douglas

Advanced
- Skin
  - Cold
  - Moist
  - Cyanosed
- Abdomen
  - Distension
  - Hyper-resonant percussion note

Abscesses

Pelvic
- Abdo wall
- Will rupture into
  - Vagina
  - Rectum
- If not treated
- Drain — Rx
- Clinical
  - Per rectum — Mucus discharge
  - Local
    - Per vaginum — Mass
    - Per rectum
    - Diarrhoea
  - General — As for all abscesses
- Commonly
  - Post-gynae infection
  - Post-appendicitis
- Rx — USS/CT guided aspiration

Subphrenic
- Ix
  - CT abdo
  - CXR
    - Air + fluid level
    - Collapse
    - Pleural
    - Effusion
    - Raised hemi-diaphragm
  - USS
  - FBC
- Rx
- Clinical
  - Nausea
  - Swinging fever
- 10–20 days — Follow peritonitis
- Referred pain from diaphragm. Shoulder-tip pain

Rx
- If indicated — Laparotomy
- Abx
- NG aspiration
- IV fluids
- Oxygen
- Resuscitation

Leads to
- Pneumonia
- Distension
  - Lung collapse
  - Protein
- Reduced
  - Electrolytes
  - Fluid
- Paralytic ileus
- Toxin absorption

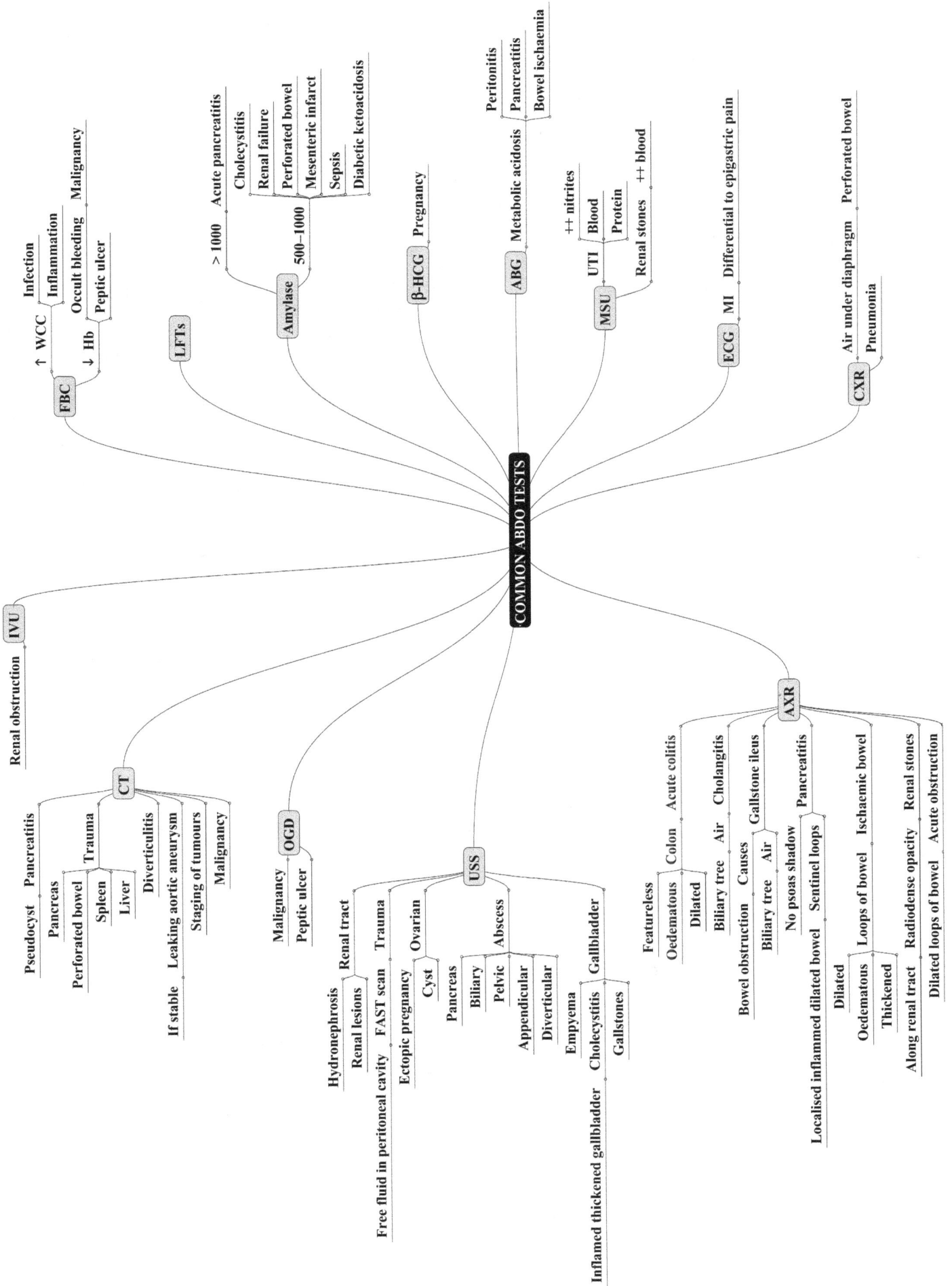

COMMON ABDO TESTS

FBC
- ↑ WCC
  - Infection
  - Inflammation
- ↓ Hb
  - Occult bleeding
  - Malignancy
  - Peptic ulcer

LFTs

Amylase
- > 1000 — Acute pancreatitis
- 500–1000
  - Cholecystitis
  - Renal failure
  - Perforated bowel
  - Mesenteric infarct
  - Sepsis
  - Diabetic ketoacidosis

β-HCG
- Pregnancy

ABG
- Metabolic acidosis
  - Peritonitis
  - Pancreatitis
  - Bowel ischaemia

MSU
- UTI
  - ++ nitrites
  - ++ Blood
  - Protein
- Renal stones — ++ blood

ECG
- MI — Differential to epigastric pain

CXR
- Air under diaphragm — Perforated bowel
- Pneumonia

IVU
- Renal obstruction

CT
- Pseudocyst — Pancreatitis
- Pancreas
- Perforated bowel — Trauma
  - Spleen
  - Liver
- Diverticulitis
- If stable — Leaking aortic aneurysm
- Staging of tumours
- Malignancy

OGD
- Malignancy
- Peptic ulcer

USS
- Hydronephrosis — Renal tract
- Renal lesions
- Free fluid in peritoneal cavity — FAST scan — Trauma
- Ectopic pregnancy — Ovarian
  - Cyst
  - Pancreas
  - Biliary
  - Pelvic
- Appendicular — Abscess
- Diverticular
- Empyema
- Inflamed thickened gallbladder — Cholecystitis — Gallbladder
- Gallstones

AXR
- Featureless — Colon — Acute colitis
- Oedematous — Dilated
- Biliary tree — Air — Cholangitis
- Bowel obstruction — Causes — Gallstone ileus
  - Biliary tree — Air
- No psoas shadow — Pancreatitis
- Localised inflammed dilated bowel — Sentinel loops
  - Dilated
  - Oedematous — Loops of bowel — Ischaemic bowel
  - Thickened
- Along renal tract — Radiodense opacity — Renal stones
- Dilated loops of bowel — Acute obstruction

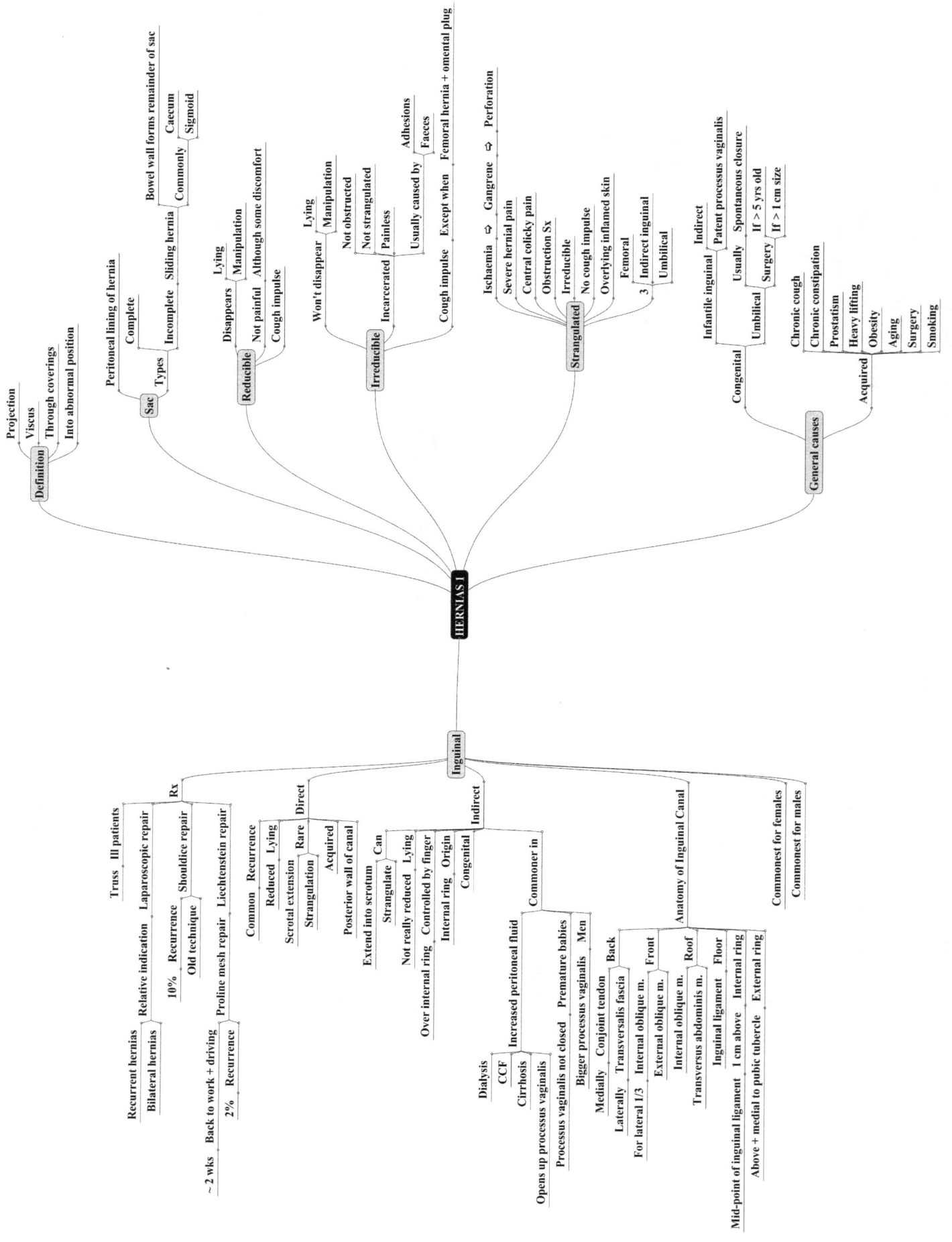

HERNIAS 1

Definition
- Projection
  - Viscus
  - Through coverings
  - Into abnormal position

Sac
- Peritoneal lining of hernia
- Types
  - Complete
  - Incomplete
  - Sliding hernia
    - Bowel wall forms remainder of sac
      - Commonly
        - Caecum
        - Sigmoid

Reducible
- Disappears
  - Lying
  - Manipulation
- Not painful — Although some discomfort
- Cough impulse

Irreducible
- Incarcerated
  - Won't disappear
    - Lying
    - Manipulation
  - Not obstructed
  - Not strangulated
  - Painless
- Usually caused by
  - Adhesions
  - Faeces
- Cough impulse — Except when — Femoral hernia + omental plug

Strangulated
- Ischaemia ⇨ Gangrene ⇨ Perforation
- Severe hernial pain
- Central colicky pain
- Obstruction Sx
- Irreducible
- No cough impulse
- Overlying inflamed skin
- Femoral
- Indirect inguinal — 3
- Umbilical

General causes
- Congenital
  - Infantile inguinal
  - Indirect
    - Patent processus vaginalis
      - Usually — Spontaneous closure
        - If > 5 yrs old
        - Surgery — If > 1 cm size
  - Umbilical
- Acquired
  - Chronic cough
  - Chronic constipation
  - Prostatism
  - Heavy lifting
  - Obesity
  - Aging
  - Surgery
  - Smoking

Inguinal
- Rx
  - Truss — Ill patients
  - Laparoscopic repair
    - Recurrent hernias
    - Bilateral hernias — Relative indication
  - Recurrence — 10%
  - Shouldice repair — Old technique
  - Liechtenstein repair
    - Proline mesh repair
    - Back to work + driving — ~ 2 wks
    - Recurrence — 2%
- Direct
  - Common — Recurrence
  - Reduced — Lying
  - Scrotal extension — Rare
  - Strangulation
  - Acquired
  - Posterior wall of canal
- Indirect
  - Can
    - Extend into scrotum
    - Strangulate
  - Not really reduced — Lying
  - Over internal ring — Controlled by finger
  - Internal ring — Origin
  - Congenital
  - Commoner in
    - Increased peritoneal fluid
      - Dialysis
      - CCF
      - Cirrhosis
    - Processus vaginalis not closed — Opens up processus vaginalis
    - Premature babies — Bigger processus vaginalis
    - Men
- Anatomy of Inguinal Canal
  - Back
    - Conjoint tendon — Medially
    - Transversalis fascia — Laterally
  - Front
    - Internal oblique m. — For lateral 1/3
    - External oblique m.
  - Roof
    - Internal oblique m.
    - Transversus abdominis m.
  - Floor — Inguinal ligament
  - Internal ring — Mid-point of inguinal ligament — 1 cm above
  - External ring — Above + medial to pubic tubercle
- Commonest for females
- Commonest for males

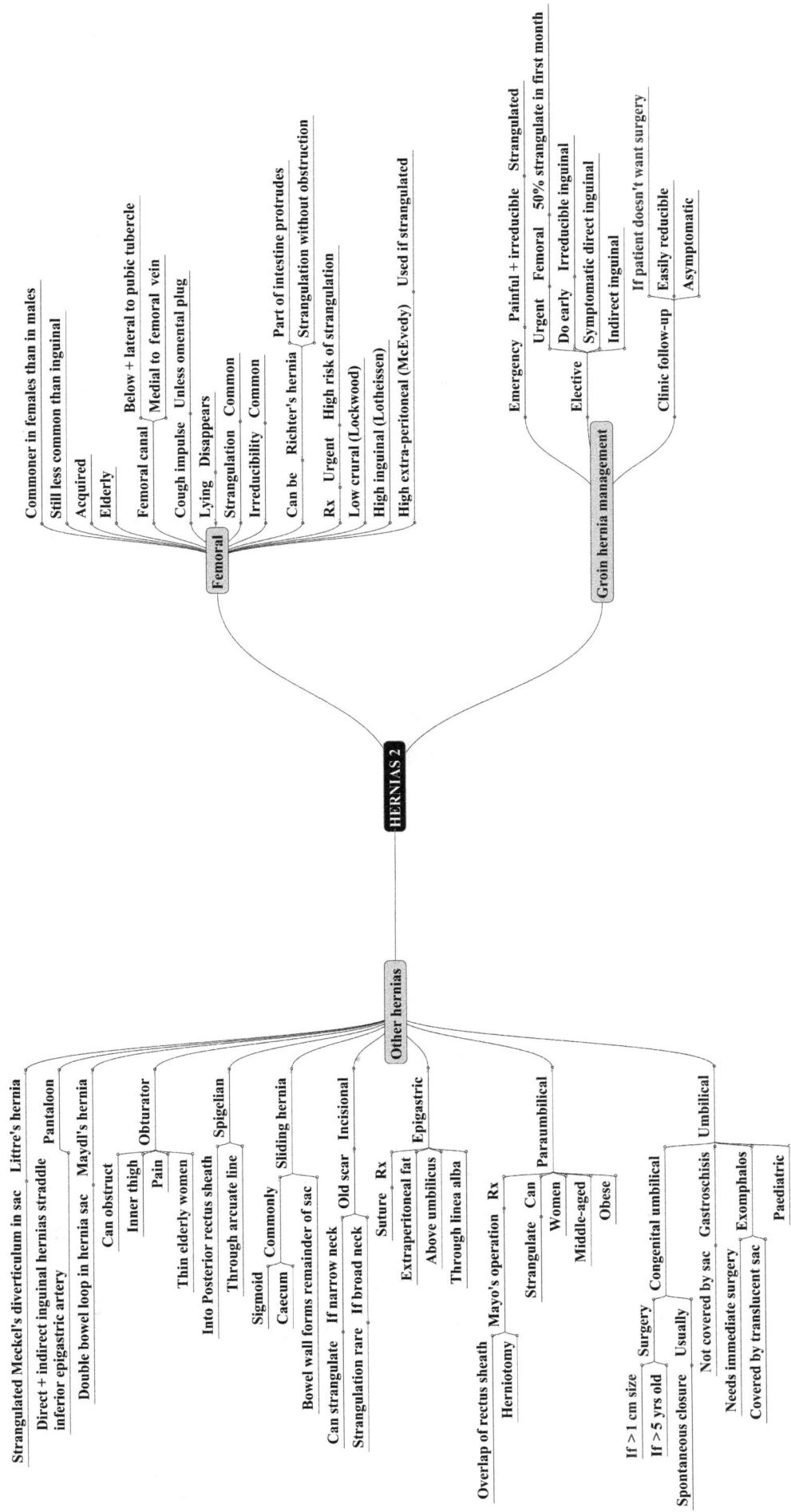

HERNIAS 2

Femoral
- Commoner in females than in males
- Still less common than inguinal
- Acquired
- Elderly
- Femoral canal
  - Below + lateral to pubic tubercle
  - Medial to femoral vein
- Cough impulse — Unless omental plug
- Lying — Disappears
- Strangulation — Common
- Irreducibility — Common
- Can be — Richter's hernia
  - Part of intestine protrudes
  - Strangulation without obstruction
- Rx — Urgent — High risk of strangulation
  - Low crural (Lockwood)
  - High inguinal (Lotheissen)
  - High extra-peritoneal (McEvedy) — Used if strangulated

Groin hernia management
- Emergency
  - Painful + irreducible
  - Strangulated
- Urgent — Femoral — 50% strangulate in first month
- Elective — Do early
  - Irreducible inguinal
  - Symptomatic direct inguinal
  - Indirect inguinal
- Clinic follow-up — If patient doesn't want surgery
  - Easily reducible
  - Asymptomatic

Other hernias
- Strangulated Meckel's diverticulum in sac — Littre's hernia
- Direct + indirect inguinal hernias straddle inferior epigastric artery — Pantaloon
- Double bowel loop in hernia sac — Maydl's hernia
  - Can obstruct
- Obturator
  - Inner thigh
  - Pain
  - Thin elderly women
- Into Posterior rectus sheath — Spigelian
  - Through arcuate line
- Sliding hernia
  - Sigmoid
  - Caecum — Commonly
  - Bowel wall forms remainder of sac
- Incisional
  - Can strangulate — If narrow neck
  - Strangulation rare — If broad neck
  - Old scar
  - Rx — Suture
- Epigastric
  - Extraperitoneal fat
  - Above umbilicus
  - Through linea alba
- Paraumbilical
  - Rx — Mayo's operation
    - Overlap of rectus sheath
    - Herniotomy
  - Can — Strangulate
  - Women
  - Middle-aged
  - Obese
- Umbilical
  - Congenital umbilical
    - If >1 cm size — Surgery
    - If >5 yrs old — Surgery
    - Spontaneous closure — Usually
  - Gastroschisis
    - Not covered by sac
    - Needs immediate surgery
  - Exomphalos
    - Covered by translucent sac
    - Paediatric

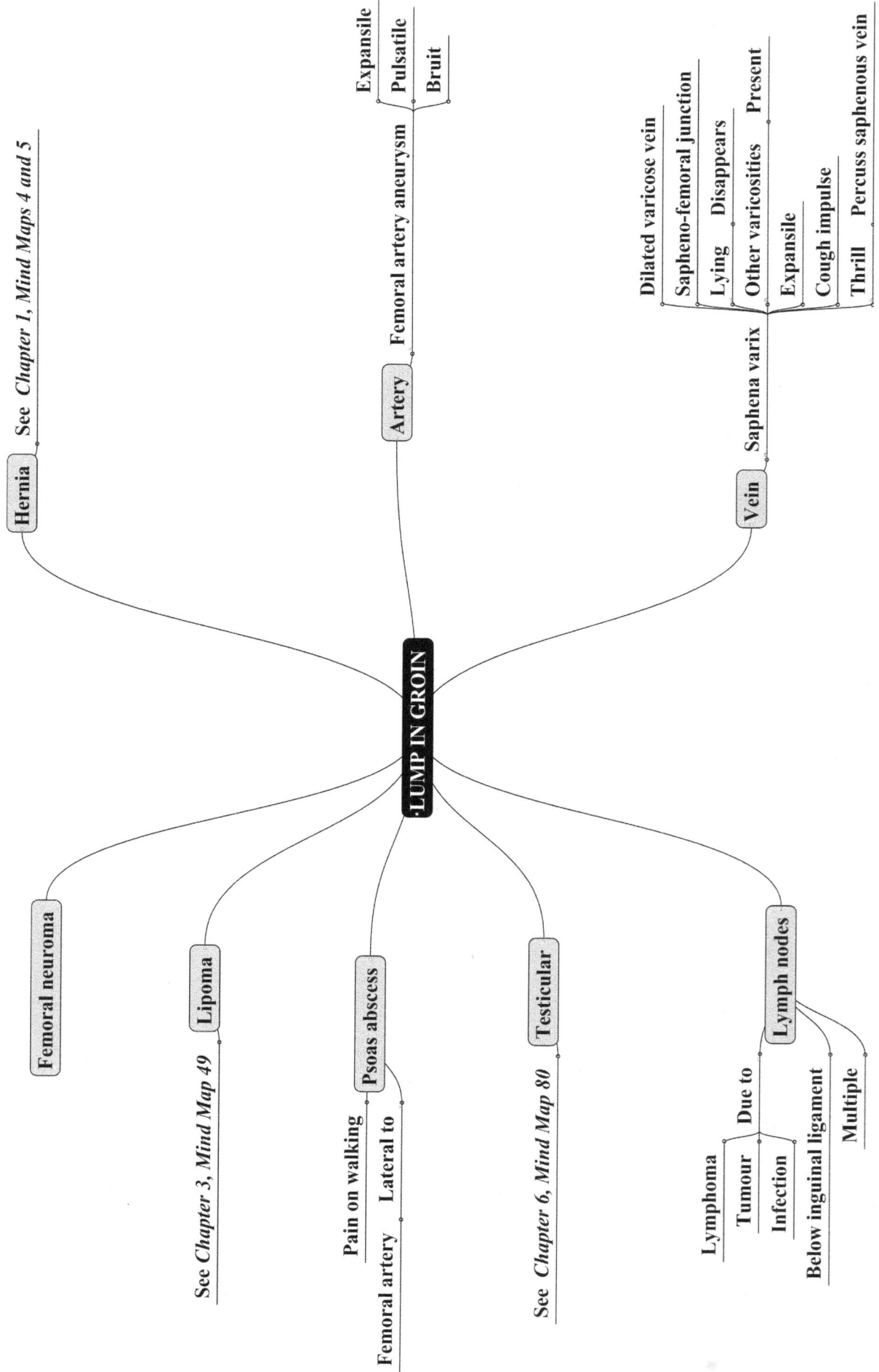

LUMP IN GROIN

Hernia — See *Chapter 1, Mind Maps 4 and 5*

Artery — Femoral artery aneurysm
- Expansile
- Pulsatile
- Bruit

Vein — Saphena varix
- Dilated varicose vein
- Sapheno-femoral junction
  - Lying
  - Disappears
- Other varicosities — Present
- Expansile
- Cough impulse
- Thrill — Percuss saphenous vein

Femoral neuroma

Lipoma — See *Chapter 3, Mind Map 49*

Psoas abscess
- Pain on walking
- Femoral artery — Lateral to

Testicular — See *Chapter 6, Mind Map 80*

Lymph nodes
- Lymphoma
- Due to
  - Tumour
  - Infection
- Below inguinal ligament
- Multiple

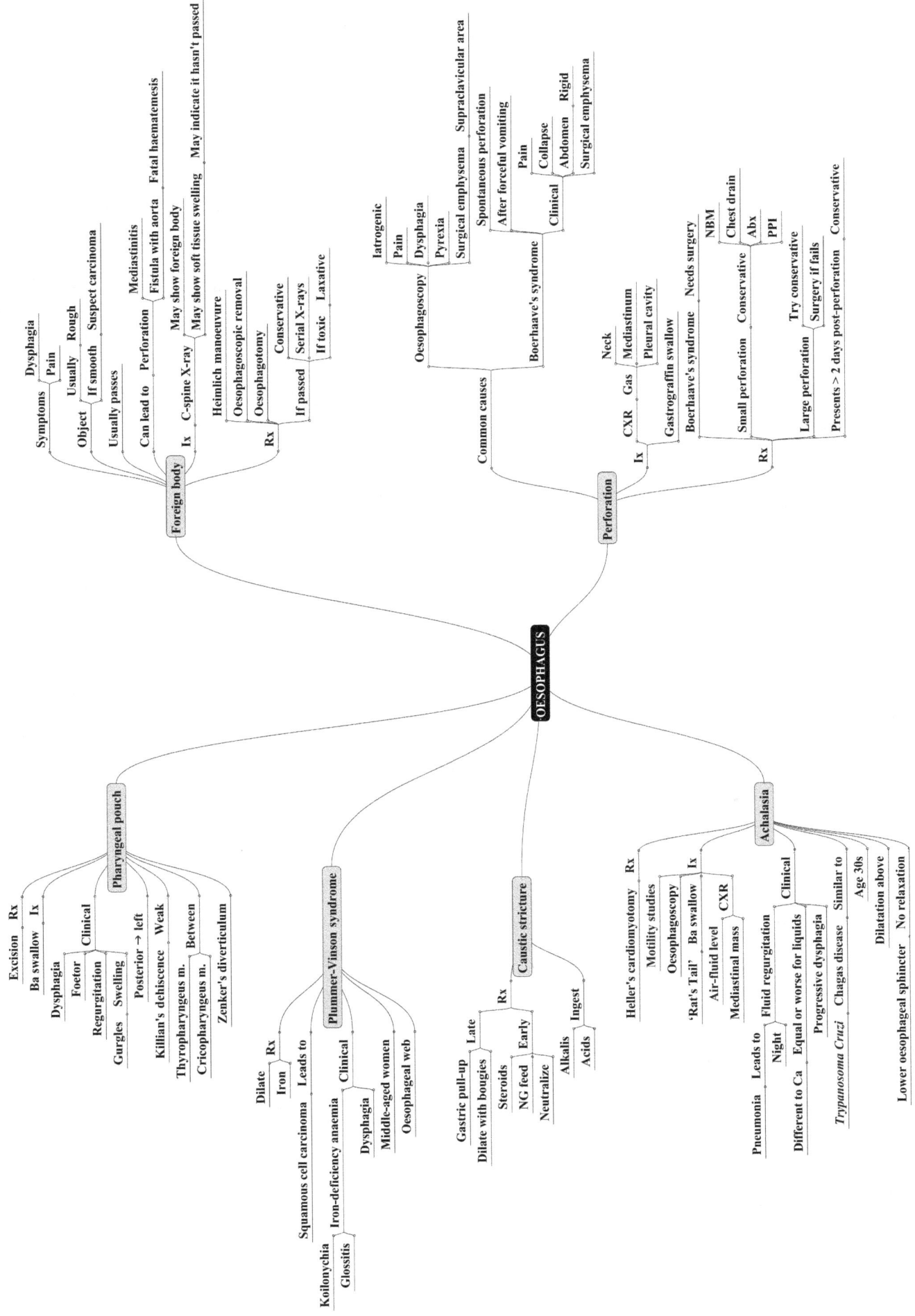

OESOPHAGUS

Foreign body

- Symptoms
  - Dysphagia
  - Pain
- Object
  - Usually
    - Rough → Suspect carcinoma
    - Smooth → Usually passes
  - If smooth
- Can lead to Perforation
  - Mediastinitis
  - Fistula with aorta → Fatal haematemesis
- Ix
  - C-spine X-ray
    - May show foreign body
    - May show soft tissue swelling → May indicate it hasn't passed
- Rx
  - Heimlich manoeuvre
  - Oesophagoscopic removal
  - Oesophagotomy
  - Conservative
    - If passed → Serial X-rays
    - If toxic → Laxative

Perforation

- Common causes
  - Iatrogenic
  - Oesophagoscopy
    - Pain
    - Dysphagia
    - Pyrexia
    - Surgical emphysema → Supraclavicular area
  - Spontaneous perforation
  - Boerhaave's syndrome
    - After forceful vomiting
    - Clinical
      - Pain
      - Collapse
      - Abdomen Rigid
      - Surgical emphysema
- Ix
  - CXR
    - Gas
      - Neck
      - Mediastinum
      - Pleural cavity
  - Gastrograffin swallow
    - Boerhaave's syndrome → Needs surgery
- Rx
  - Small perforation → Conservative
    - NBM
    - Chest drain
    - Abx
    - PPI
  - Large perforation → Try conservative
    - Surgery if fails
  - Presents > 2 days post-perforation → Conservative

Pharyngeal pouch

- Excision Rx
- Ba swallow Ix
- Clinical
  - Dysphagia
  - Foetor
  - Regurgitation
  - Gurgles
  - Swelling
  - Posterior → left
  - Killian's dehiscence
    - Weak
    - Between
      - Thyropharyngeus m.
      - Cricopharyngeus m.
  - Zenker's diverticulum

Plummer-Vinson syndrome

- Dilate Rx
- Iron
- Leads to Squamous cell carcinoma
- Iron-deficiency anaemia
  - Koilonychia
  - Glossitis
- Clinical
  - Dysphagia
  - Middle-aged women
  - Oesophageal web

Caustic stricture

- Rx
  - Gastric pull-up
  - Late → Dilate with bougies
  - Steroids
  - NG feed
  - Early → Neutralize
- Ingest
  - Alkalis
  - Acids

Achalasia

- Rx → Heller's cardiomyotomy
- Ix
  - Motility studies
  - Oesophagoscopy
  - Ba swallow → 'Rat's Tail'
  - CXR
    - Air-fluid level
    - Mediastinal mass
- Clinical
  - Fluid regurgitation
    - Leads to
      - Pneumonia
      - Night
  - Different to Ca → Equal or worse for liquids
  - Progressive dysphagia
  - Age 30s
- Similar to Chagas disease → *Trypanosoma Cruzi*
- Dilatation above
- Lower oesophageal sphincter → No relaxation

OESOPHAGEAL CANCER

Benign
- Leiomyoma

Malignant
- **Primary**
  - Carcinoma
    - SCC
      - 90% of worldwide oesophageal Ca
      - Japan
      - Common
    - Adenocarcinoma
      - Westerners
      - 65% of UK oesophageal Ca
  - Leiomyosarcoma
  - Oat cell carcinoma
- **Secondary**
  - Liver
  - Stomach

Common sites
- Middle — 50%
- Lower — 30%
- Upper — 20%
- Adenocarcinoma — Lower third

Risk factors
- **Common risk factors**
  - Smoking
  - Alcohol
  - Diet — Nitrosamines — Pickled foods
- **SCC risk factors**
  - Achalasia
  - Vitamin C deficiency
  - Vitamin A deficiency
  - Coeliac
  - Strictures
  - Plummer–Vinson syndrome
- **AdenoCa risk factors**
  - Barret's oesophagus
  - Oesophagitis
  - Obesity

Barret's oesophagus
- Lower oesophagus — Site
- Adenocarcinoma — Leads to
- Chronic reflux — Cause
- Metaplasia

Rx
- Prognosis
  - 25% — Average 5 year survival
- **Palliative**
  - Laser
  - Stent
  - Intubation
- **Curative**
  - Pre-op chemo
  - Gastric pull-up
  - Resection
    - Transhiatal
    - Transthoracic
    - If localized
  - Ivor-Lewis resection

Ix
- Laparoscopy — For staging — Peritoneal seeds/mets
- Endoscopic USS — Look for local invasion
- CT — For staging
- Oesophagoscopy — Biopsy
- Ba swallow — Shouldered stricture

Clinical
- If upper 1/3 — Cough
- Hoarse voice
- Hepatomegaly
- ↓ weight
- Enlarged neck nodes
- Dysphagia
  - Solids first
  - Progressive

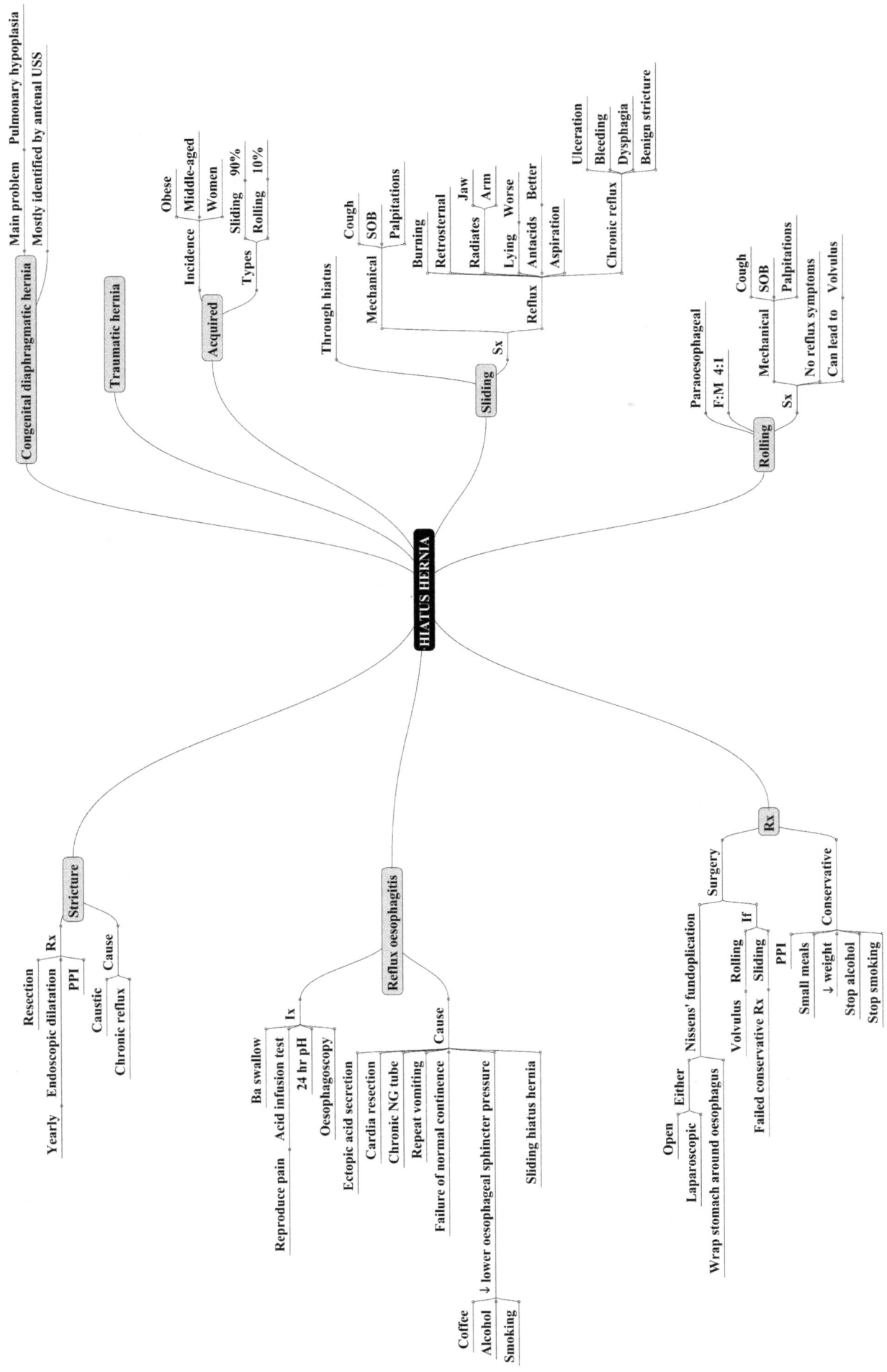

HIATUS HERNIA

Congenital diaphragmatic hernia
- Main problem — Pulmonary hypoplasia
- Mostly identified by antenal USS

Traumatic hernia

Acquired
- Incidence
  - Obese
  - Middle-aged
  - Women
- Types
  - Sliding 90%
  - Rolling 10%

Sliding
- Through hiatus
- Sx
  - Mechanical
    - Cough
    - SOB
    - Palpitations
  - Burning
    - Retrosternal
    - Radiates
      - Jaw
      - Arm
    - Lying — Worse
    - Antacids — Better
    - Aspiration
  - Reflux
    - Chronic reflux
      - Ulceration
      - Bleeding
      - Dysphagia
      - Benign stricture

Rolling
- Paraoesophageal
- F:M 4:1
- Sx
  - Mechanical
    - Cough
    - SOB
    - Palpitations
  - No reflux symptoms
  - Can lead to — Volvulus

Stricture
- Rx
  - Resection
  - Endoscopic dilatation — Yearly
  - PPI
- Cause
  - Caustic
  - Chronic reflux

Reflux oesophagitis
- Ix
  - Ba swallow
  - Acid infusion test — Reproduce pain
  - 24 hr pH
  - Oesophagoscopy
- Cause
  - Ectopic acid secretion
  - Cardia resection
  - Chronic NG tube
  - Repeat vomiting
  - Failure of normal continence
    - ↓ lower oesophageal sphincter pressure
      - Coffee
      - Alcohol
      - Smoking
  - Sliding hiatus hernia

Rx
- Surgery
  - Nissens' fundoplication
    - Either
      - Open
      - Laparoscopic
    - Wrap stomach around oesophagus
  - If
    - Rolling
      - Volvulus
      - Failed conservative Rx
    - Sliding
      - PPI
- Conservative
  - Small meals
  - ↓ weight
  - Stop alcohol
  - Stop smoking

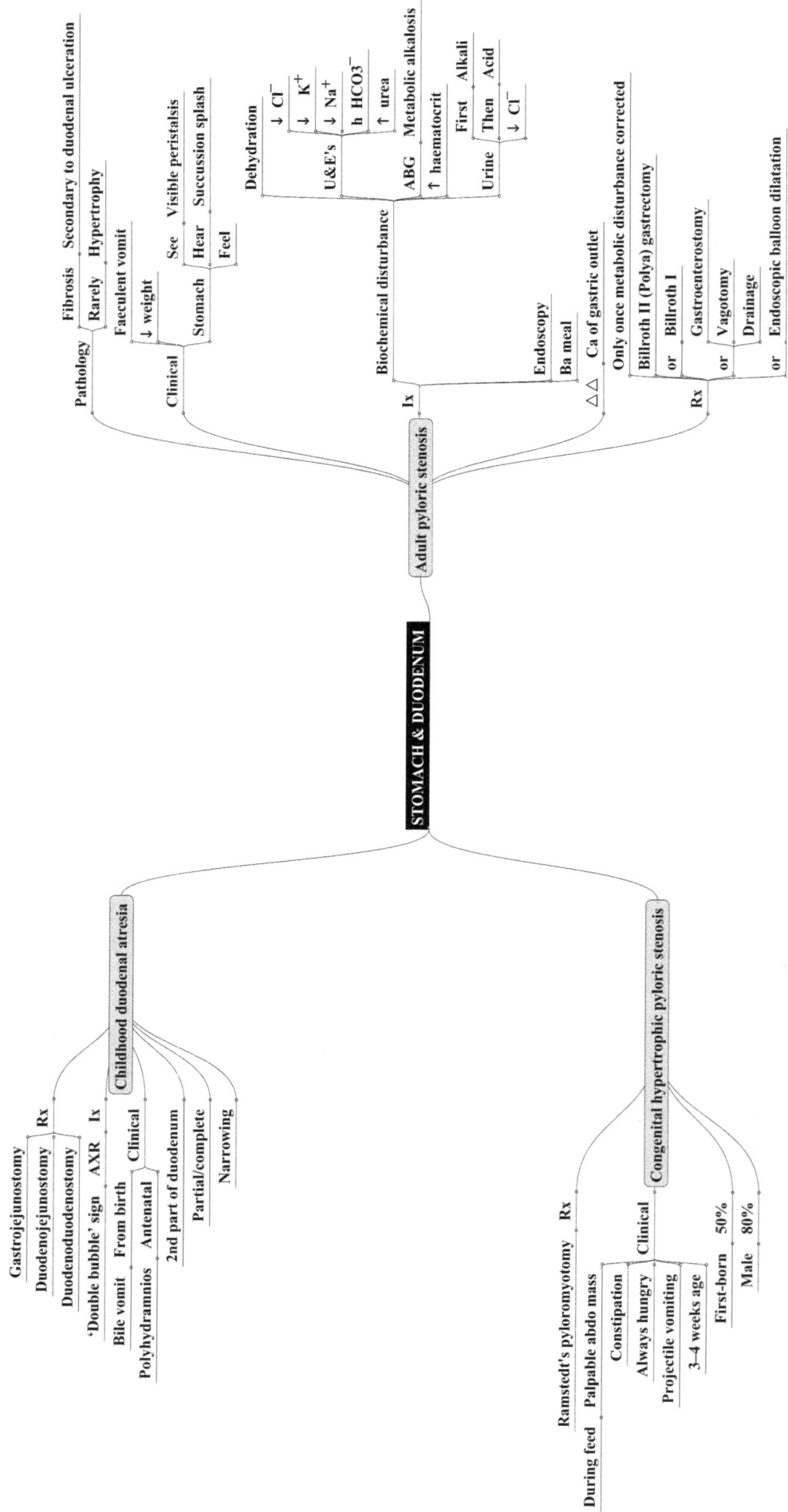

STOMACH & DUODENUM

Adult pyloric stenosis

Pathology
- Fibrosis
- Secondary to duodenal ulceration
- Rarely — Hypertrophy

Clinical
- Faeculent vomit
- ↓ weight
- See — Visible peristalsis
- Stomach
  - Hear — Succussion splash
  - Feel

Ix
- Biochemical disturbance
  - Dehydration
  - U&E's
    - ↓ Cl⁻
    - ↓ K⁺
    - ↓ Na⁺
    - h HCO3⁻
    - ↑ urea
  - ABG — Metabolic alkalosis
  - ↑ haematocrit
  - Urine
    - First — Alkali
    - Then — Acid
    - ↓ Cl⁻
- Endoscopy
- Ba meal
- ΔΔ — Ca of gastric outlet

Rx
- Only once metabolic disturbance corrected
- Billroth II (Polya) gastrectomy
  - or — Billroth I
- Gastroenterostomy
- Vagotomy
  - or — Drainage
- or — Endoscopic balloon dilatation

Childhood duodenal atresia

Rx
- Gastrojejunostomy
- Duodenojejunostomy
- Duodenoduodenostomy

Ix
- 'Double bubble' sign — AXR

Clinical
- From birth
- Bile vomit
- Antenatal — Polyhydramnios
- 2nd part of duodenum
- Partial/complete
- Narrowing

Congenital hypertrophic pyloric stenosis

Rx
- Ramstedt's pyloromyotomy
- Palpable abdo mass

Clinical
- During feed
- Constipation
- Always hungry
- Projectile vomiting
- 3–4 weeks age
- First-born — 50%
- Male — 80%

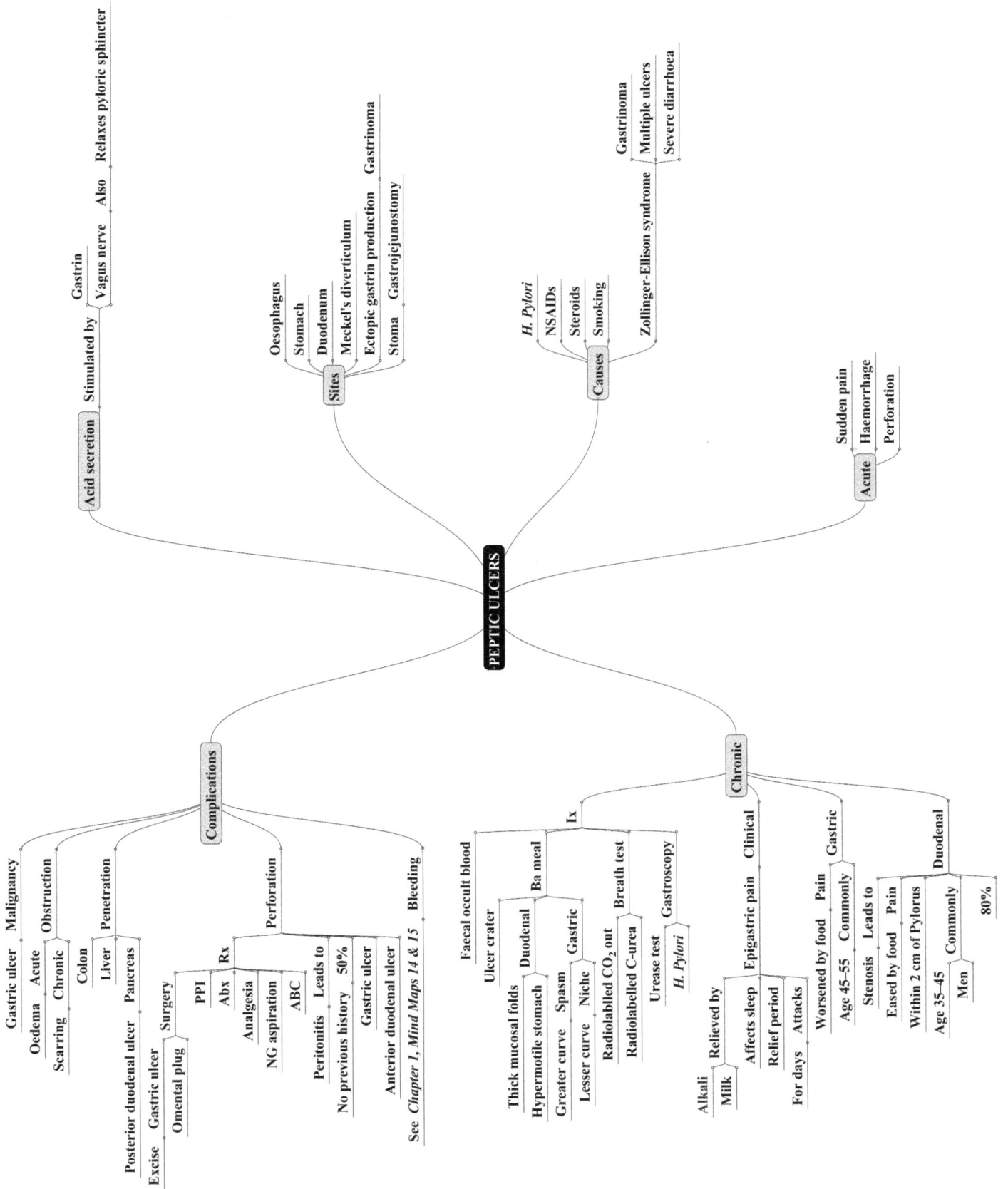

PEPTIC ULCERS

Acid secretion

Stimulated by — **Gastrin**
- **Vagus nerve**
- **Also** — **Relaxes pyloric sphincter**

Sites

- Oesophagus
- Stomach
- Duodenum — Meckel's diverticulum
- Ectopic gastrin production — Gastrinoma
- Stoma — Gastrojejunostomy

Causes

- *H. Pylori*
- NSAIDs
- Steroids
- Smoking
- Zollinger-Ellison syndrome
  - Gastrinoma
  - Multiple ulcers
  - Severe diarrhoea

Acute

- Sudden pain
- Haemorrhage
- Perforation

Complications

- Gastric ulcer — Malignancy
- Oedema — Acute — Obstruction
- Scarring — Chronic
- Penetration
  - Colon
  - Liver
  - Pancreas
- Posterior duodenal ulcer
- Gastric ulcer — Excise
  - Omental plug — Surgery
- Perforation — Rx
  - PPI
  - Abx
  - Analgesia
  - NG aspiration
  - ABC
  - Peritonitis — Leads to
  - No previous history — 50%
  - Gastric ulcer
  - Anterior duodenal ulcer
- Bleeding — See *Chapter 1, Mind Maps 14 & 15*

Chronic

Ix
- Faecal occult blood
- Ba meal
  - Ulcer crater
  - Duodenal — Thick mucosal folds
    - Hypermotile stomach
  - Gastric — Spasm — Greater curve
    - Niche — Lesser curve
- Breath test
  - Radiolabelled CO$_2$ out
  - Urease test — Radiolabelled C-urea
- Gastroscopy — *H. Pylori*

Clinical
- Epigastric pain
  - Relieved by — Alkali
    - Milk
  - Affects sleep
  - Relief period — For days
  - Attacks

Gastric
- Pain — Worsened by food
- Age 45–55 — Commonly
- Stenosis — Leads to

Duodenal
- Pain — Eased by food
- Within 2 cm of Pylorus — Commonly
- Age 35–45
- Men
- 80%

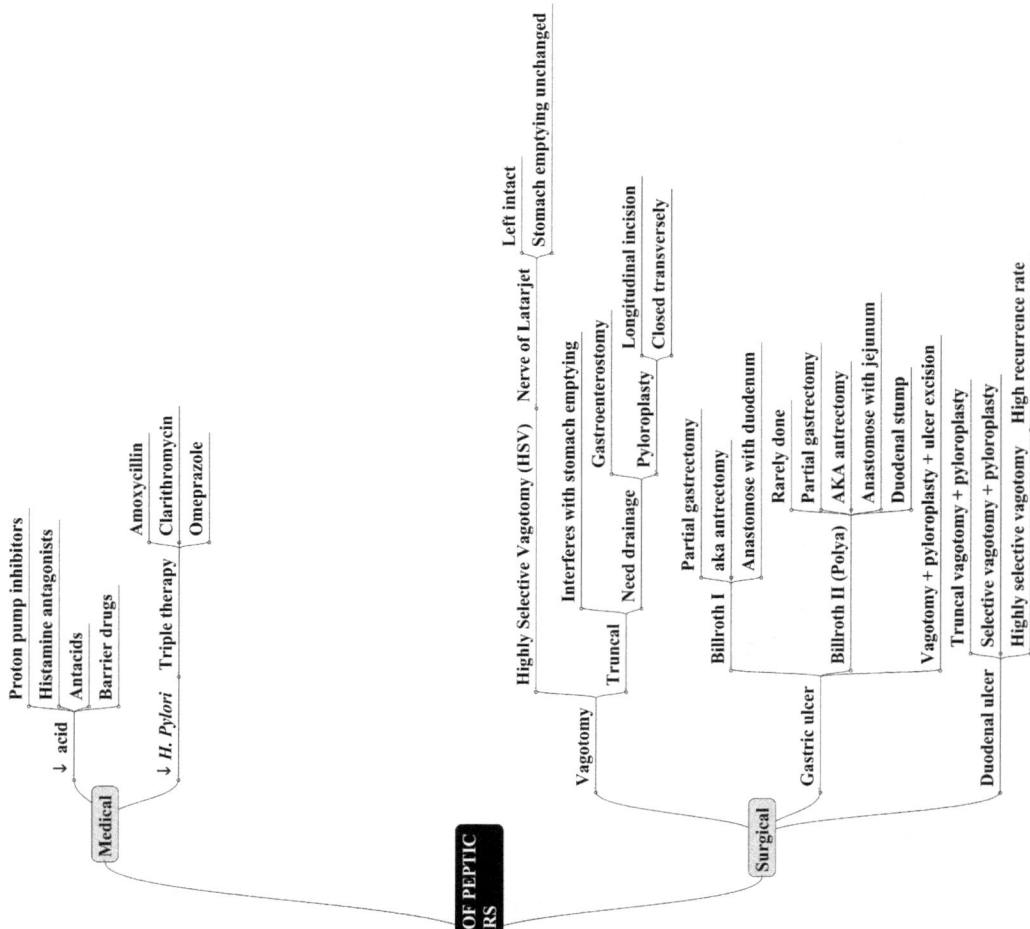

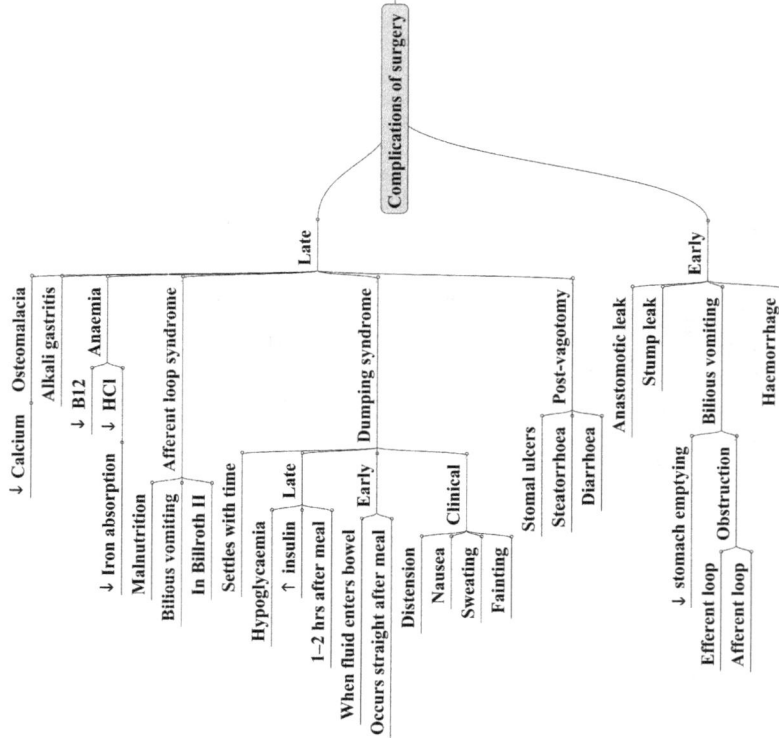

TREATMENT OF PEPTIC ULCERS

Medical

↓ acid
- Proton pump inhibitors
- Histamine antagonists
- Antacids
- Barrier drugs

↓ *H. Pylori* — Triple therapy
- Amoxycillin
- Clarithromycin
- Omeprazole

Surgical

Vagotomy
- Highly Selective Vagotomy (HSV) — Nerve of Latarjet — Left intact — Stomach emptying unchanged
- Truncal
  - Interferes with stomach emptying
  - Need drainage
    - Gastroenterostomy
    - Pyloroplasty — Longitudinal incision — Closed transversely

Gastric ulcer
- Billroth I
  - Partial gastrectomy
  - aka antrectomy
  - Anastomose with duodenum
- Billroth II (Polya)
  - Rarely done
  - Partial gastrectomy
  - AKA antrectomy
  - Anastomose with jejunum
  - Duodenal stump

Duodenal ulcer
- Vagotomy + pyloroplasty + ulcer excision
- Truncal vagotomy + pyloroplasty
- Selective vagotomy + pyloroplasty
- Highly selective vagotomy — High recurrence rate

Complications of surgery

Late
- ↓ Calcium — Osteomalacia
- Alkali gastritis
- ↓ B12 — Anaemia
- ↓ HCl
- ↓ Iron absorption
- Malnutrition
- Bilious vomiting — In Billroth II
- Afferent loop syndrome — Settles with time
- Hypoglycaemia — ↑ insulin — Late — 1–2 hrs after meal
- Dumping syndrome
  - Early — Occurs straight after meal — When fluid enters bowel
    - Distension
    - Clinical
      - Nausea
      - Sweating
      - Fainting
- Stomal ulcers
- Post-vagotomy
  - Steatorrhoea
  - Diarrhoea

Early
- Anastomotic leak — Stump leak
- Bilious vomiting — Obstruction
  - ↓ stomach emptying
  - Efferent loop
  - Afferent loop
- Haemorrhage

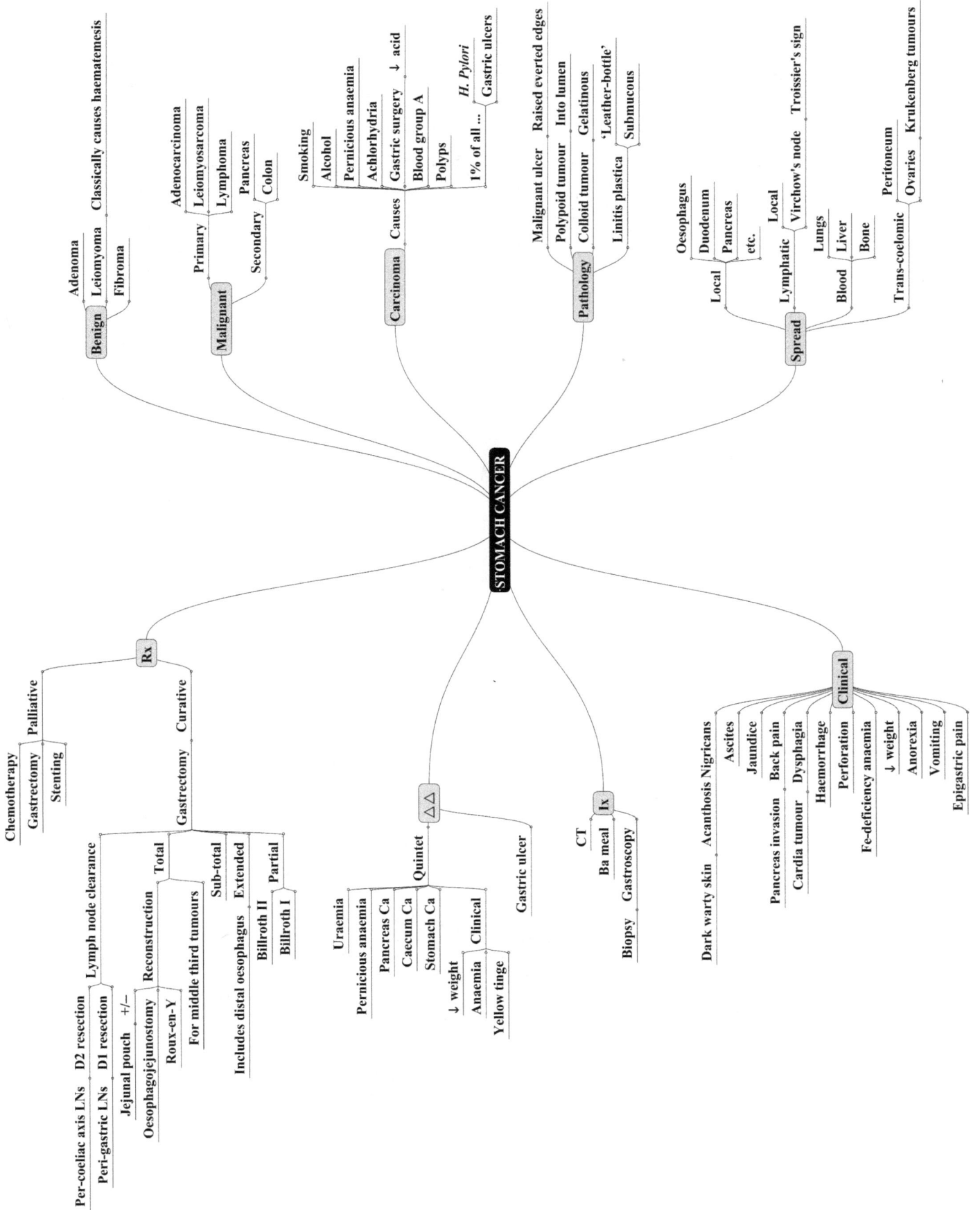

STOMACH CANCER

Benign
- Adenoma
- Leiomyoma
- Fibroma — Classically causes haematemesis

Malignant
- Primary
  - Adenocarcinoma
  - Leiomyosarcoma
  - Lymphoma
- Secondary
  - Pancreas
  - Colon

Carcinoma
- Causes
  - Smoking
  - Alcohol
  - Pernicious anaemia
  - Achlorhydria
  - Gastric surgery — ↓ acid
  - Blood group A
  - Polyps
  - *H. Pylori*
  - Gastric ulcers — 1% of all ...

Pathology
- Malignant ulcer — Raised everted edges
- Polypoid tumour — Into lumen
- Colloid tumour — Gelatinous
- Linitis plastica — 'Leather-bottle' — Submucous

Spread
- Local
  - Oesophagus
  - Duodenum
  - Pancreas
  - etc.
- Lymphatic
  - Local
  - Virchow's node — Troissier's sign
- Blood
  - Lungs
  - Liver
  - Bone
- Trans-coelomic
  - Peritoneum
  - Ovaries — Krukenberg tumours

Rx
- Palliative
  - Chemotherapy
  - Gastrectomy
  - Stenting
- Curative
  - Gastrectomy
    - Lymph node clearance
      - Per-coeliac axis LNs — D2 resection
      - Peri-gastric LNs — D1 resection
    - +/−
      - Jejunal pouch
      - Oesophagojejunostomy
      - Roux-en-Y
    - Reconstruction
    - Total
      - For middle third tumours
      - Includes distal oesophagus
    - Sub-total
    - Extended
    - Partial
      - Billroth II
      - Billroth I

ΔΔ
- Quintet
  - Uraemia
  - Pernicious anaemia
  - Pancreas Ca
  - Caecum Ca
  - Stomach Ca
    - Clinical
      - ↓ weight
      - Anaemia
      - Yellow tinge
- Gastric ulcer

Ix
- CT
- Ba meal
- Gastroscopy
  - Biopsy

Clinical
- Dark warty skin — Acanthosis Nigricans
- Ascites
- Jaundice
- Back pain — Pancreas invasion
- Dysphagia — Cardia tumour
- Haemorrhage
- Perforation
- Fe-deficiency anaemia
- ↓ weight
- Anorexia
- Vomiting
- Epigastric pain

GI HAEMORRHAGE 1

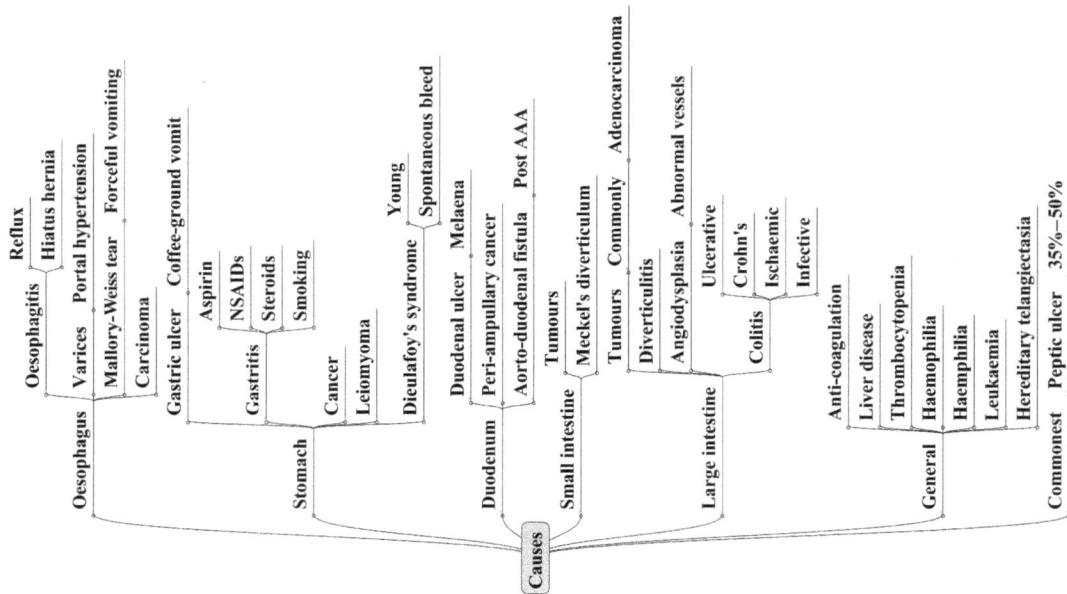

Causes

Oesophagus
- Oesophagitis
  - Reflux
  - Hiatus hernia
- Varices — Portal hypertension
- Mallory-Weiss tear — Forceful vomiting
- Carcinoma

Stomach
- Gastric ulcer — Coffee-ground vomit
- Gastritis
  - Aspirin
  - NSAIDs
  - Steroids
  - Smoking
- Cancer
- Leiomyoma
- Dieulafoy's syndrome
  - Young
  - Spontaneous bleed

Duodenum
- Duodenal ulcer — Melaena
- Peri-ampullary cancer
- Aorto-duodenal fistula — Post AAA

Small intestine
- Tumours
- Meckel's diverticulum

Large intestine
- Tumours — Commonly — Adenocarcinoma
- Diverticulitis
- Angiodysplasia — Abnormal vessels
- Colitis
  - Ulcerative
  - Crohn's
  - Ischaemic
  - Infective

General
- Anti-coagulation
- Liver disease
- Thrombocytopenia
- Haemophilia
- Haemphilia
- Leukaemia
- Hereditary telangiectasia

Commonest — Peptic ulcer — 35%–50%

Initial management

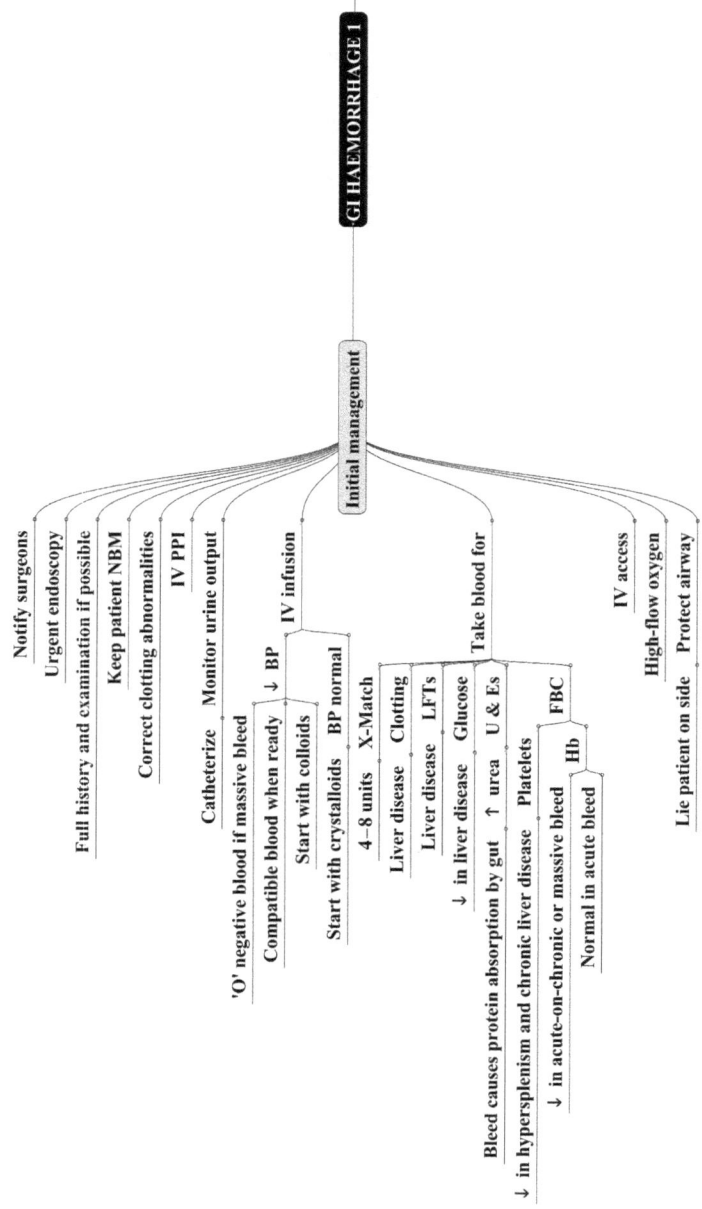

- Notify surgeons
- Urgent endoscopy
- Full history and examination if possible
- Keep patient NBM
- Correct clotting abnormalities
- IV PPI
- Catheterize — Monitor urine output
- IV infusion
  - ↓ BP
    - 'O' negative blood if massive bleed
    - Compatible blood when ready
    - Start with colloids
  - BP normal
    - Start with crystalloids
- Take blood for
  - X-Match — 4–8 units
  - Clotting — Liver disease
  - LFTs — Liver disease
  - Glucose — ↓ in liver disease
  - U & Es — ↑ urea — ↑ in acute-on-chronic or massive bleed
  - Platelets — ↓ in hypersplenism and chronic liver disease
  - FBC — Hb — Normal in acute bleed
- IV access
- High-flow oxygen
- Lie patient on side
- Protect airway

Bleed causes protein absorption by gut

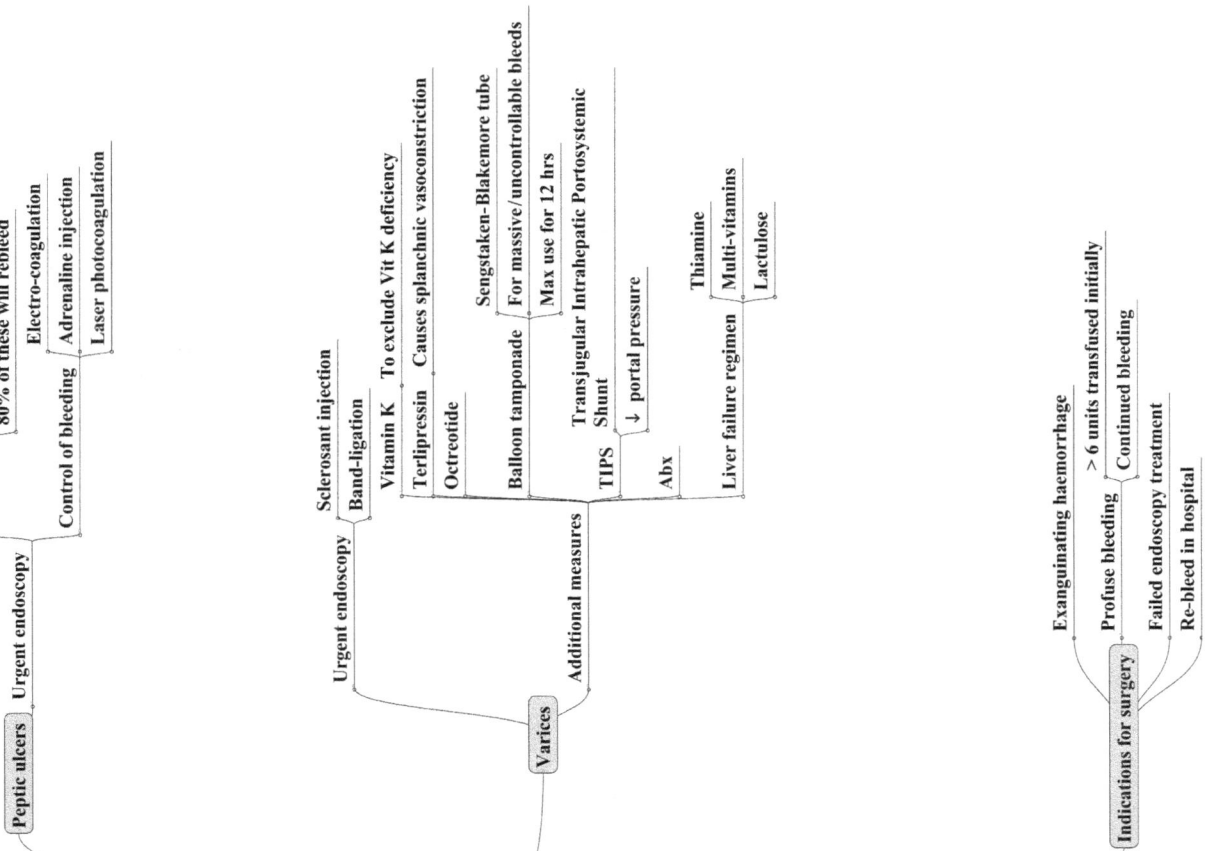

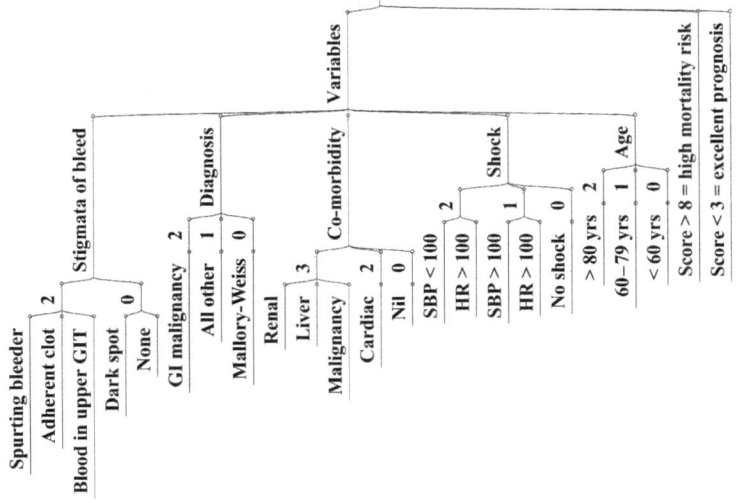

GI HAEMORRHAGE 2

Peptic ulcers
- **Urgent endoscopy**
  - **Diagnosis**
    - **Bleeding vessel**
    - **Adherent clot** — 80% of these will rebleed
  - **Control of bleeding**
    - Electro-coagulation
    - Adrenaline injection
    - Laser photocoagulation

Varices
- **Urgent endoscopy**
  - Sclerosant injection
  - Band-ligation
- **Additional measures**
  - Vitamin K — To exclude Vit K deficiency
  - Terlipressin — Causes splanchnic vasoconstriction
  - Octreotide
  - Balloon tamponade
    - Sengstaken–Blakemore tube
    - For massive/uncontrollable bleeds
    - Max use for 12 hrs
  - TIPS — Transjugular Intrahepatic Portosystemic Shunt — ↓ portal pressure
  - Abx
  - Liver failure regimen
    - Thiamine
    - Multi-vitamins
    - Lactulose

Indications for surgery
- Exsanguinating haemorrhage
- Profuse bleeding — > 6 units transfused initially
- Continued bleeding
- Failed endoscopy treatment
- Re-bleed in hospital

Prognosis
- **Rockall's score**
  - **Variables**
    - **Stigmata of bleed**
      - Spurting bleeder — 2
      - Adherent clot — 2
      - Blood in upper GIT
      - Dark spot — 0
      - None — 0
    - **Diagnosis**
      - GI malignancy — 2
      - All other — 1
      - Mallory–Weiss — 0
    - **Co-morbidity**
      - Renal — 3
      - Liver — 3
      - Malignancy — 3
      - Cardiac — 2
      - Nil — 0
    - **Shock**
      - SBP < 100 — 2
      - HR > 100 — 2
      - SBP > 100 — 1
      - HR > 100 — 1
      - No shock — 0
    - **Age**
      - > 80 yrs — 2
      - 60–79 yrs — 1
      - < 60 yrs — 0
    - Score > 8 = high mortality risk
    - Score < 3 = excellent prognosis

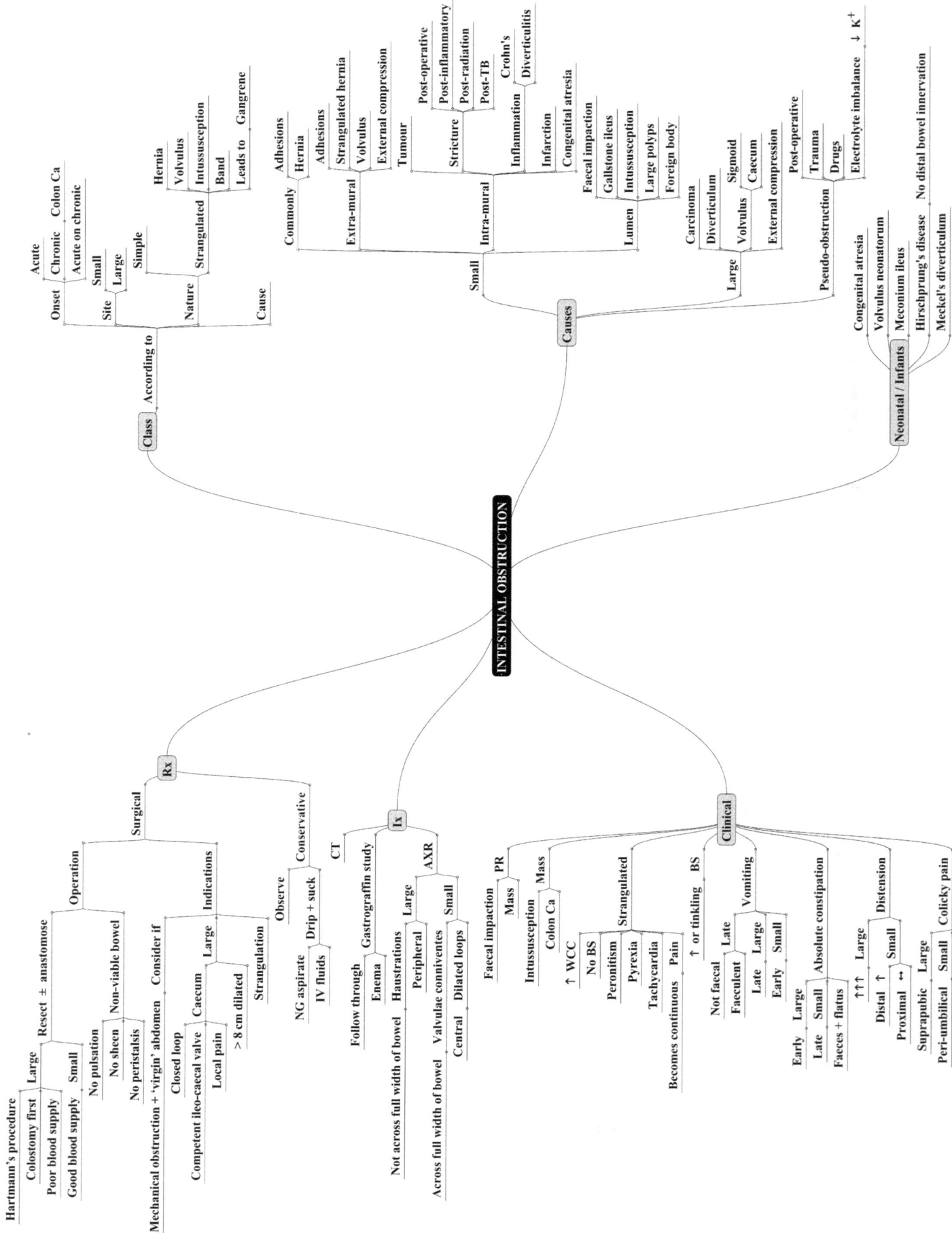

INTESTINAL OBSTRUCTION

Class — According to
- **Onset**: Acute · Chronic · Acute on chronic
  - Acute: Colon Ca
- **Site**: Small · Large
- **Nature**: Simple · Strangulated
  - Strangulated: Hernia · Volvulus · Intussusception · Band → Leads to Gangrene
- **Cause**

Hartmann's procedure

Causes
Small
- **Extra-mural**
  - Commonly: Adhesions · Hernia
  - Adhesions
  - Strangulated hernia
  - Volvulus
  - External compression
  - Tumour
- **Intra-mural**
  - Stricture: Post-operative · Post-inflammatory · Post-radiation · Post-TB
  - Inflammation: Crohn's · Diverticulitis
  - Infarction
  - Congenital atresia
- **Lumen**
  - Faecal impaction
  - Gallstone ileus
  - Intussusception
  - Large polyps
  - Foreign body

Large
- Carcinoma
- Diverticulum
- Volvulus: Sigmoid · Caecum
- External compression
- Pseudo-obstruction: Post-operative · Trauma · Drugs · Electrolyte imbalance ↓ K⁺

Neonatal / Infants
- Congenital atresia
- Volvulus neonatorum
- Meconium ileus
- Hirschprung's disease — No distal bowel innervation
- Meckel's diverticulum

Clinical
- **PR**: Faecal impaction · Mass
- **Mass**: Intussusception · Colon Ca
- ↑ WCC
- No BS
- **Strangulated**: Peritonitis · Pyrexia · Tachycardia · Pain (Becomes continuous)
- **BS**: ↑ or tinkling
- **Vomiting**: Late (Faeculent) · Not faecal — Late / Early
- **Absolute constipation**: Large (Late) · Small (Early) · Faeces + flatus
- **Distension**: Large — Distal ↑↑ / Proximal ↑ — Small
- **Colicky pain**: Large (Suprapubic) · Small (Peri-umbilical)

Ix
- **CT**
- **Gastrografin study**: Follow through · Enema
- **AXR**
  - Large: Haustrations · Peripheral · Not across full width of bowel
  - Small: Valvulae conniventes · Central · Dilated loops · Across full width of bowel

Rx
Surgical
- **Operation**
  - Large: Hartmann's procedure · Colostomy first (Poor blood supply) · Resect ± anastomose (Good blood supply) — Small
  - Non-viable bowel: No pulsation · No sheen · No peristalsis
- **Consider if** 'virgin' abdomen · Mechanical obstruction
- **Indications**
  - Closed loop
  - Competent ileo-caecal valve
  - Caecum — Large — Local pain — > 8 cm dilated
  - Strangulation

Conservative
- Observe
- Drip + suck: NG aspirate · IV fluids

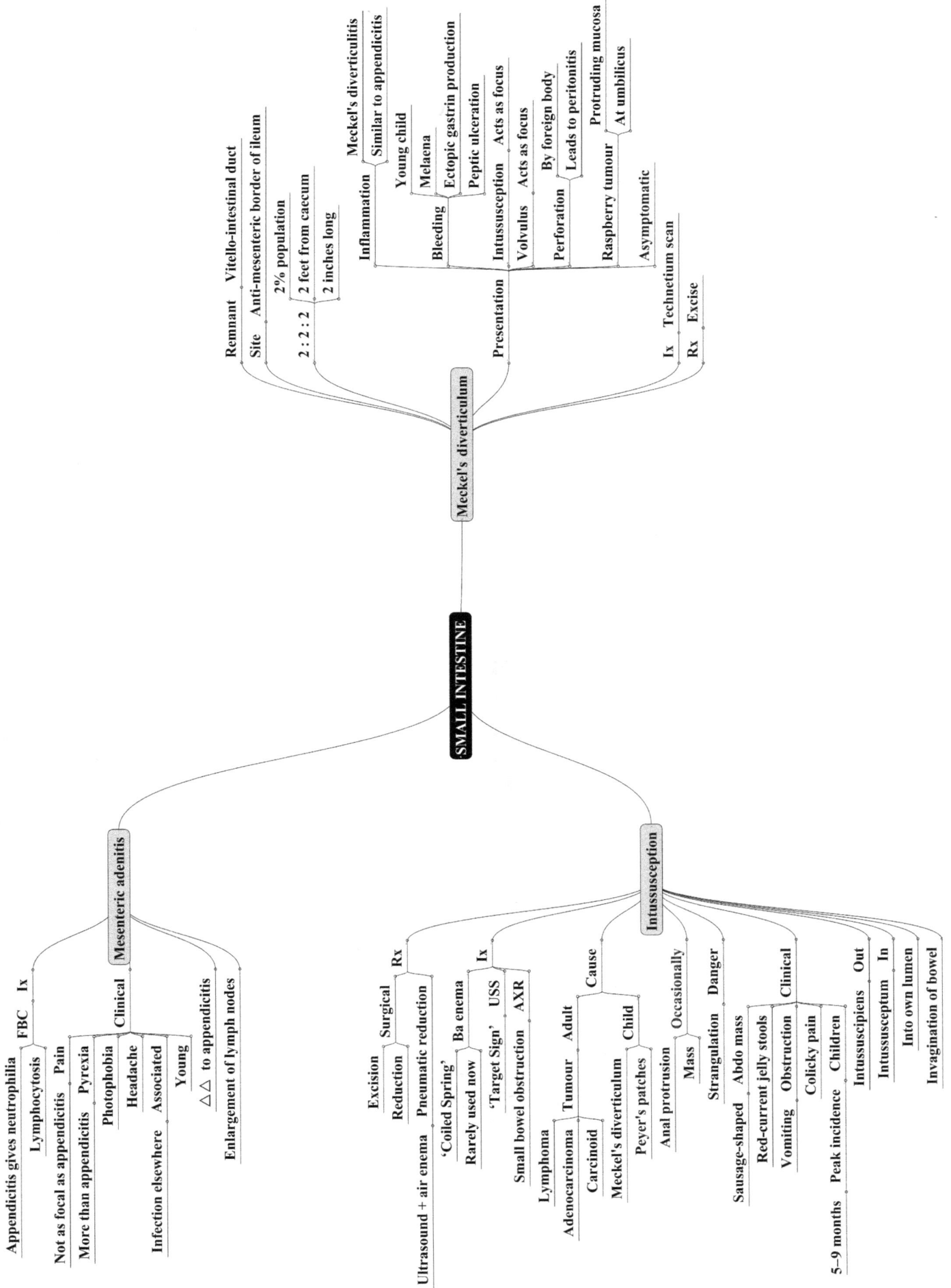

SMALL INTESTINE

Meckel's diverticulum

- Remnant — Vitello-intestinal duct
- Site — Anti-mesenteric border of ileum
- 2 : 2 : 2
  - 2% population
  - 2 feet from caecum
  - 2 inches long
- Presentation
  - Inflammation — Meckel's diverticulitis — Similar to appendicitis
  - Bleeding — Young child
    - Melaena
    - Ectopic gastrin production
    - Peptic ulceration
  - Intussusception — Acts as focus
  - Volvulus — Acts as focus
  - Perforation — By foreign body — Leads to peritonitis
  - Raspberry tumour — Protruding mucosa — At umbilicus
  - Asymptomatic
- Ix — Technetium scan
- Rx — Excise

Mesenteric adenitis

- Ix — FBC
  - Appendicitis gives neutrophilia
  - Lymphocytosis
- Clinical
  - Pain — Not as focal as appendicitis
  - Pyrexia — More than appendicitis
  - Photophobia
  - Headache
  - Associated — Infection elsewhere
  - Young
  - ΔΔ to appendicitis
  - Enlargement of lymph nodes

Intussusception

- Rx
  - Surgical — Excision
  - Reduction — Pneumatic reduction — Ultrasound + air enema
- Ix
  - Ba enema — 'Coiled Spring' — Rarely used now
  - USS — 'Target Sign'
  - AXR — Small bowel obstruction
- Cause
  - Adult — Tumour — Lymphoma / Adenocarcinoma / Carcinoid
  - Child — Meckel's diverticulum / Peyer's patches
- Clinical
  - Occasionally — Anal protrusion
  - Mass — Abdo mass — Sausage-shaped
  - Danger — Strangulation
  - Obstruction — Red-current jelly stools — Vomiting
  - Colicky pain
- Peak incidence — 5–9 months — Children
- Intussuscipiens — Out
- Intussusceptum — In — Into own lumen
- Invagination of bowel

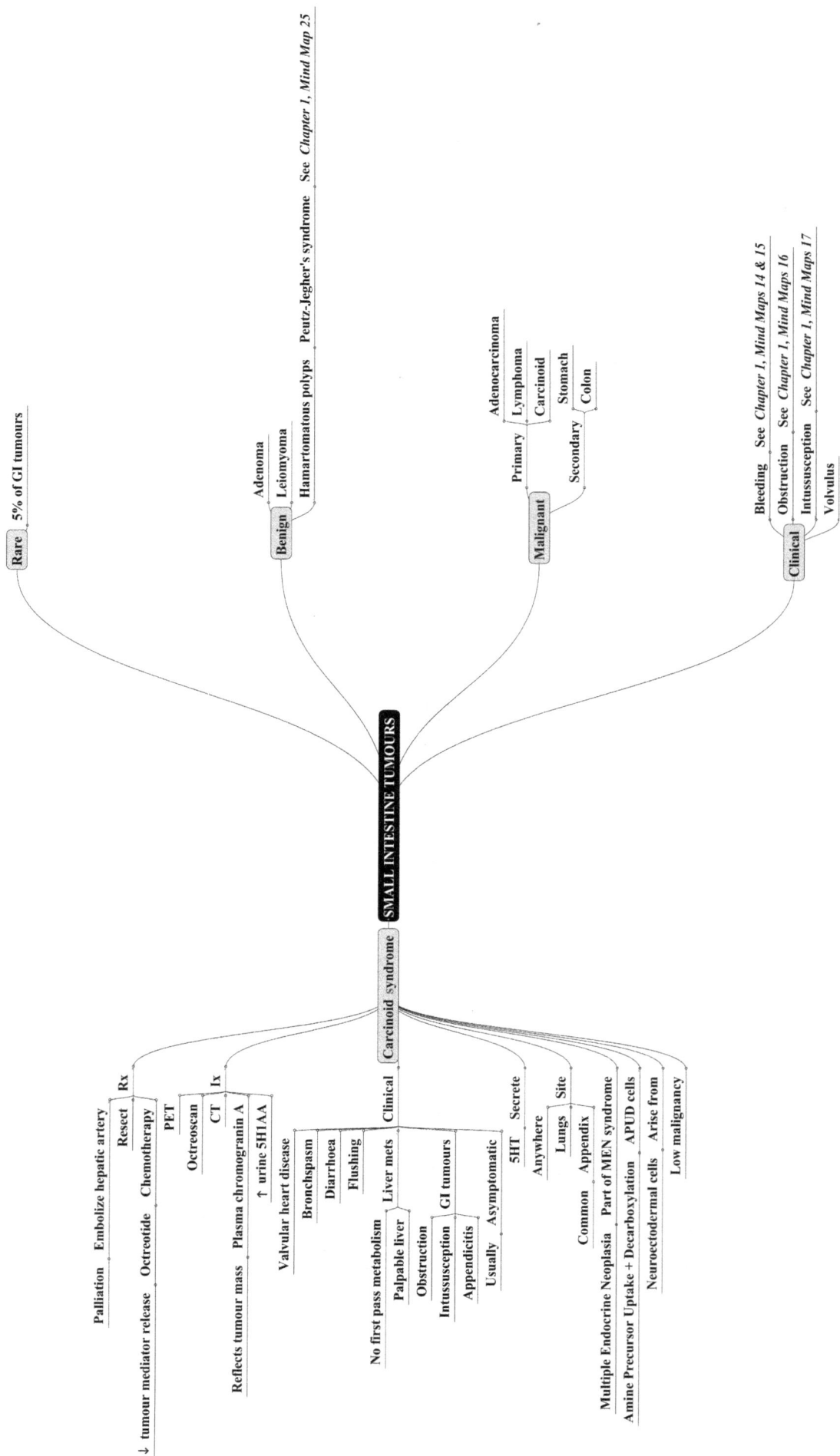

SMALL INTESTINE TUMOURS

Rare — 5% of GI tumours

Benign
- Adenoma
- Leiomyoma
- Hamartomatous polyps — Peutz-Jegher's syndrome   See *Chapter 1, Mind Map 25*

Malignant
- Primary
  - Adenocarcinoma
  - Lymphoma
  - Carcinoid
- Secondary
  - Stomach
  - Colon

Clinical
- Bleeding   See *Chapter 1, Mind Maps 14 & 15*
- Obstruction   See *Chapter 1, Mind Maps 16*
- Intussusception   See *Chapter 1, Mind Maps 17*
- Volvulus

Carcinoid syndrome

Rx
- Palliation — Embolize hepatic artery
- Resect
- → tumour mediator release — Octreotide
- Chemotherapy

Ix
- PET
- Octreoscan
- CT
- Plasma chromogranin A — Reflects tumour mass
- ↑ urine 5H1AA

Clinical
- Valvular heart disease
- Bronchspasm
- Diarrhoea
- Flushing
- Liver mets
  - No first pass metabolism
  - Palpable liver
- Obstruction
- Intussusception
- Appendicitis
  - GI tumours
- Usually Asymptomatic

Secrete
- 5HT

Site
- Anywhere
- Lungs
- Appendix — Common

- Part of MEN syndrome — Multiple Endocrine Neoplasia
- APUD cells — Amine Precursor Uptake + Decarboxylation
- Arise from — Neuroectodermal cells
- Low malignancy

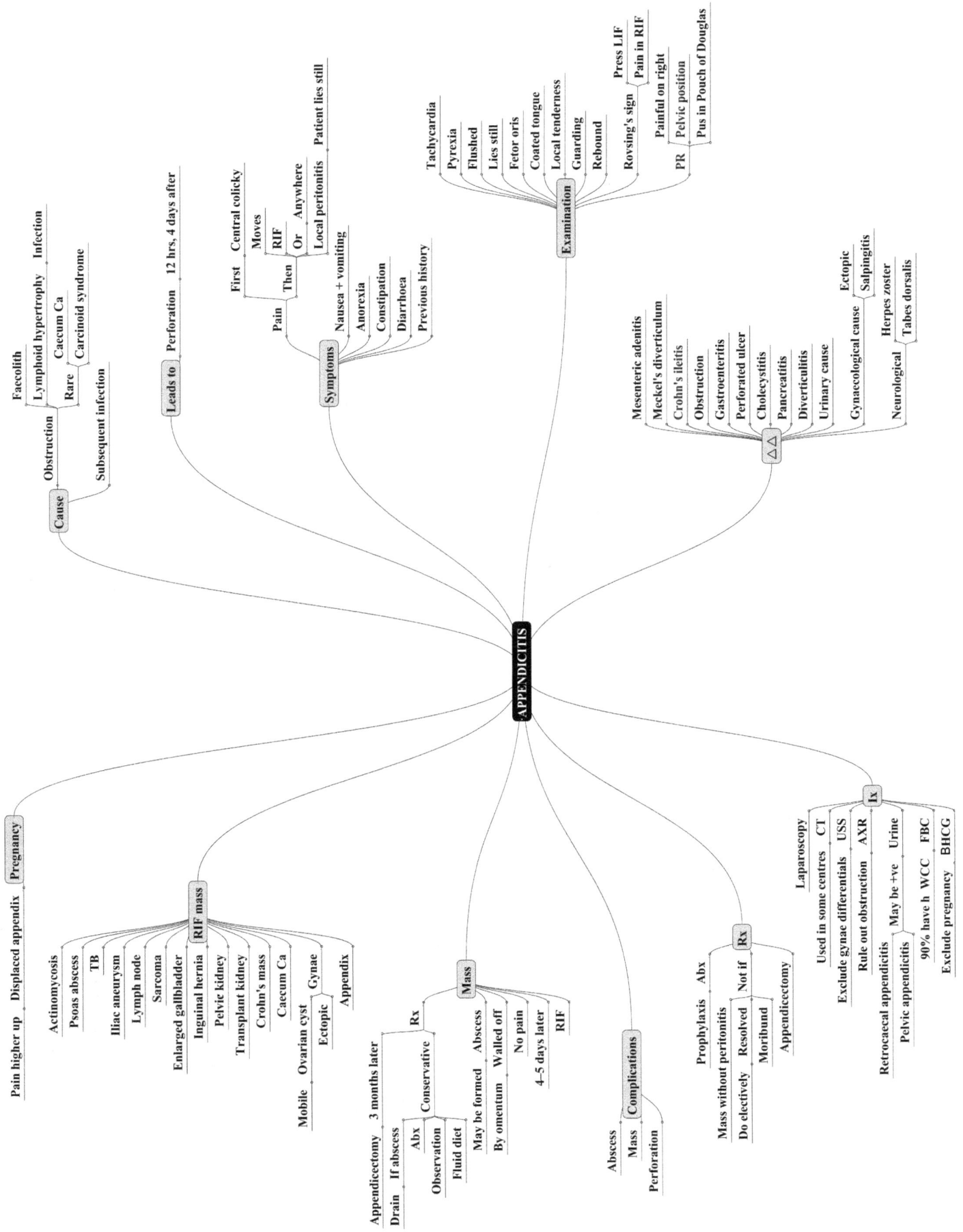

APPENDICITIS

Cause
- Obstruction
  - Faecolith
  - Lymphoid hypertrophy — Infection
  - Rare
    - Caecum Ca
    - Carcinoid syndrome
- Subsequent infection

Leads to
- Perforation — 12 hrs, 4 days after

Symptoms
- Pain
  - First — Central colicky
  - Then
    - Moves
      - RIF
      - Or — Anywhere
    - Local peritonitis — Patient lies still
- Nausea + vomiting
- Anorexia
- Constipation
- Diarrhoea
- Previous history

Examination
- Tachycardia
- Pyrexia
- Flushed
- Lies still
- Fetor oris
- Coated tongue
- Local tenderness
- Guarding
- Rebound
- Rovsing's sign
  - Press LIF
  - Pain in RIF
- PR
  - Painful on right
  - Pelvic position
  - Pus in Pouch of Douglas

ΔΔ
- Mesenteric adenitis
- Meckel's diverticulum
- Crohn's ileitis
- Obstruction
- Gastroenteritis
- Perforated ulcer
- Cholecystitis
- Pancreatitis
- Diverticulitis
- Urinary cause
- Gynaecological cause
  - Ectopic
  - Salpingitis
- Neurological
  - Herpes zoster
  - Tabes dorsalis

Pregnancy
- Pain higher up
- Displaced appendix

RIF mass
- Actinomycosis
- Psoas abscess
- TB
- Iliac aneurysm
- Lymph node
- Sarcoma
- Enlarged gallbladder
- Inguinal hernia
- Pelvic kidney
- Transplant kidney
- Crohn's mass
- Caecum Ca
- Gynae
  - Ovarian cyst
    - Mobile
  - Ectopic
- Appendix

Mass
- Rx
  - Appendicectomy — 3 months later
  - Drain — If abscess
  - Conservative
    - Abx
    - Observation
    - Fluid diet
- May be formed
  - By omentum
  - Abscess — Walled off
- No pain
- 4–5 days later
- RIF

Complications
- Abscess
- Mass
- Perforation

Rx
- Abx
  - Prophylaxis
  - Mass without peritonitis
- Appendicectomy
  - Do electively
  - Not if
    - Resolved
    - Moribund

Ix
- Laparoscopy
  - Used in some centres
- CT
  - Exclude gynae differentials
- USS
- AXR
  - Rule out obstruction
  - May be +ve
    - Retrocaecal appendicitis
    - Pelvic appendicitis
- Urine
- WCC — 90% have ↑
- FBC
- BHCG — Exclude pregnancy

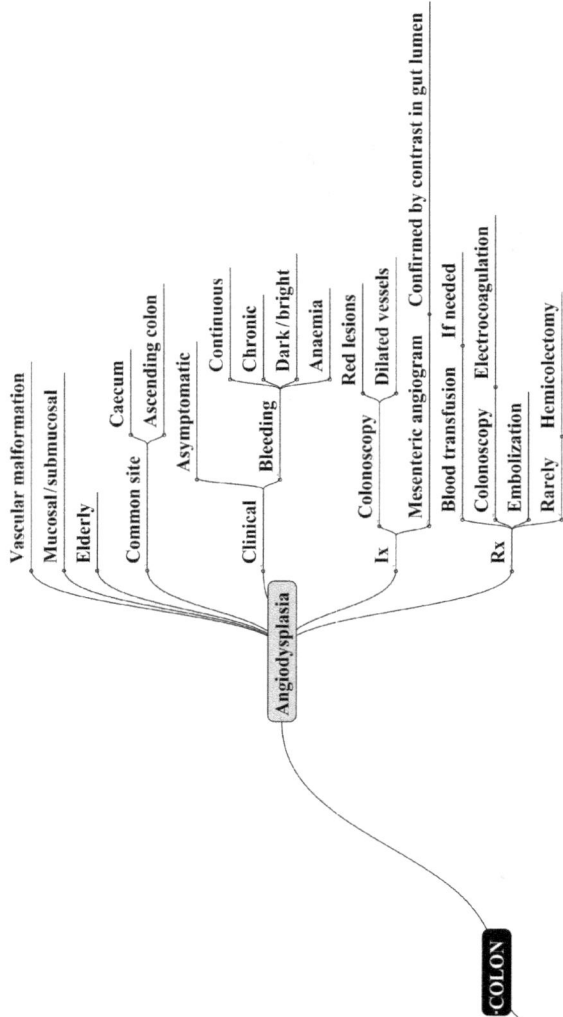

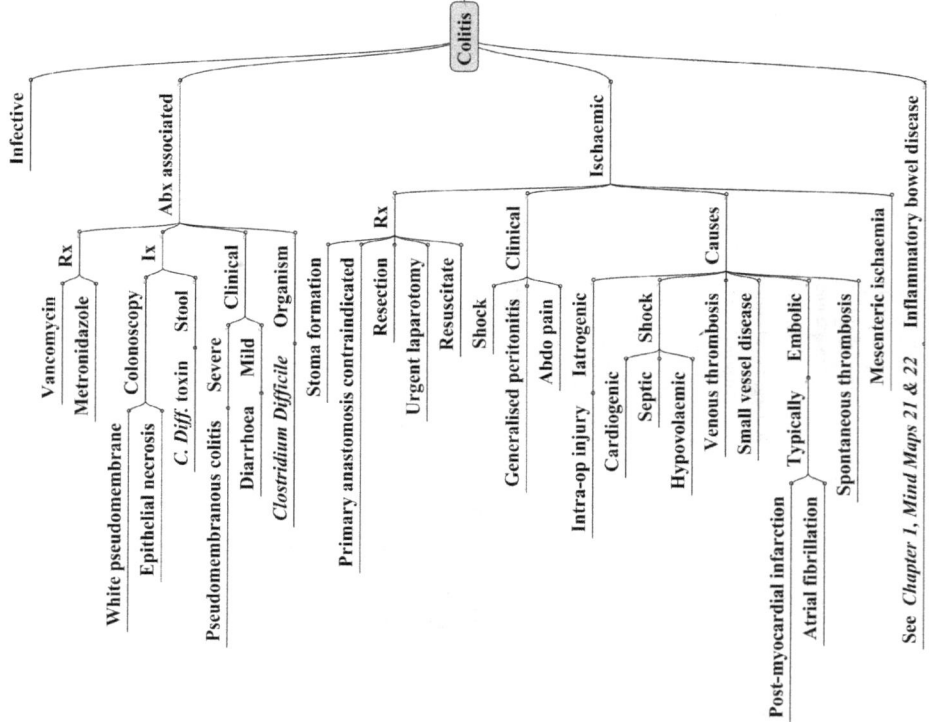

COLON

Angiodysplasia

- Vascular malformation
- Mucosal/submucosal
- Elderly
- Common site
  - Caecum
  - Ascending colon
- Clinical
  - Asymptomatic
  - Bleeding
    - Continuous
    - Chronic
    - Dark/bright
    - Anaemia
- Ix
  - Colonoscopy
    - Red lesions
    - Dilated vessels
  - Mesenteric angiogram — Confirmed by contrast in gut lumen
- Rx
  - Blood transfusion — If needed
  - Colonoscopy — Electrocoagulation
  - Embolization
  - Rarely — Hemicolectomy

Colitis

- Infective
- Abx associated
  - Rx
    - Vancomycin
    - Metronidazole
  - Ix
    - Colonoscopy
      - White pseudomembrane
      - Epithelial necrosis
    - C. Diff. toxin
    - Stool
  - Clinical
    - Pseudomembranous colitis
    - Severe
    - Mild
    - Diarrhoea
  - Clostridium Difficile
  - Organism
- Ischaemic
  - Rx
    - Stoma formation
    - Primary anastomosis contraindicated
    - Resection
    - Urgent laparotomy
    - Resuscitate
  - Clinical
    - Shock
    - Generalised peritonitis
    - Abdo pain
  - Causes
    - Iatrogenic
      - Intra-op injury
    - Cardiogenic
      - Septic
        - Shock
      - Hypovolaemic
    - Venous thrombosis
    - Small vessel disease
    - Post-myocardial infarction
    - Atrial fibrillation
      - Typically
      - Embolic
      - Spontaneous thrombosis
    - Mesenteric ischaemia
- Inflammatory bowel disease

See *Chapter 1, Mind Maps 21 & 22*

CROHN'S

Incidence
- Commonest age group — 15–40 yrs old
- Smokers

Pathology
- Skip lesions
- Whole GIT
- Commonly — Terminal ileum
- Transmural lesions
- Granulomas
- Fistulas
- Risk of — Peri-anal involvement — 75%
- Perforation

Clinical
- Diarrhoea — Painful — Bloody — Less common than ulcerative colitis
- Abdo pain
- ↓ weight
- RIF mass
- Peri-anal fistula
- Bowel obstruction — Inflammatory strictures

Can lead to — Extra-GIT
- Clubbing
- Aphthous ulcers
- Erythema nodosum
- Pyoderma gangrenosum
- Arthritis
- Uveitis
- Kidney stones
- Gallstones

Rx

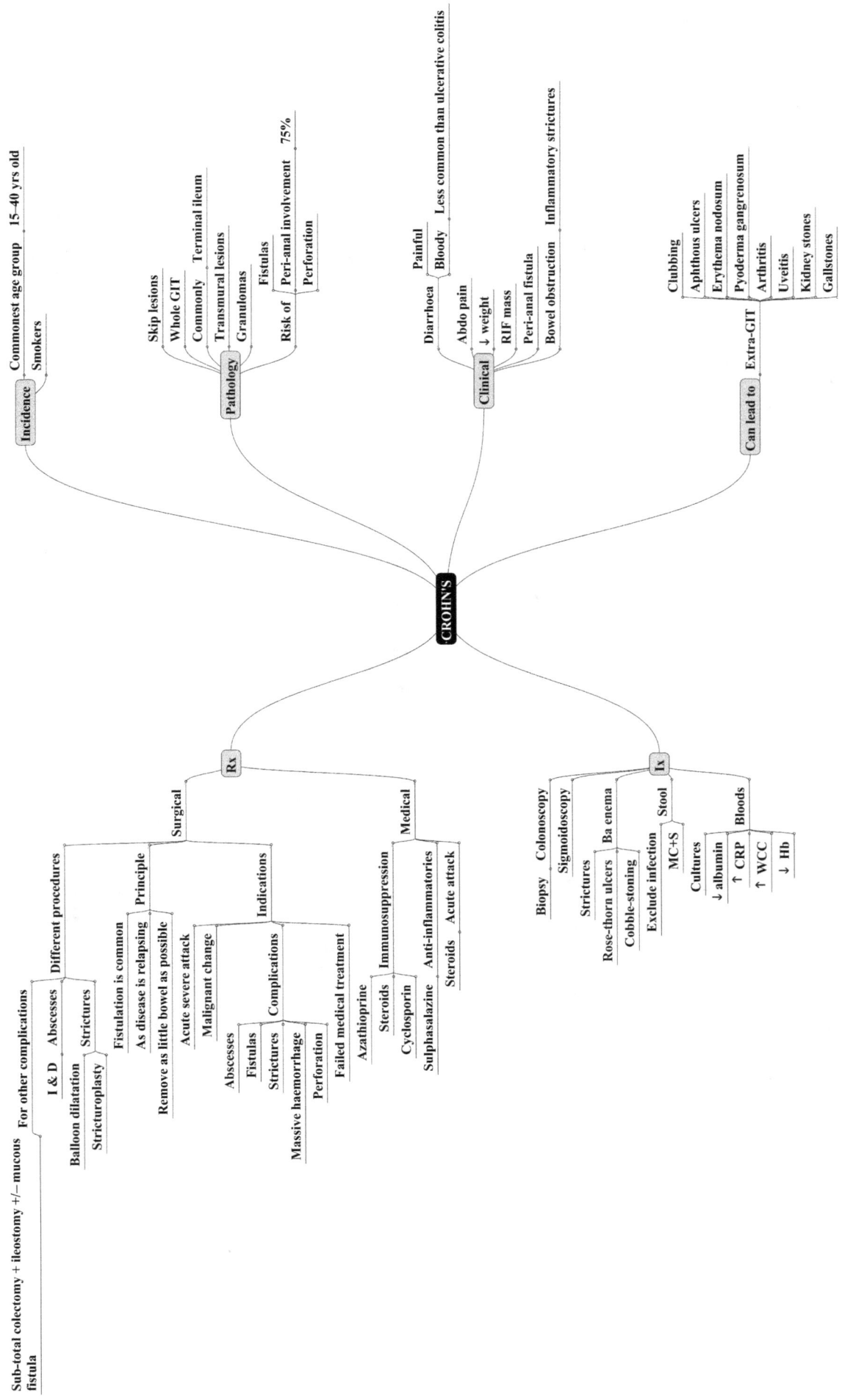

Surgical
- Different procedures
  - Abscesses — I & D
  - Strictures — Balloon dilatation, Stricturoplasty
  - For other complications — Sub-total colectomy + ileostomy +/– mucous fistula
- Principle
  - Fistulation is common
  - As disease is relapsing
  - Remove as little bowel as possible
- Indications
  - Acute severe attack
  - Malignant change
  - Complications
    - Abscesses
    - Fistulas
    - Strictures
    - Massive haemorrhage
    - Perforation
  - Failed medical treatment

Medical
- Immunosuppression
  - Azathioprine
  - Steroids
  - Cyclosporin
- Anti-inflammatories — Sulphasalazine
- Acute attack — Steroids

Ix
- Colonoscopy
  - Biopsy
  - Sigmoidoscopy
- Ba enema
  - Strictures
  - Rose-thorn ulcers
  - Cobble-stoning
- Stool
  - Exclude infection
  - MC+S
  - Cultures
- Bloods
  - ↓ albumin
  - ↑ CRP
  - ↑ WCC
  - ↓ Hb

ULCERATIVE COLITIS

Incidence
- Commonest age group 20–40 yrs old
- Non-smokers

Pathology
- Site Rectum → proximal
- Continuous
- Occasional 'backwash ileitis'
- Affects mucosa
- Forms pseudopolyps
- Toxic megacolon
- Risk of Malignancy

Clinical
- Diarrhoea
  - Periodic
  - Bloody More common than Crohn's dz
  - Slime
- Abdo pain
  - LIF
  - Eased by defaecation
- Fever
- Remissions
- Acute attack
  - Very ill
  - Vomiting
  - Diarrhoea Bloody
  - Systemic signs
  - Toxic megacolon
    - AXR Colon diameter > 6 cm
  - Perforation Peritonitis
  - Haemorrhage

Can lead to
- Colorectal Ca 10%
- Extra-GIT
  - Clubbing
  - Aphthous ulcers
  - Erythema nodosum
  - Pyoderma gangrenosum
  - Ankylosing spondylitis
  - Conjunctivitis
  - Sclerosing cholangitis

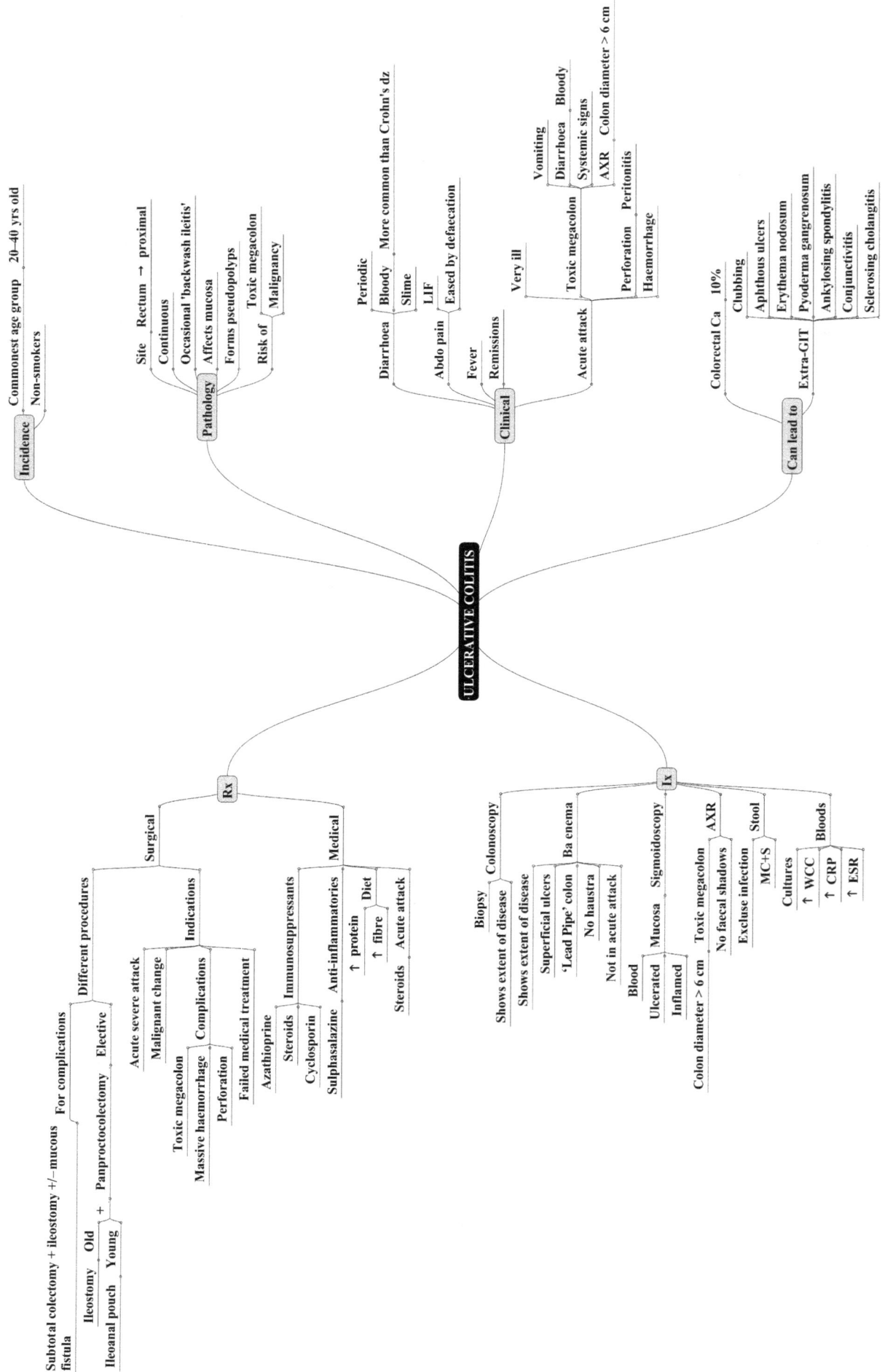

Rx
Surgical
- Different procedures
  - Subtotal colectomy + ileostomy +/– mucous fistula For complications
  - Panproctocolectomy Elective
    - + Ileostomy Old
    - + Ileoanal pouch Young
- Indications
  - Acute severe attack
  - Malignant change
  - Complications
    - Toxic megacolon
    - Massive haemorrhage
    - Perforation
  - Failed medical treatment

Medical
- Immunosuppressants
  - Azathioprine
  - Steroids
  - Cyclosporin
- Anti-inflammatories
  - Sulphasalazine
- Diet
  - ↑ protein
  - ↑ fibre
- Acute attack
  - Steroids

Ix
- Colonoscopy
  - Biopsy
  - Shows extent of disease
- Ba enema
  - Shows extent of disease
  - Superficial ulcers
  - 'Lead Pipe' colon
  - No haustra
  - Not in acute attack
- Sigmoidoscopy
  - Mucosa
    - Blood
    - Ulcerated
    - Inflamed
- AXR
  - Toxic megacolon
    - Colon diameter > 6 cm
  - No faecal shadows
- Stool
  - Excluse infection
  - MC+S
  - Cultures
- Bloods
  - ↑ WCC
  - ↑ CRP
  - ↑ ESR

DIVERTICULAR DISEASE

Definition
- Mucosal outpouchings
- Anti-mesenteric border
- Diverticulosis — Diverticula present
- Diverticular disease — Symptomatic
- Diverticulitis — Inflammation

Incidence
- Very common

Cause
- Low fibre
- ↑ colonic pressure

Clinical
- Diverticular disease
  - Asymptomatic
  - Abdo pain
  - Diarrhoea
  - Constipation
  - Bleeding — Commonest cause
- Diverticulitis
  - LIF pain — 'Left appendicitis'
  - Mucus PR
  - Pyrexia
  - LIF mass
  - Pericolic abscess
  - Peritonism

Can lead to
- Perforation
- Fistulas to
  - Small bowel
  - Vagina
  - Bladder — Pneumaturia — Bubbling in urine
  - Faeces in urine
- Strictures — Bowel obstruction
- Abscess — Due to localized perforation

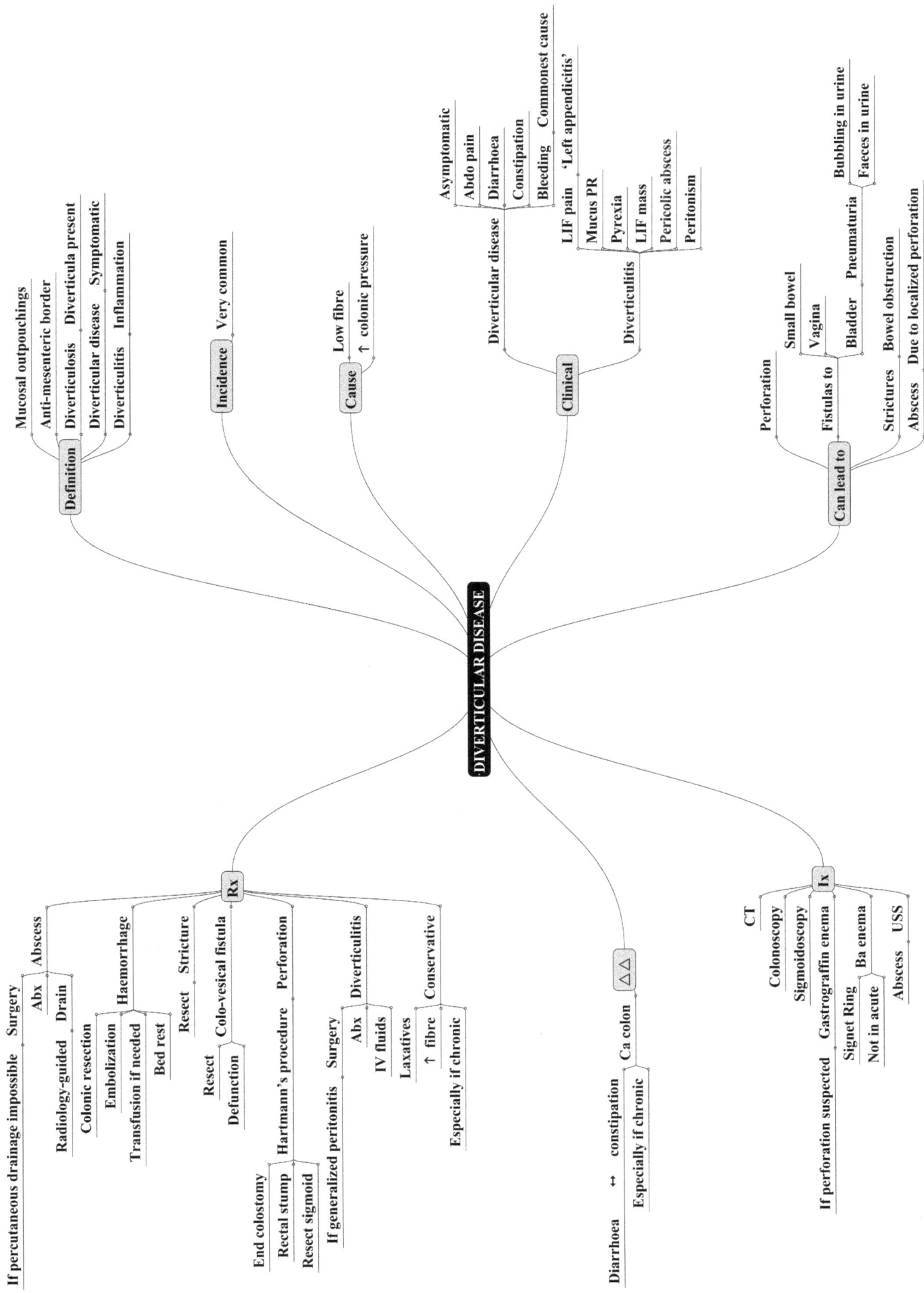

Rx
- Abscess
  - If percutaneous drainage impossible — Surgery
  - Abx
  - Drain — Radiology-guided
- Haemorrhage
  - Colonic resection
  - Embolization
  - Transfusion if needed
  - Bed rest
- Stricture — Resect
- Colo-vesical fistula
  - Resect
  - Defunction
- Perforation
  - End colostomy
  - Rectal stump — Hartmann's procedure
  - Resect sigmoid
  - If generalized peritonitis — Surgery
- Diverticulitis
  - Abx
  - IV fluids
  - Laxatives
- Conservative
  - ↑ fibre
  - Especially if chronic

ΔΔ
- Diarrhoea ↔ constipation
- Ca colon
  - Especially if chronic

Ix
- CT
- Colonoscopy
- Sigmoidoscopy
- Gastrograffin enema — If perforation suspected
- Ba enema
  - Signet Ring
  - Not in acute
- Abscess
- USS

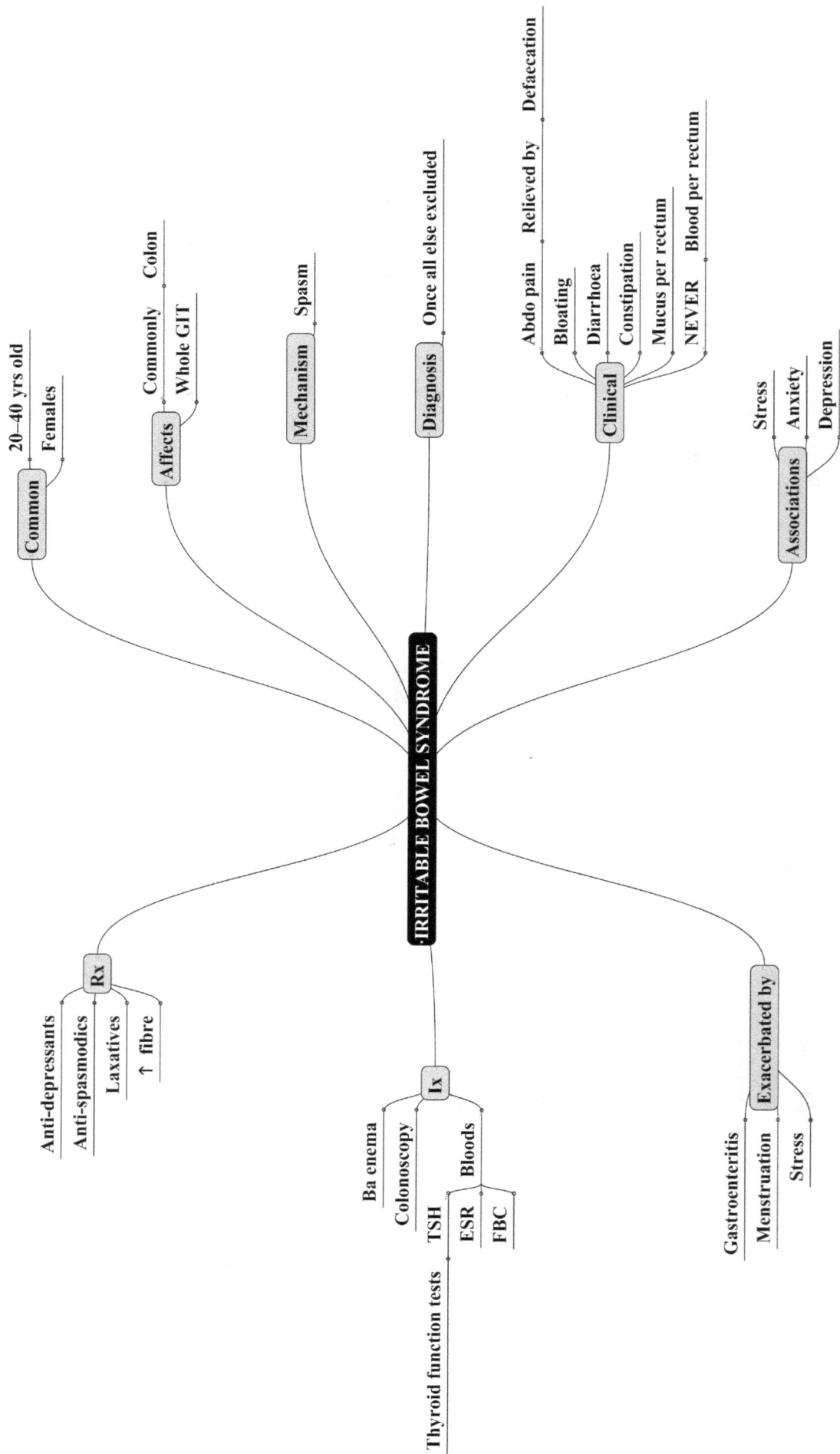

IRRITABLE BOWEL SYNDROME

Common
- 20–40 yrs old
- Females

Affects
- Commonly Colon
- Whole GIT

Mechanism
- Spasm

Diagnosis
- Once all else excluded

Clinical
- Abdo pain
- Relieved by Defaecation
- Bloating
- Diarrhoea
- Constipation
- Mucus per rectum
- NEVER Blood per rectum

Associations
- Stress
- Anxiety
- Depression

Rx
- Anti-depressants
- Anti-spasmodics
- Laxatives
- ↑ fibre

Ix
- Ba enema
- Colonoscopy
- Bloods
  - TSH Thyroid function tests
  - ESR
  - FBC

Exacerbated by
- Gastroenteritis
- Menstruation
- Stress

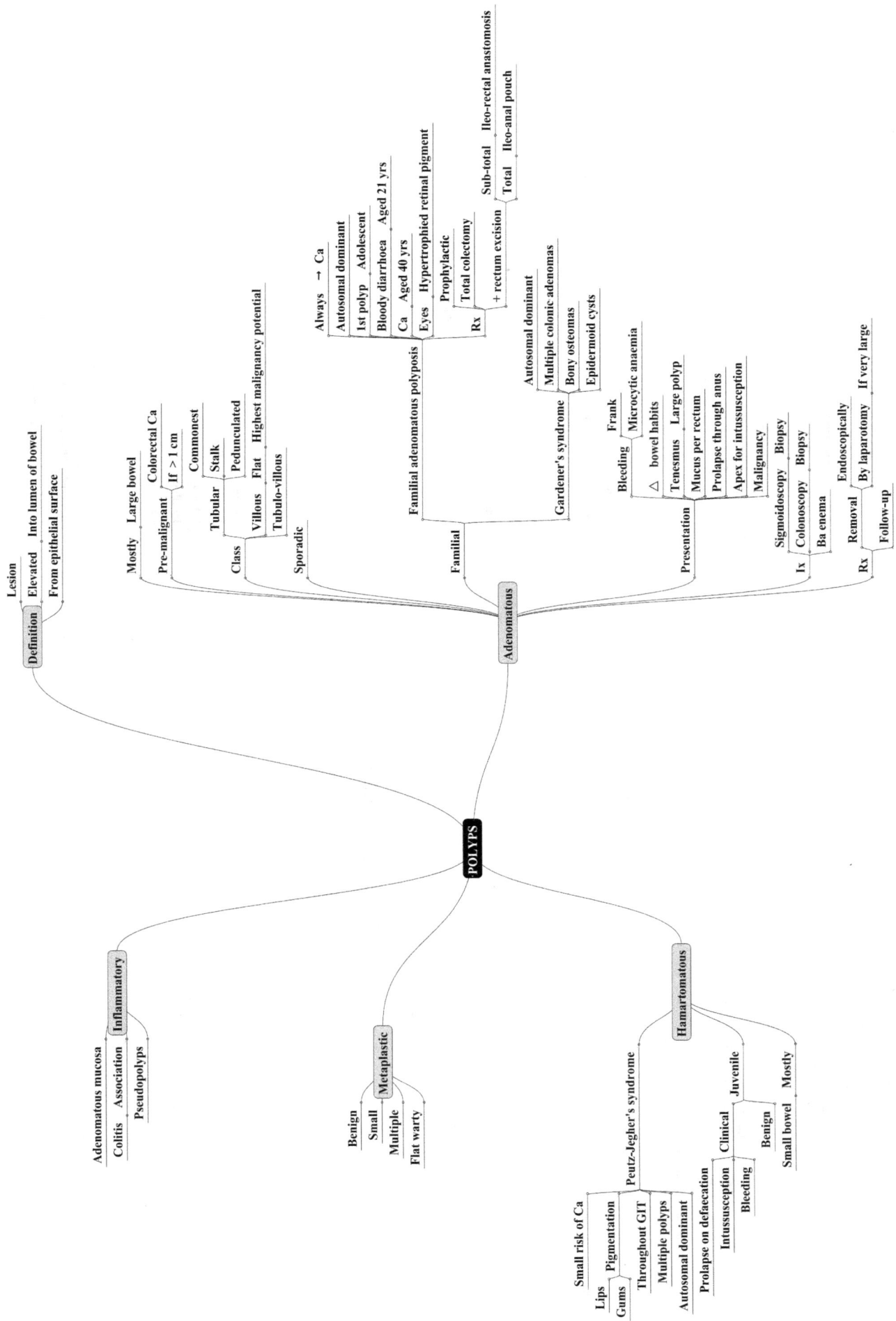

POLYPS

Definition
- Lesion
- Elevated
- Into lumen of bowel
- From epithelial surface

Inflammatory
- Adenomatous mucosa
- Association — Colitis
- Pseudopolyps

Metaplastic
- Benign
- Small
- Multiple
- Flat warty

Adenomatous

Mostly Large bowel
- Pre-malignant
  - Colorectal Ca
  - If > 1 cm
- Class
  - Tubular — Commonest
    - Stalk
    - Pedunculated
  - Villous — Highest malignancy potential
    - Flat
  - Tubulo-villous
- Sporadic

Familial
Familial adenomatous polyposis
- Always → Ca
- Autosomal dominant
- 1st polyp — Adolescent
- Bloody diarrhoea — Aged 21 yrs
- Ca — Aged 40 yrs
- Eyes — Hypertrophied retinal pigment
- Rx
  - Prophylactic
  - Total colectomy
  - + rectum excision
    - Sub-total — Ileo-rectal anastomosis
    - Total — Ileo-anal pouch

Gardener's syndrome
- Autosomal dominant
- Multiple colonic adenomas
- Bony osteomas
- Epidermoid cysts

Presentation
- Bleeding — Frank / Microcytic anaemia
- Δ bowel habits
- Tenesmus — Large polyp
- Mucus per rectum
- Prolapse through anus
- Apex for intussusception
- Malignancy

Ix
- Sigmoidoscopy — Biopsy
- Colonoscopy — Biopsy
- Ba enema

Rx
- Removal
  - Endoscopically
  - By laparotomy — If very large
- Follow-up

Hamartomatous

Peutz–Jegher's syndrome
- Small risk of Ca
- Pigmentation — Lips / Gums
- Throughout GIT
- Multiple polyps
- Autosomal dominant

Juvenile
- Clinical
  - Prolapse on defaecation
  - Intussusception
  - Bleeding
- Benign
- Small bowel — Mostly

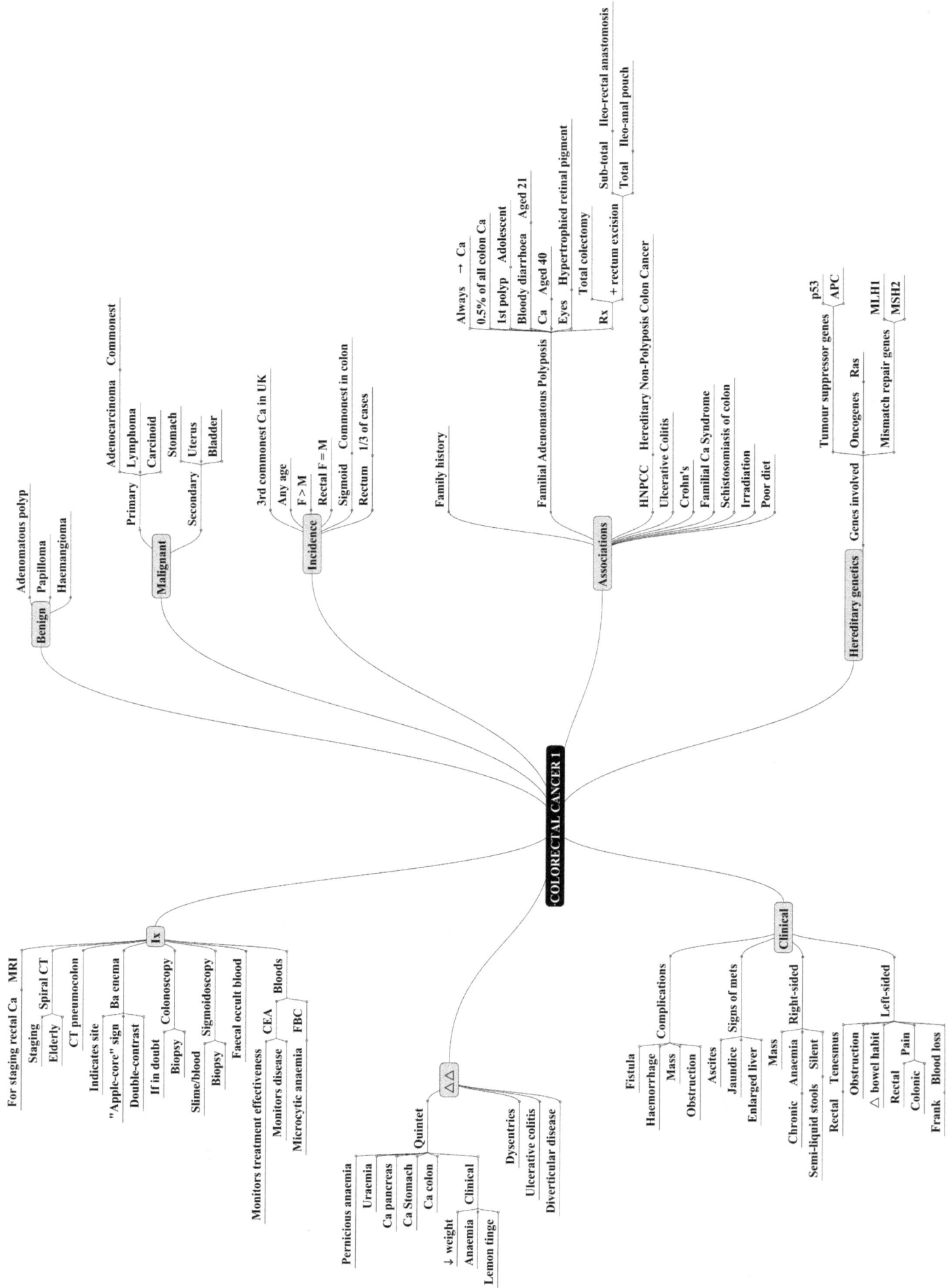

COLORECTAL CANCER 1

Benign
- Adenomatous polyp
- Papilloma
- Haemangioma

Malignant
- Primary
  - Adenocarcinoma — Commonest
  - Lymphoma
  - Carcinoid
- Secondary
  - Stomach
  - Uterus
  - Bladder

Incidence
- 3rd commonest Ca in UK
- Any age
- F > M
- Rectal F = M
- Sigmoid — Commonest in colon
- Rectum — 1/3 of cases

Associations
- Family history
- Familial Adenomatous Polyposis
  - Always → Ca
  - 0.5% of all colon Ca
  - 1st polyp — Adolescent
  - Bloody diarrhoea — Aged 21
  - Ca — Aged 40
  - Eyes — Hypertrophied retinal pigment
  - Rx — Total colectomy + rectum excision
    - Sub-total — Ileo-rectal anastomosis
    - Total — Ileo-anal pouch
- HNPCC — Hereditary Non-Polyposis Colon Cancer
- Ulcerative Colitis
- Crohn's
- Familial Ca Syndrome
- Schistosomiasis of colon
- Irradiation
- Poor diet

Hereditary genetics
- Genes involved
  - Tumour suppressor genes
    - p53
    - APC
  - Oncogenes — Ras
  - Mismatch repair genes
    - MLH1
    - MSH2

Ix
- For staging rectal Ca — MRI
- Staging — Spiral CT
- Elderly — CT pneumocolon
- Ba enema
  - Indicates site
  - "Apple-core" sign
  - Double-contrast
- Colonoscopy
  - If in doubt
  - Biopsy
- Sigmoidoscopy
  - Slime/blood
  - Biopsy
- Faecal occult blood
- CEA
  - Monitors treatment effectiveness
  - Monitors disease
- Bloods
  - Microcytic anaemia
  - FBC

ΔΔ
- Quintet
  - Pernicious anaemia
  - Uraemia
  - Ca pancreas
  - Ca Stomach
  - Ca colon
  - Clinical
    - ↓ weight
    - Anaemia
    - Lemon tinge
- Dysentries
- Ulcerative colitis
- Diverticular disease

Clinical
- Complications
  - Fistula
  - Haemorrhage
  - Mass
  - Obstruction
- Signs of mets
  - Ascites
  - Jaundice
  - Enlarged liver
- Right-sided
  - Mass
  - Chronic Anaemia
  - Silent
- Left-sided
  - Semi-liquid stools
  - Rectal Tenesmus
  - Obstruction
  - Δ bowel habit
  - Rectal Pain
  - Colonic Pain
  - Frank Blood loss

COLORECTAL CANCER 2

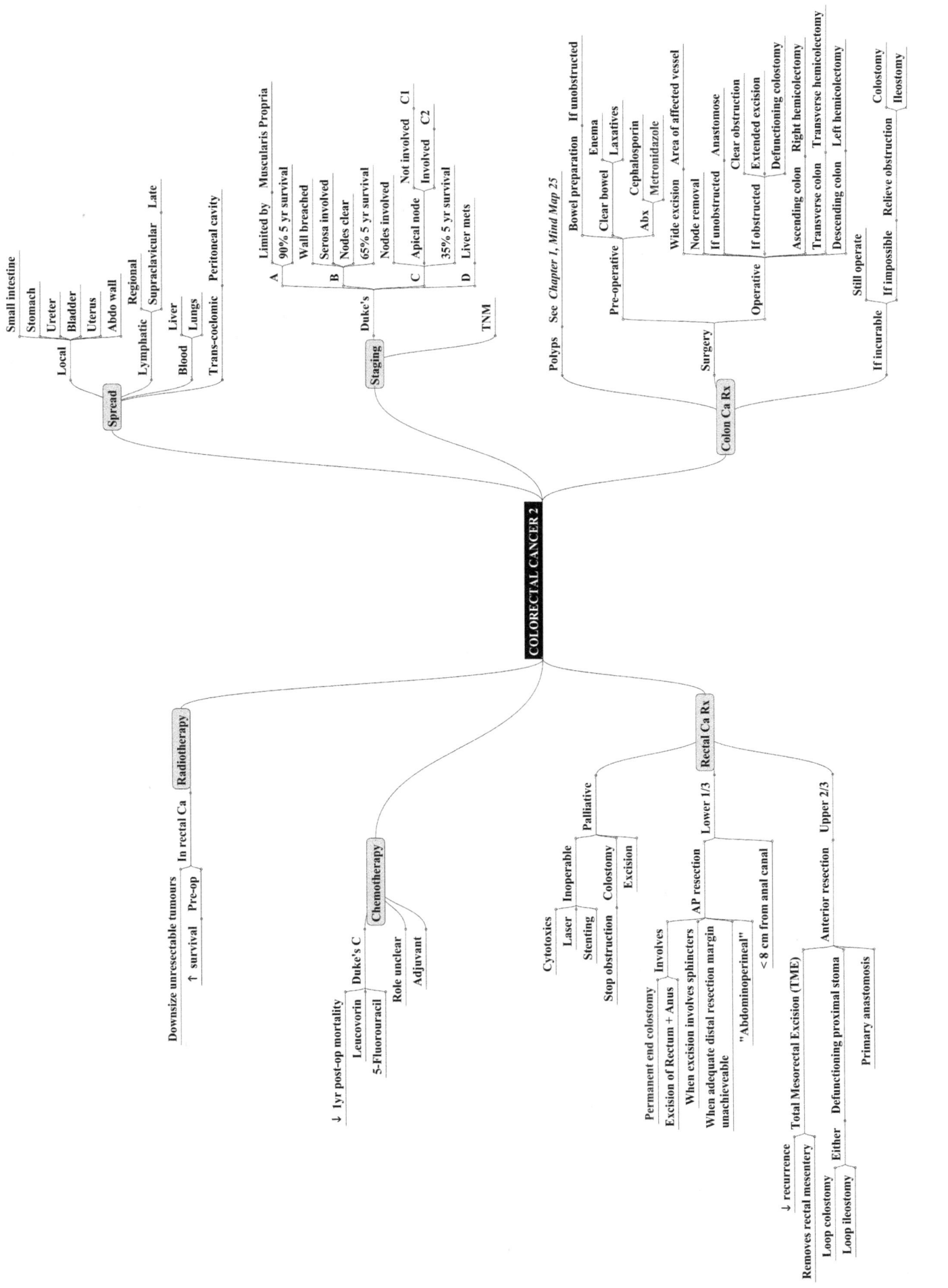

Spread

- **Local**
  - Small intestine
  - Stomach
  - Ureter
  - Bladder
  - Uterus
  - Abdo wall
- **Lymphatic**
  - Regional
  - Supraclavicular
  - Late
- **Blood**
  - Liver
  - Lungs
- Trans-coelomic — Peritoneal cavity

Staging

- **Duke's**
  - **A** — Limited by — Muscularis Propria — 90% 5 yr survival
  - **B**
    - Wall breached
    - Serosa involved
    - Nodes clear — 65% 5 yr survival
  - **C**
    - Nodes involved
    - Apical node — Not involved **C1** / Involved **C2** — 35% 5 yr survival
  - **D** — Liver mets
- TNM

Colon Ca Rx

- Polyps — See *Chapter 1, Mind Map 25*
- **Surgery**
  - **Pre-operative**
    - Bowel preparation — If unobstructed
    - Clear bowel
      - Enema
      - Laxatives
    - Abx
      - Cephalosporin
      - Metronidazole
  - **Operative**
    - Wide excision — Area of affected vessel
    - Node removal
    - If unobstructed — Anastomose
    - If obstructed
      - Clear obstruction
      - Extended excision
      - Defunctioning colostomy
    - Ascending colon — Right hemicolectomy
    - Transverse colon — Transverse hemicolectomy
    - Descending colon — Left hemicolectomy
  - **If incurable**
    - Still operate
    - If impossible — Relieve obstruction
      - Colostomy
      - Ileostomy

Radiotherapy

- Downsize unresectable tumours — In rectal Ca
- ↑ survival — Pre-op

Chemotherapy

- ↓ 1yr post-op mortality — Duke's C
  - Leucovorin
  - 5-Fluorouracil
- Role unclear — Adjuvant

Rectal Ca Rx

- **Palliative**
  - Cytotoxics
  - Inoperable
    - Laser
    - Stenting
  - Stop obstruction
    - Colostomy
    - Excision
- **Lower 1/3**
  - Involves
    - Permanent end colostomy
    - Excision of Rectum + Anus
    - When excision involves sphincters
    - When adequate distal resection margin unachieveable
  - **AP resection** — "Abdominoperineal" — < 8 cm from anal canal
- **Upper 2/3**
  - **Anterior resection**
    - Total Mesorectal Excision (TME)
      - ↓ recurrence
      - Removes rectal mesentery
    - Defunctioning proximal stoma
      - Either
        - Loop colostomy
        - Loop ileostomy
    - Primary anastomosis

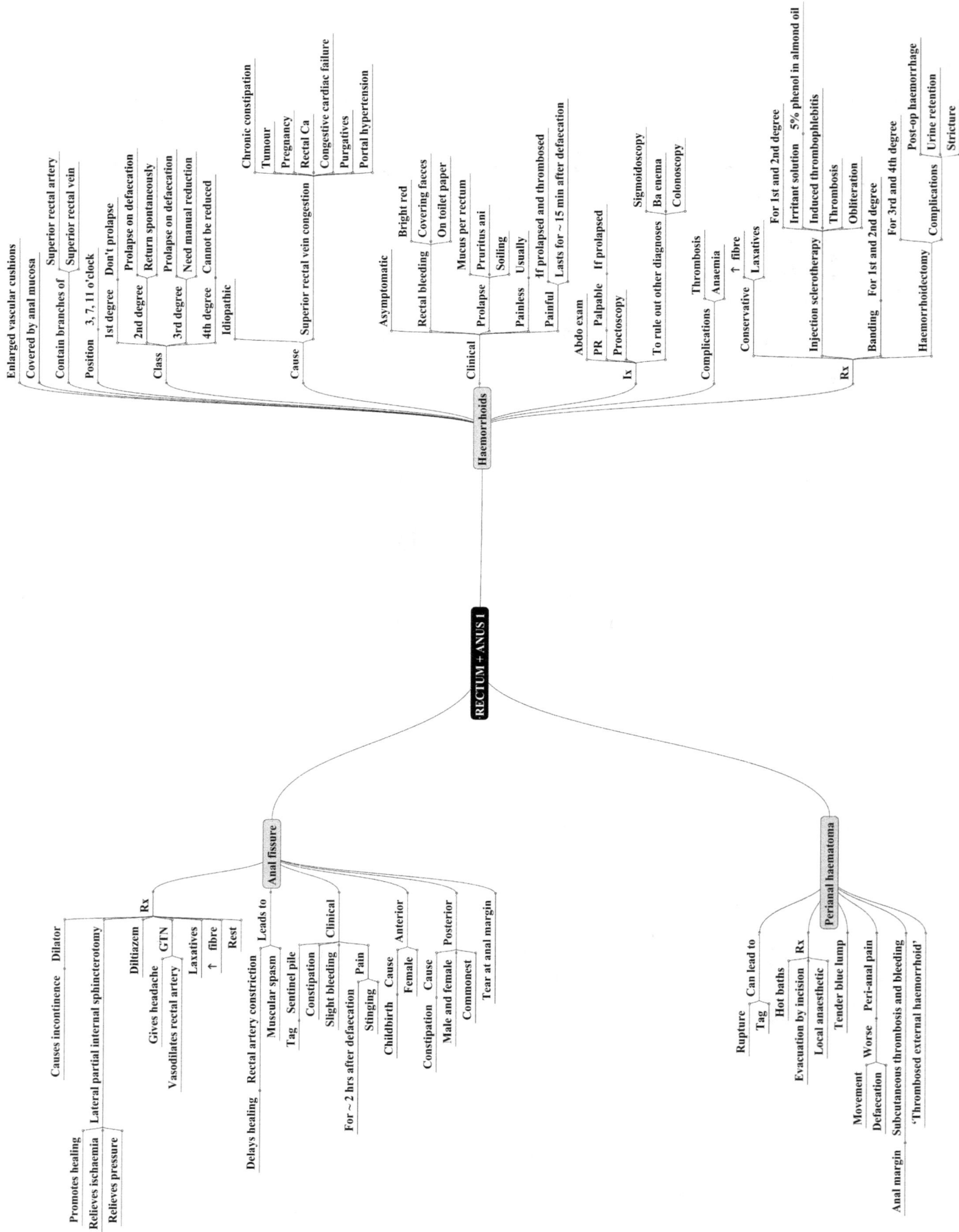

RECTUM + ANUS 1

Haemorrhoids

- Enlarged vascular cushions
- Covered by anal mucosa
- Contain branches of — Superior rectal artery / Superior rectal vein
- Position 3, 7, 11 o'clock
- Class
  - 1st degree — Don't prolapse
  - 2nd degree — Prolapse on defaecation / Return spontaneously
  - 3rd degree — Prolapse on defaecation / Need manual reduction
  - 4th degree — Cannot be reduced
- Cause
  - Idiopathic
  - Superior rectal vein congestion
    - Chronic constipation
    - Tumour
    - Pregnancy
    - Rectal Ca
    - Congestive cardiac failure
    - Purgatives
    - Portal hypertension
- Clinical
  - Asymptomatic
  - Rectal bleeding — Bright red / Covering faeces / On toilet paper
  - Prolapse — Mucus per rectum / Pruritus ani / Soiling
  - Painless — Usually
  - Painful — If prolapsed and thrombosed / Lasts for ~ 15 min after defaecation
- Ix
  - Abdo exam
  - PR — Palpable / If prolapsed
  - Proctoscopy
  - To rule out other diagnoses — Sigmoidoscopy / Ba enema / Colonoscopy
- Complications
  - Thrombosis
  - Anaemia
- Rx
  - Conservative — ↑ fibre / Laxatives
  - Injection sclerotherapy
    - For 1st and 2nd degree
    - Irritant solution — 5% phenol in almond oil
    - Induced thrombophlebitis — Thrombosis / Obliteration
  - Banding — For 1st and 2nd degree
  - Haemorrhoidectomy
    - For 3rd and 4th degree
    - Complications — Post-op haemorrhage / Urine retention / Stricture

Anal fissure

- Rx
  - Dilator — Causes incontinence
  - Lateral partial internal sphincterotomy — Promotes healing / Relieves ischaemia / Relieves pressure
  - Diltiazem
  - GTN — Gives headache / Vasodilates rectal artery
  - Laxatives — ↑ fibre
  - Rest
- Leads to
  - Rectal artery constriction — Delays healing
  - Muscular spasm
  - Sentinel pile — Tag
- Clinical
  - Constipation
  - Slight bleeding
  - Pain — Stinging / For ~ 2 hrs after defaecation
- Cause
  - Anterior — Female — Childbirth
  - Posterior — Male and female — Commonest — Constipation
- Tear at anal margin

Perianal haematoma

- Can lead to
  - Rupture
  - Tag
- Rx
  - Hot baths
  - Evacuation by incision — Local anaesthetic
- Tender blue lump
- Peri-anal pain — Worse — Movement / Defaecation
- Subcutaneous thrombosis and bleeding
- 'Thrombosed external haemorrhoid'
- Anal margin

RECTUM + ANUS 2

Fistula-in-ano

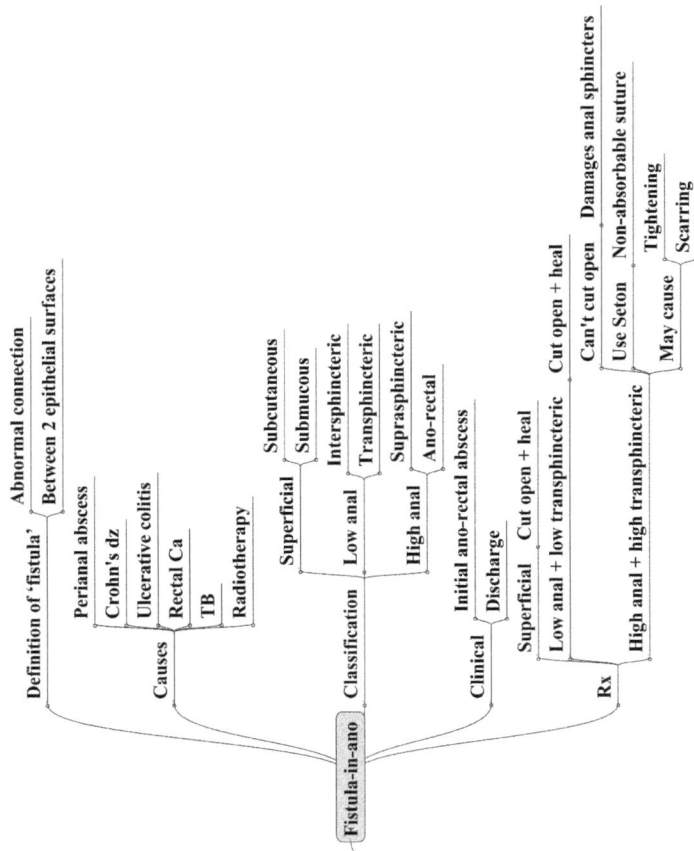

Definition of 'fistula'
- Abnormal connection
- Between 2 epithelial surfaces

Causes
- Perianal abscess
- Crohn's dz
- Ulcerative colitis
- Rectal Ca
- TB
- Radiotherapy

Classification
- Subcutaneous
- Submucous
- Intersphincteric
- Superficial
- Low anal — Transsphincteric
- High anal — Suprasphincteric
- Ano-rectal

Clinical
- Initial ano-rectal abscess
- Discharge

Rx
- Superficial — Cut open + heal
- Low anal + low transphincteric — Cut open + heal
- High anal + high transphincteric
  - Can't cut open — Damages anal sphincters
  - Use Seton — Non-absorbable suture
  - May cause — Tightening — Scarring

Ano-rectal abscess

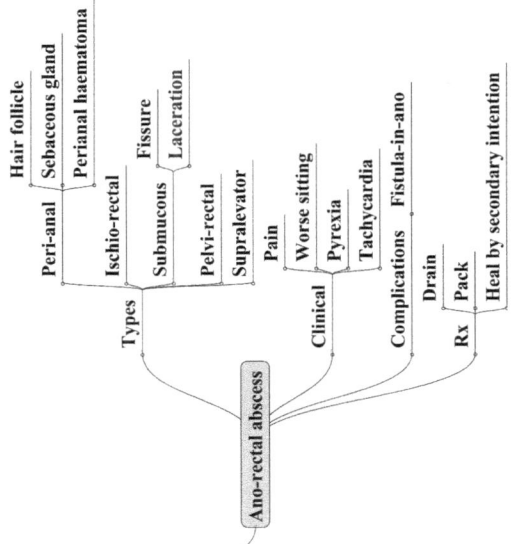

Types
- Peri-anal
  - Hair follicle
  - Sebaceous gland
  - Perianal haematoma
- Ischio-rectal
  - Fissure
  - Laceration
- Submucous
- Pelvi-rectal
- Supralevator

Clinical
- Pain — Worse sitting
- Pyrexia
- Tachycardia

Complications
- Fistula-in-ano

Rx
- Drain
- Pack
- Heal by secondary intention

Pilonidal abscess / sinus

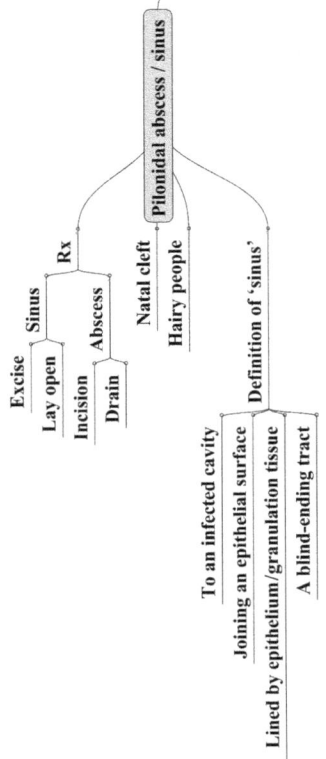

Rx
- Sinus — Excise — Lay open
- Abscess — Incision — Drain

- Natal cleft
- Hairy people

Definition of 'sinus'
- To an infected cavity
- Joining an epithelial surface
- Lined by epithelium/granulation tissue
- A blind-ending tract

Rectal prolapse

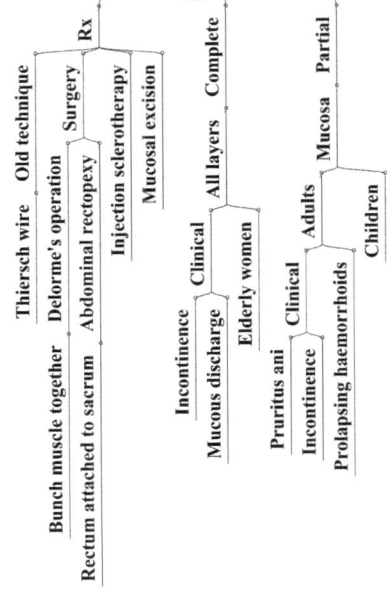

Rx
- Old technique
  - Thiersch wire — Bunch muscle together
  - Delorme's operation
- Surgery
  - Abdominal rectopexy — Rectum attached to sacrum
  - Injection sclerotherapy
  - Mucosal excision

Complete
- All layers
- Clinical
  - Incontinence
  - Mucous discharge
- Elderly women

Partial
- Mucosa
- Adults — Clinical
  - Pruritus ani
  - Incontinence
  - Prolapsing haemorrhoids
- Children

Chapter 2

HEPATOBILIARY

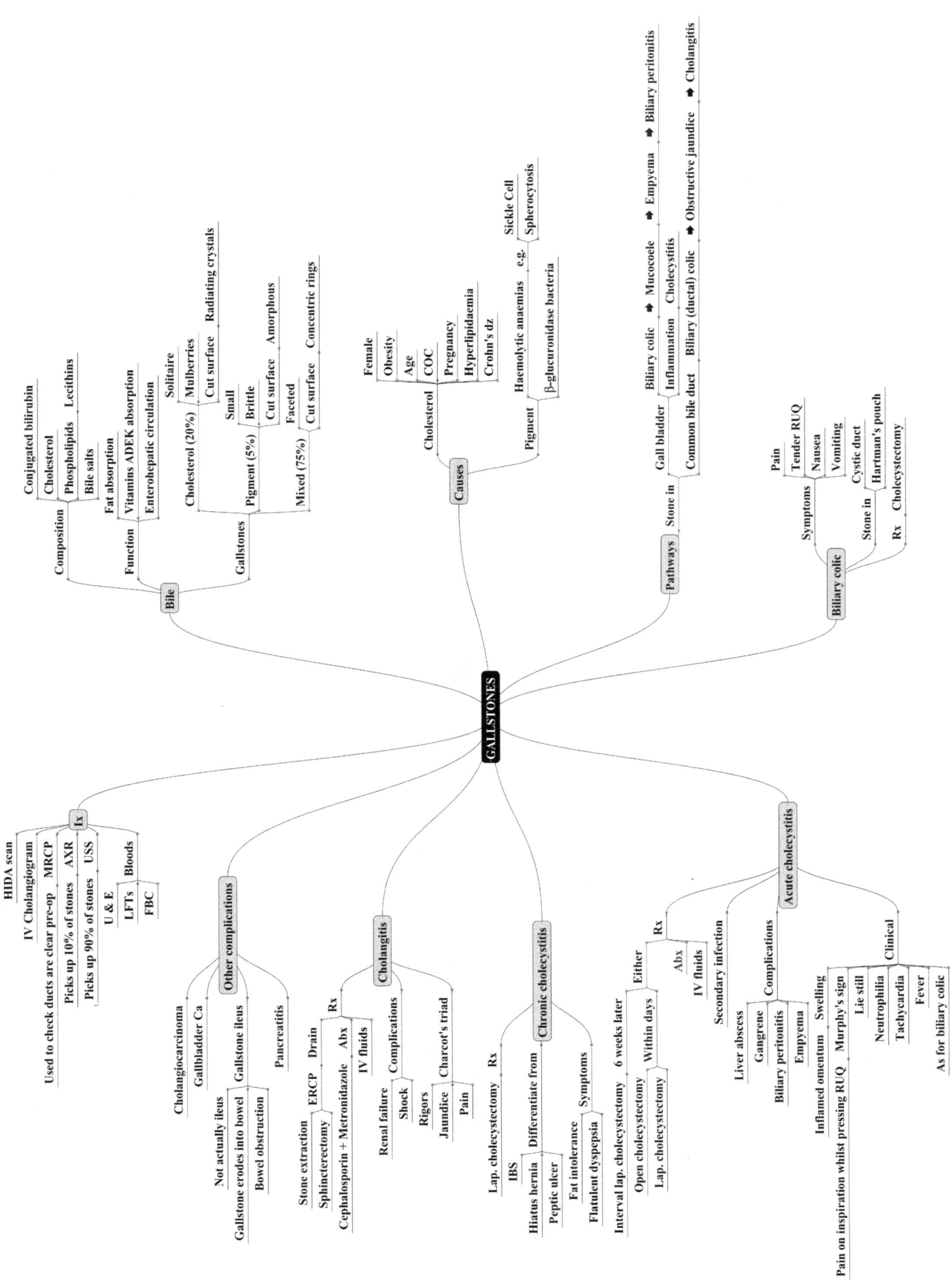

GALLSTONES

Bile

Composition
- Conjugated bilirubin
- Cholesterol
- Phospholipids — Lecithins
- Bile salts

Function
- Fat absorption
- Vitamins ADEK absorption
- Enterohepatic circulation

Gallstones
- Cholesterol (20%)
  - Solitaire
  - Mulberries
  - Cut surface — Radiating crystals
- Pigment (5%)
  - Small
  - Brittle
  - Cut surface — Amorphous
- Mixed (75%)
  - Faceted
  - Cut surface — Concentric rings

Causes

Cholesterol
- Female
- Obesity
- Age
- COC
- Pregnancy
- Hyperlipidaemia
- Crohn's dz

Pigment
- Haemolytic anaemias e.g. Sickle Cell / Spherocytosis
- β-glucuronidase bacteria

Pathways

Stone in
- Gall bladder
  - Biliary colic
  - ↑ Mucocoele
  - Inflammation — ↑ Empyema
  - Cholecystitis
- Common bile duct
  - Biliary (ductal) colic
  - ↑ Obstructive jaundice — ↑ Biliary peritonitis
  - ↑ Cholangitis

Biliary colic

Symptoms
- Pain
- Tender RUQ
- Nausea
- Vomiting

Stone in — Cystic duct / Hartman's pouch

Rx — Cholecystectomy

Ix
- HIDA scan
- IV Cholangiogram
  - Used to check ducts are clear pre-op
- MRCP
- AXR — Picks up 10% of stones
- USS — Picks up 90% of stones
- Bloods
  - U & E
  - LFTs
  - FBC

Other complications
- Cholangiocarcinoma
- Gallbladder Ca
- Gallstone ileus
  - Not actually ileus
  - Gallstone erodes into bowel
  - Bowel obstruction
- Pancreatitis

Cholangitis
- Rx
  - Stone extraction
    - ERCP
    - Sphincterectomy
  - Abx — Cephalosporin + Metronidazole
  - IV fluids
- Complications
  - Renal failure
  - Shock
- Charcot's triad
  - Rigors
  - Jaundice
  - Pain

Chronic cholecystitis
- Rx — Lap. cholecystectomy
- Differentiate from
  - IBS
  - Hiatus hernia
  - Peptic ulcer
- Symptoms
  - Fat intolerance
  - Flatulent dyspepsia

Acute cholecystitis
- Rx
  - Either
    - Interval lap. cholecystectomy — 6 weeks later
    - Open cholecystectomy — Within days
    - Lap. cholecystectomy
  - Abx
  - IV fluids
- Complications
  - Secondary infection
  - Liver abscess
  - Gangrene
  - Biliary peritonitis
  - Empyema
- Clinical
  - Murphy's sign
    - Inflamed omentum pressing RUQ
    - Swelling
    - Pain on inspiration whilst pressing RUQ
  - Lie still
  - Neutrophilia
  - Tachycardia
  - Fever
  - As for biliary colic

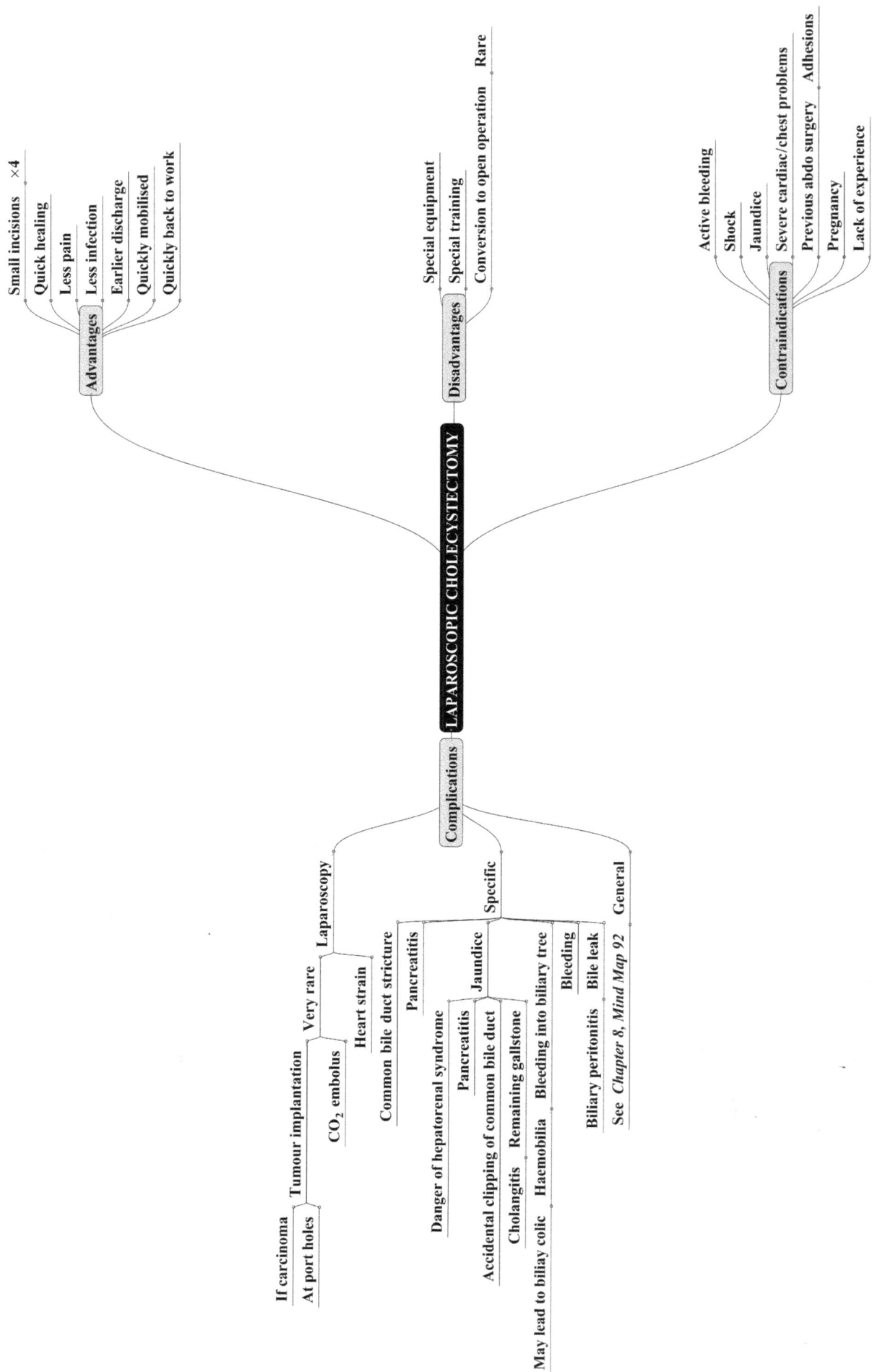

LAPAROSCOPIC CHOLECYSTECTOMY

Advantages

- Small incisions ×4
- Quick healing
- Less pain
- Less infection
- Earlier discharge
- Quickly mobilised
- Quickly back to work

Disadvantages

- Special equipment
- Special training
- Conversion to open operation   Rare

Contraindications

- Active bleeding
- Shock
- Jaundice
- Severe cardiac/chest problems   Adhesions
- Previous abdo surgery
- Pregnancy
- Lack of experience

Complications

Laparoscopy

- If carcinoma
- Tumour implantation
  - At port holes
- Very rare
- CO_2 embolus
- Heart strain

Specific

- Common bile duct stricture
- Pancreatitis
- Danger of hepatorenal syndrome
- Accidental clipping of common bile duct
  - Pancreatitis
  - Jaundice
  - Cholangitis   Remaining gallstone
  - May lead to biliay colic   Haemobilia   Bleeding into biliary tree
- Bleeding
- Bile leak
  - Biliary peritonitis

General

See *Chapter 8, Mind Map 92*

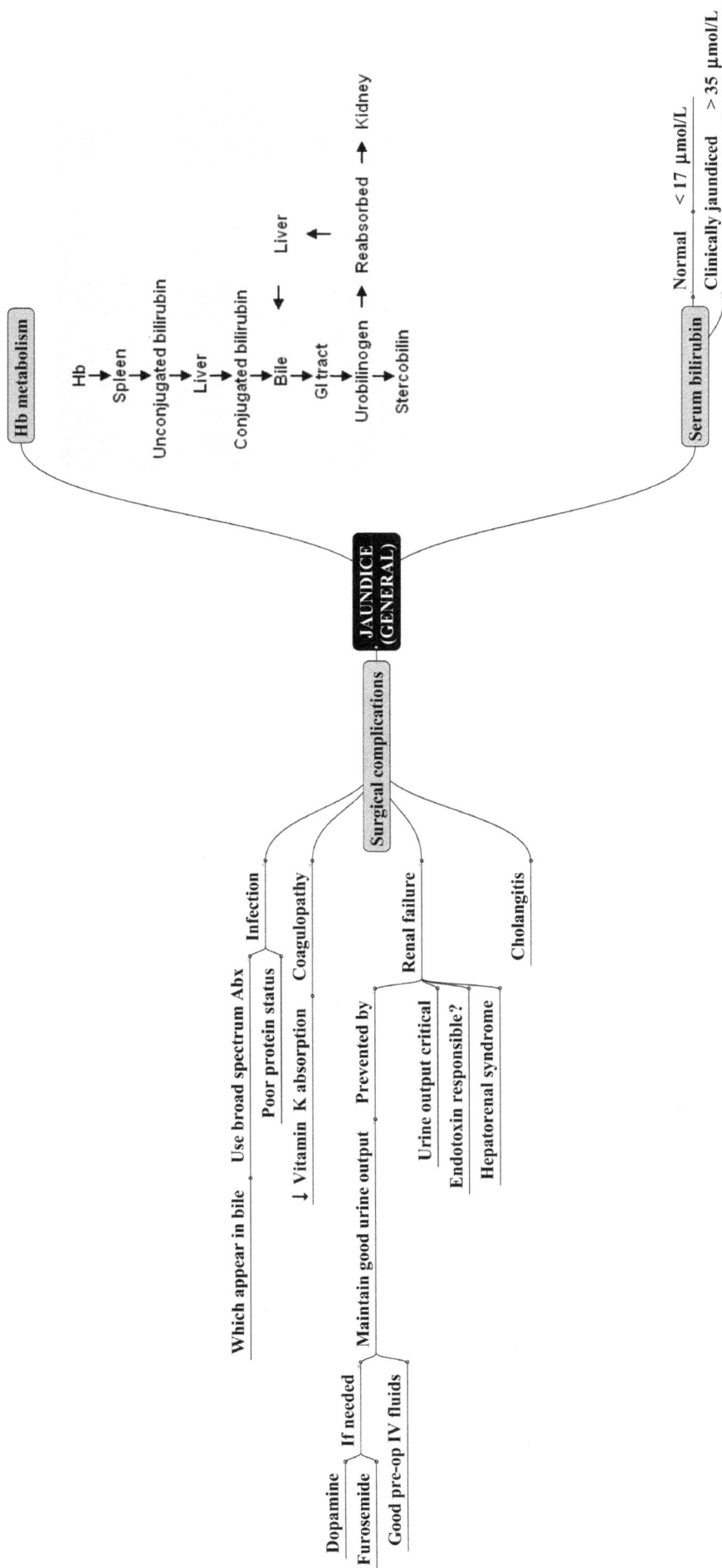

Hb metabolism

Hb → Spleen → Unconjugated bilirubin → Liver → Conjugated bilirubin → Bile → GI tract

Bile → Liver ↑ ← Liver

Urobilinogen → Reabsorbed → Kidney

Stercobilin

Serum bilirubin

Normal <17 μmol/L

Clinically jaundiced >35 μmol/L

JAUNDICE (GENERAL)

Surgical complications

Infection
- Which appear in bile — Use broad spectrum Abx
- Poor protein status
- ↓ Vitamin K absorption

Coagulopathy

Maintain good urine output — Prevented by

Renal failure
- Urine output critical
- Endotoxin responsible?
- Hepatorenal syndrome

Cholangitis

Dopamine — If needed

Furosemide

Good pre-op IV fluids

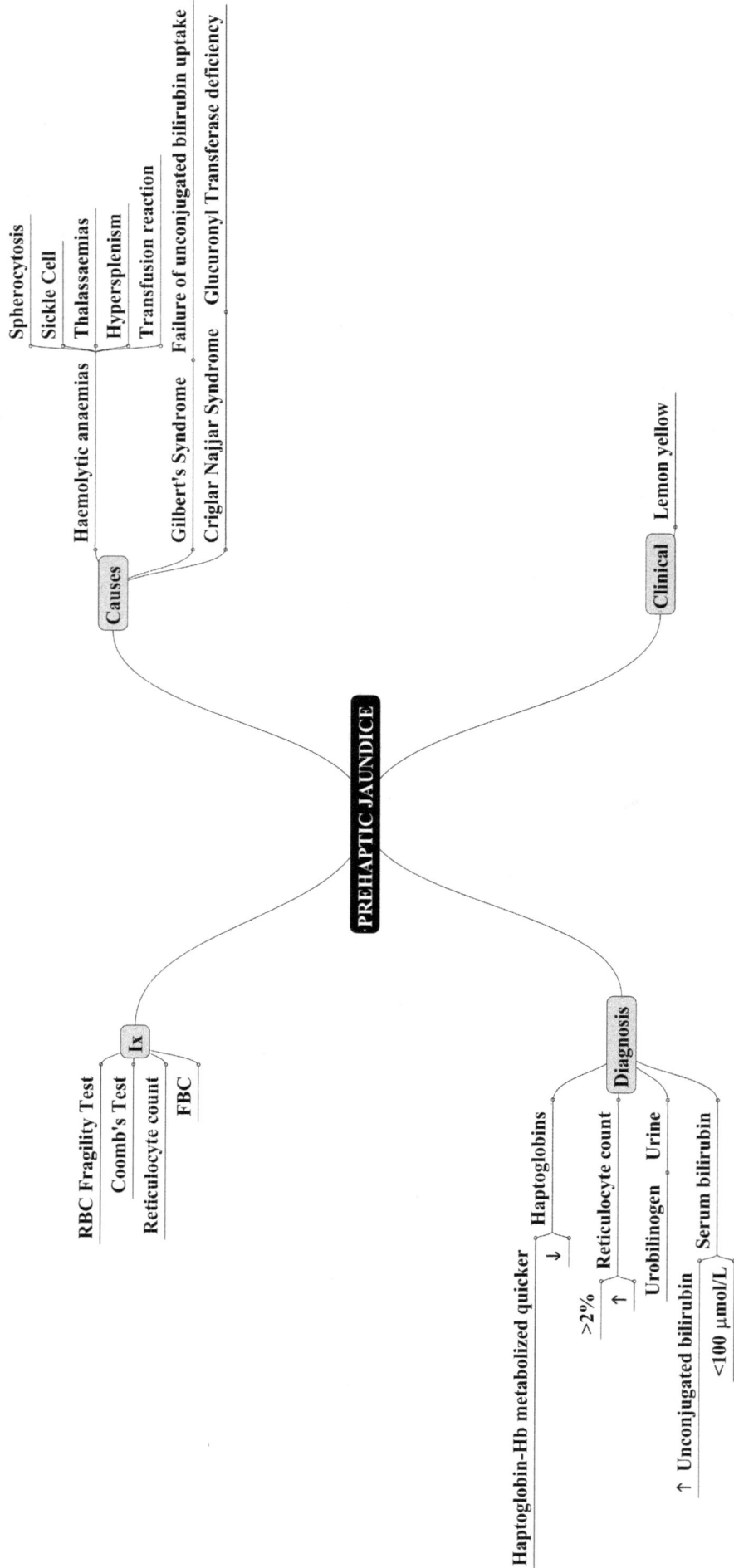

PREHAPTIC JAUNDICE

Causes

- Haemolytic anaemias
  - Spherocytosis
  - Sickle Cell
  - Thalassaemias
  - Hypersplenism
  - Transfusion reaction
- Failure of unconjugated bilirubin uptake
- Gilbert's Syndrome
- Criglar Najjar Syndrome — Glucuronyl Transferase deficiency

Clinical

- Lemon yellow

Ix

- RBC Fragility Test
- Coomb's Test
- Reticulocyte count
- FBC

Diagnosis

- Haptoglobins — Haptoglobin-Hb metabolized quicker ↓
- Reticulocyte count — >2% ↑
- Urine
  - Urobilinogen
  - Serum bilirubin — Unconjugated bilirubin ↑ — <100 μmol/L

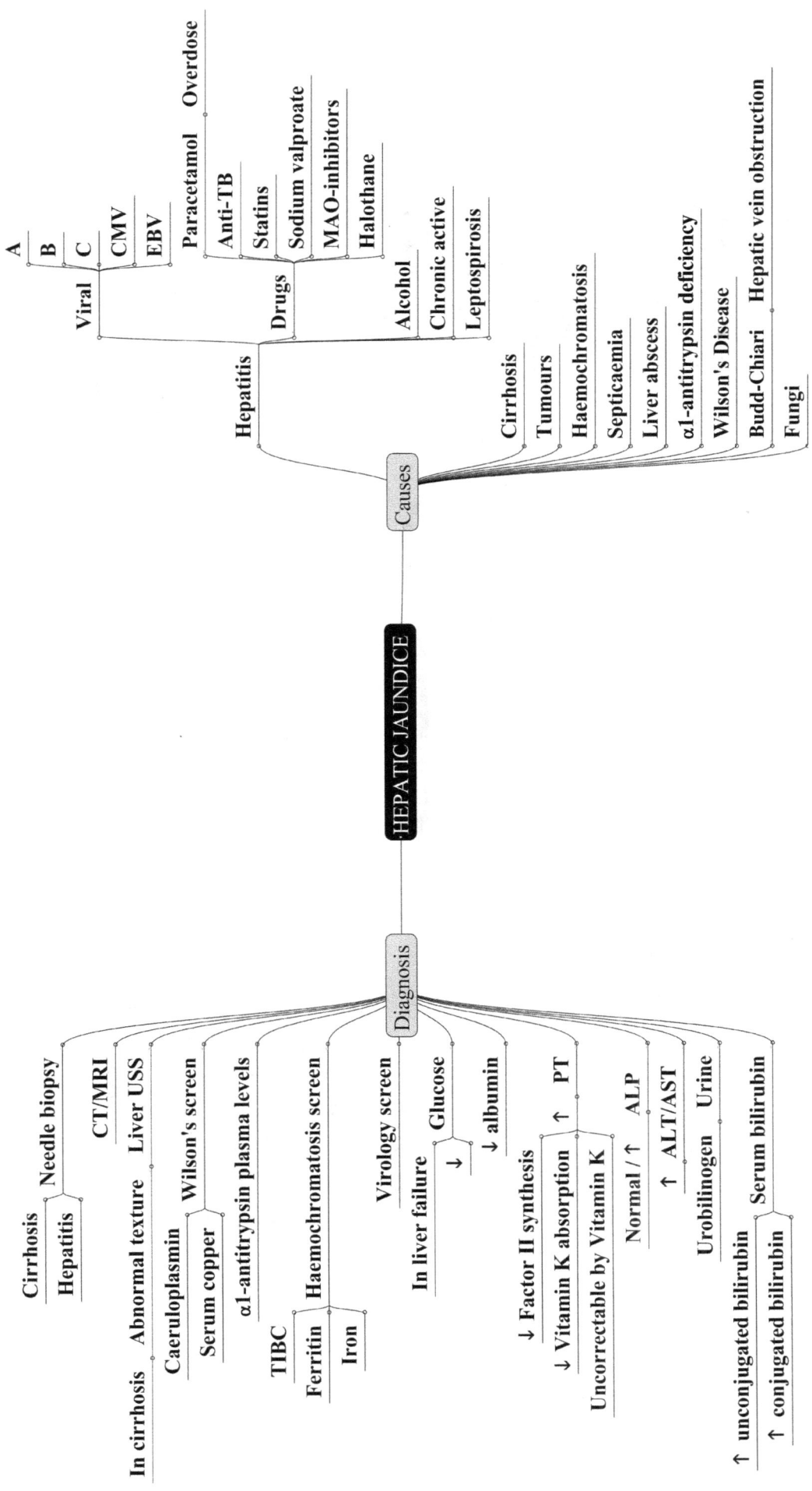

HEPATIC JAUNDICE

Causes

- Hepatitis
  - Viral
    - A
    - B
    - C
    - CMV
    - EBV
  - Drugs
    - Paracetamol — Overdose
    - Anti-TB
    - Statins
    - Sodium valproate
    - MAO-inhibitors
    - Halothane
  - Alcohol
  - Chronic active
  - Leptospirosis
- Cirrhosis
- Tumours
- Haemochromatosis
- Septicaemia
- Liver abscess
- α1-antitrypsin deficiency
- Wilson's Disease
- Budd-Chiari — Hepatic vein obstruction
- Fungi

Diagnosis

- Needle biopsy
  - Cirrhosis
  - Hepatitis
- CT/MRI
  - In cirrhosis — Abnormal texture
- Liver USS
- Wilson's screen
  - Caeruloplasmin
  - Serum copper
- α1-antitrypsin plasma levels
- Haemochromatosis screen
  - TIBC
  - Ferritin
  - Iron
- Virology screen
- Glucose
  - In liver failure — ↓
- ↓ albumin
- PT
  - ↓ Factor II synthesis
  - ↓ Vitamin K absorption
  - Uncorrectable by Vitamin K
- ALP
  - Normal / ↑
- ALT/AST
  - ↑
- Urine
  - ↑ Urobilinogen
- Serum bilirubin
  - ↑ unconjugated bilirubin
  - ↑ conjugated bilirubin

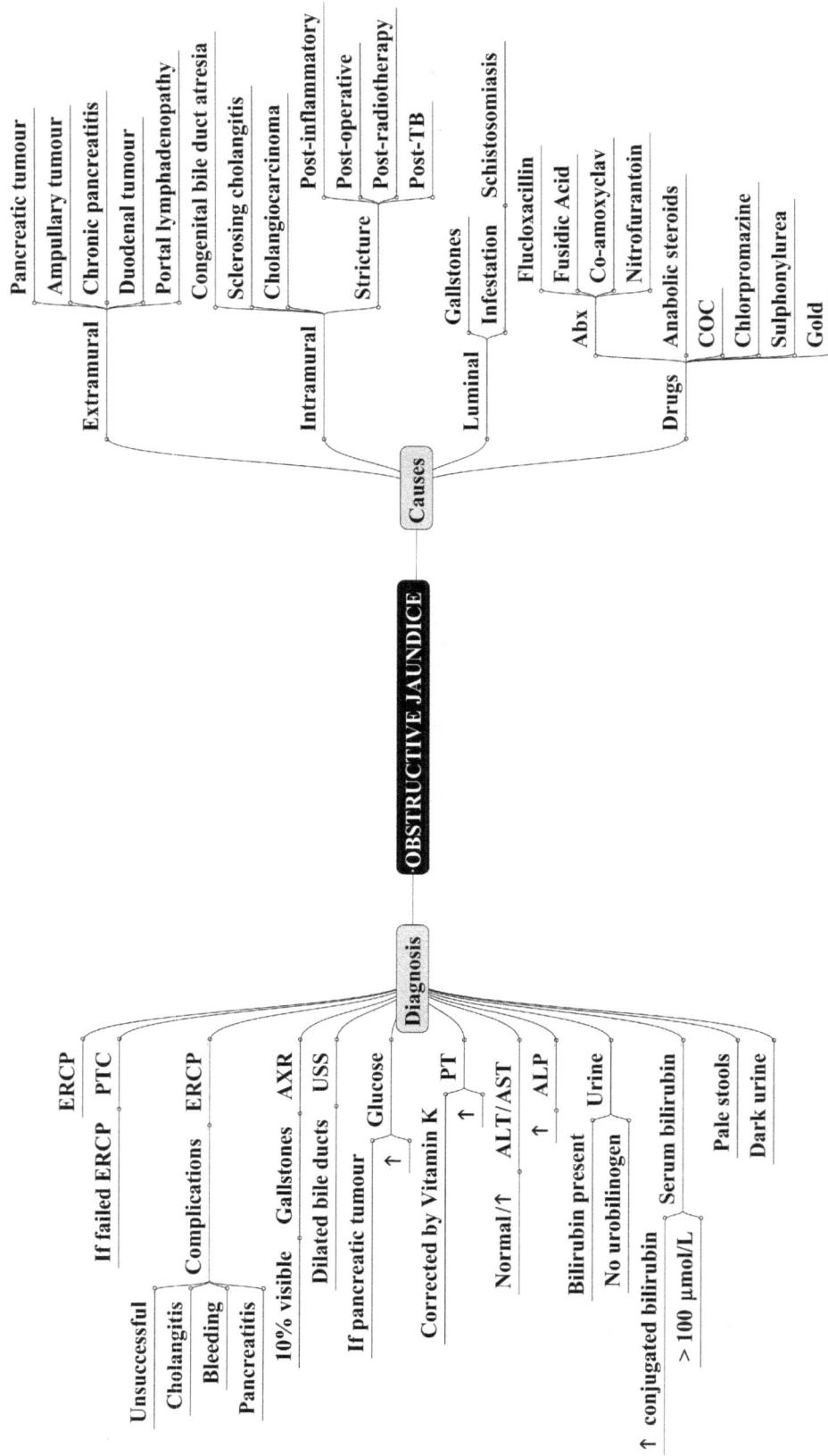

OBSTRUCTIVE JAUNDICE

Causes

- **Extramural**
  - Pancreatic tumour
  - Ampullary tumour
  - Chronic pancreatitis
  - Duodenal tumour
  - Portal lymphadenopathy
- **Intramural**
  - Congenital bile duct atresia
  - Sclerosing cholangitis
  - Cholangiocarcinoma
  - Stricture
    - Post-inflammatory
    - Post-operative
    - Post-radiotherapy
    - Post-TB
- **Luminal**
  - Gallstones
  - Infestation
    - Schistosomiasis
- **Drugs**
  - Abx
    - Flucloxacillin
    - Fusidic Acid
    - Co-amoxyclav
    - Nitrofurantoin
  - Anabolic steroids
  - COC
  - Chlorpromazine
  - Sulphonylurea
  - Gold

Diagnosis

- **ERCP**
  - PTC — If failed ERCP
  - Unsuccessful
  - Complications ERCP
    - Cholangitis
    - Bleeding
    - Pancreatitis
- **AXR** — Gallstones 10% visible
- **USS**
  - Dilated bile ducts
  - If pancreatic tumour
- **Glucose** ↑
- **PT** — Corrected by Vitamin K ↑
- **ALT/AST** — Normal/↑
- **ALP** ↑
- **Urine**
  - Bilirubin present
  - No urobilinogen
- **Serum bilirubin** — ↑ conjugated bilirubin, > 100 μmol/L
- Pale stools
- Dark urine

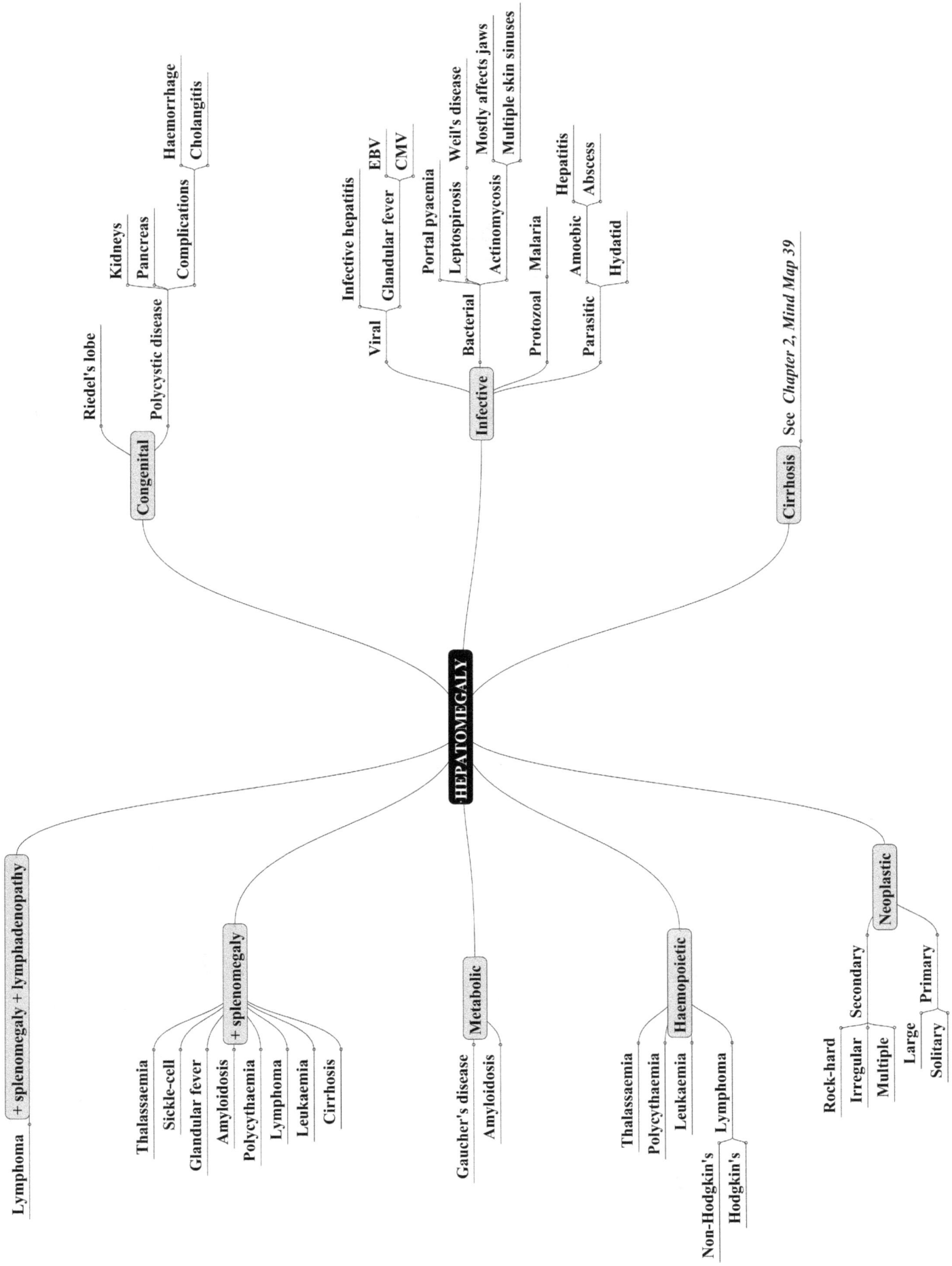

HEPATOMEGALY

Congenital

- Riedel's lobe
- Polycystic disease
  - Kidneys
  - Pancreas
  - Complications
    - Haemorrhage
    - Cholangitis

Infective

- Viral
  - Infective hepatitis
  - Glandular fever
    - EBV
    - CMV
- Bacterial
  - Portal pyaemia
  - Leptospirosis — Weil's disease
  - Actinomycosis
    - Mostly affects jaws
    - Multiple skin sinuses
- Protozoal
  - Malaria
- Parasitic
  - Amoebic
    - Hepatitis
    - Abscess
  - Hydatid

Cirrhosis

See *Chapter 2, Mind Map 39*

Lymphoma + splenomegaly + lymphadenopathy

- + splenomegaly
  - Thalassaemia
  - Sickle-cell
  - Glandular fever
  - Amyloidosis
  - Polycythaemia
  - Lymphoma
  - Leukaemia
  - Cirrhosis

Metabolic

- Gaucher's disease
- Amyloidosis

Haemopoietic

- Thalassaemia
- Polycythaemia
- Leukaemia
- Lymphoma
  - Non-Hodgkin's
  - Hodgkin's

Neoplastic

- Secondary
  - Rock-hard
  - Irregular
  - Multiple
- Primary
  - Large
  - Solitary

SPLENOMEGALY

Commonly
- Portal hypertension
- Myelofibrosis
- Massive splenomegaly
- Chronic myeloproliferative leukaemia
- Lymphoma
- Polycythaemia

Infections
- Bacterial
  - Septicaemia
  - Typhus
- Viral
  - Glandular fever
- Protozoal
  - Malaria
- Parasitic
  - Schistosomiasis
  - Hydatid

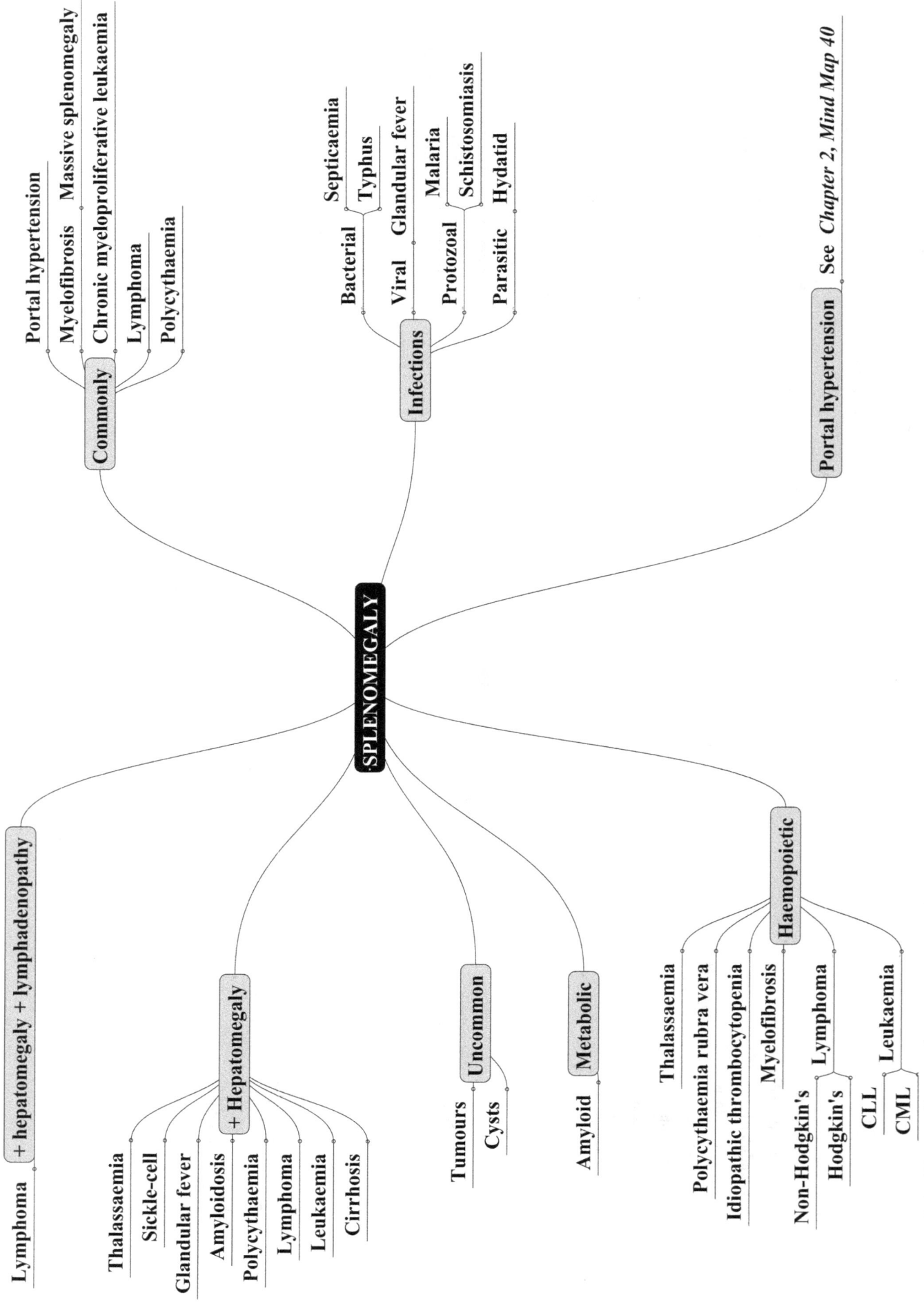

Portal hypertension
See *Chapter 2, Mind Map 40*

+ hepatomegaly + lymphadenopathy
- Lymphoma
- Thalassaemia
- Sickle-cell
- Glandular fever

+ Hepatomegaly
- Amyloidosis
- Polycythaemia
- Lymphoma
- Leukaemia
- Cirrhosis

Uncommon
- Tumours
- Cysts

Metabolic
- Amyloid

Haemopoietic
- Thalassaemia
- Polycythaemia rubra vera
- Idiopathic thrombocytopenia
- Myelofibrosis
- Lymphoma
  - Non-Hodgkin's
  - Hodgkin's
- Leukaemia
  - CLL
  - CML

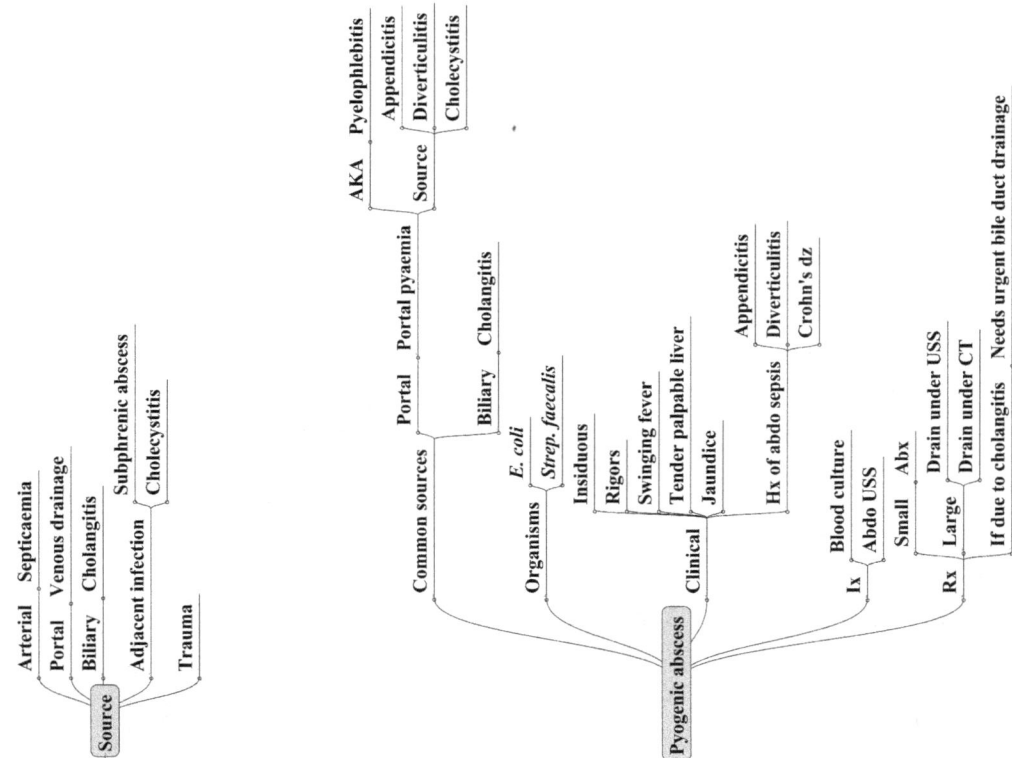

LIVER INFECTIONS

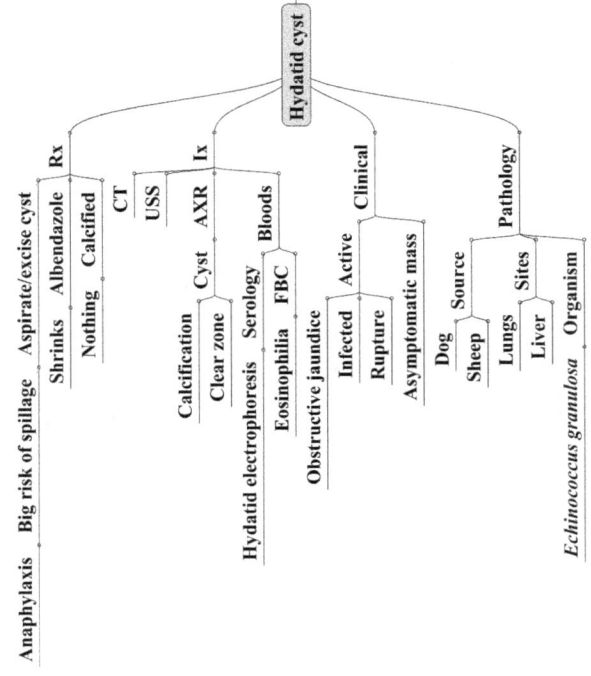

Source

- Arterial — Septicaemia
- Portal — Venous drainage
- Biliary — Cholangitis
- Adjacent infection
  - Subphrenic abscess
  - Cholecystitis
- Trauma

Pyogenic abscess

- AKA — Pyelophlebitis
- Source
  - Appendicitis
  - Diverticulitis
  - Cholecystitis
- Common sources
  - Portal — Portal pyaemia
  - Biliary — Cholangitis
- Organisms
  - *E. coli*
  - *Strep. faecalis*
- Clinical
  - Insidious
  - Rigors
  - Swinging fever
  - Tender palpable liver
  - Jaundice
  - Hx of abdo sepsis
    - Appendicitis
    - Diverticulitis
    - Crohn's dz
- Ix
  - Blood culture
  - Abdo USS
- Rx
  - Small — Abx
  - Large
    - Drain under USS
    - Drain under CT
  - If due to cholangitis — Needs urgent bile duct drainage

Hydatid cyst

- Rx
  - Aspirate/excise cyst
    - Anaphylaxis
    - Big risk of spillage
  - Albendazole
    - Shrinks
    - Calcified — Nothing
- Ix
  - CT
  - USS
    - Calcification
    - Cyst — Clear zone
  - AXR
  - Bloods
    - Serology — Hydatid electrophoresis
    - FBC — Eosinophilia
- Clinical
  - Active
    - Obstructive jaundice
    - Infected
    - Rupture
  - Asymptomatic mass
- Pathology
  - Source
    - Dog
    - Sheep
  - Sites
    - Lungs
    - Liver
  - Organism — *Echinococcus granulosa*

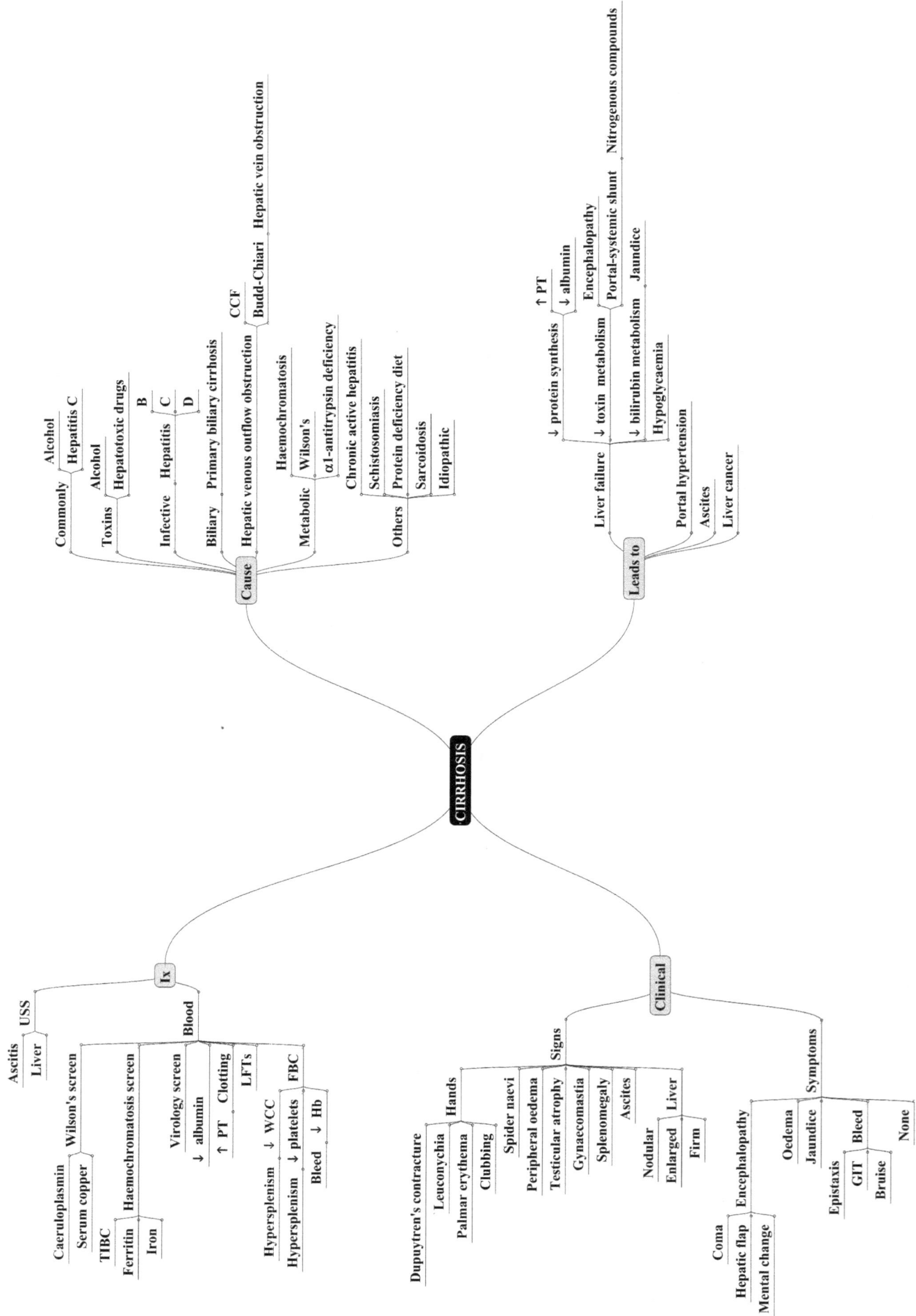

CIRRHOSIS

Cause

- Commonly
  - Alcohol
  - Hepatitis C
- Toxins
  - Alcohol
  - Hepatotoxic drugs
- Infective
  - Hepatitis
    - B
    - C
    - D
- Biliary — Primary biliary cirrhosis
- Hepatic venous outflow obstruction
  - CCF
  - Budd-Chiari
  - Hepatic vein obstruction
- Metabolic
  - Haemochromatosis
  - Wilson's
  - α1-antitrypsin deficiency
- Others
  - Chronic active hepatitis
  - Schistosomiasis
  - Protein deficiency diet
  - Sarcoidosis
  - Idiopathic

Leads to

- Liver failure
  - ↓ protein synthesis
    - ↑ PT
    - ↓ albumin
  - ↓ toxin metabolism
    - Encephalopathy
    - Portal-systemic shunt — Nitrogenous compounds
  - ↓ bilirubin metabolism — Jaundice
  - Hypoglycaemia
- Portal hypertension
- Ascites
- Liver cancer

Ix

- USS
  - Ascitis
  - Liver
- Blood
  - Wilson's screen
    - Caeruloplasmin
    - Serum copper
  - Haemochromatosis screen
    - TIBC
    - Ferritin
    - Iron
  - Virology screen
  - Clotting
    - ↓ albumin
    - ↑ PT
  - LFTs
  - FBC
    - Hypersplenism — ↓ WCC
    - Hypersplenism — ↓ platelets
    - Bleed — ↓ Hb

Clinical

- Signs
  - Hands
    - Dupuytren's contracture
    - Leuconychia
    - Palmar erythema
    - Clubbing
  - Spider naevi
  - Peripheral oedema
  - Testicular atrophy
  - Gynaecomastia
  - Splenomegaly
  - Ascites
  - Liver
    - Nodular
    - Enlarged
    - Firm
- Symptoms
  - Encephalopathy
    - Coma
    - Hepatic flap
    - Mental change
  - Oedema
  - Jaundice
  - Bleed
    - Epistaxis
    - GIT
    - Bruise
  - None

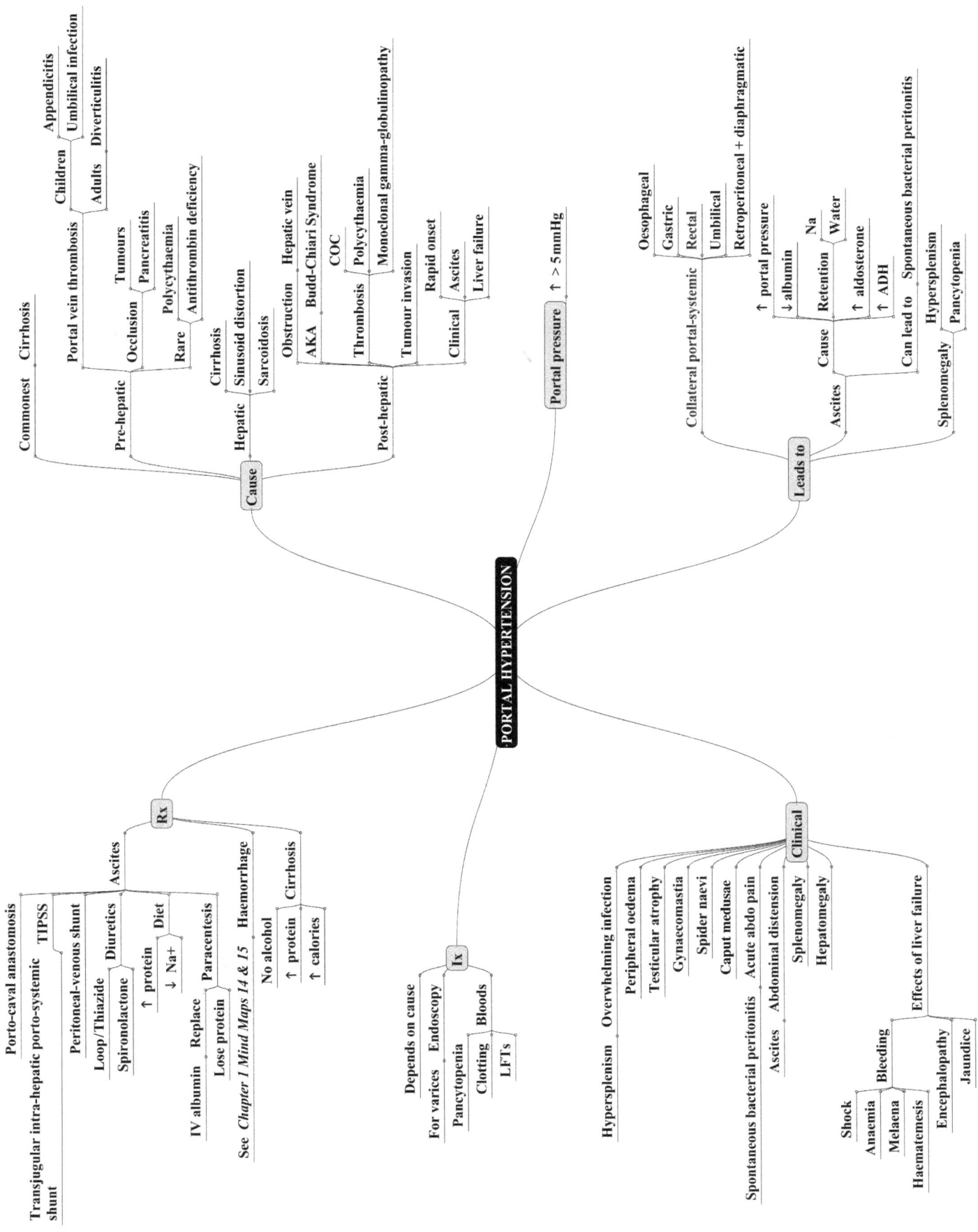

PORTAL HYPERTENSION

Cause

Pre-hepatic
- Commonest — Cirrhosis
- Portal vein thrombosis
  - Occlusion
    - Tumours
    - Pancreatitis
    - Polycythaemia
  - Rare — Antithrombin deficiency
  - Children
    - Appendicitis
    - Umbilical infection
  - Adults — Diverticulitis

Hepatic
- Cirrhosis
- Sinusoid distortion
- Sarcoidosis

Post-hepatic
- Obstruction
  - Hepatic vein
  - AKA Budd-Chiari Syndrome
  - COC
- Thrombosis
  - Polycythaemia
  - Monoclonal gamma-globulinopathy
- Tumour invasion
- Rapid onset
- Clinical
  - Ascites
  - Liver failure

Portal pressure

↑ > 5mmHg

Leads to

Collateral portal-systemic
- Oesophageal
- Gastric
- Rectal
- Umbilical
- Retroperitoneal + diaphragmatic

Ascites
- Cause
  - ↑ portal pressure
  - ↓ albumin
  - Retention
    - Na
    - Water
    - ↑ aldosterone
    - ↑ ADH
- Can lead to Spontaneous bacterial peritonitis

Splenomegaly
- Hypersplenism
- Pancytopenia

Rx

Ascites
- Porto-caval anastomosis
- Transjugular intra-hepatic porto-systemic shunt — TIPSS
- Peritoneal-venous shunt
- Diuretics
  - Loop/Thiazide
  - Spironolactone
- Diet
  - ↑ protein
  - ↓ Na+
- IV albumin
- Replace
  - Lose protein
- Paracentesis

Haemorrhage
- See *Chapter 1 Mind Maps 14 & 15*

Cirrhosis
- No alcohol
- ↑ protein
- ↑ calories

Ix

- Depends on cause
- Endoscopy
  - For varices
- Bloods
  - Pancytopenia
  - Clotting
  - LFTs

Clinical

- Hypersplenism — Overwhelming infection
- Peripheral oedema
- Testicular atrophy
- Gynaecomastia
- Spider naevi
- Caput medusae
- Acute abdo pain
- Abdominal distension
- Splenomegaly
- Hepatomegaly
- Spontaneous bacterial peritonitis
- Ascites
- Effects of liver failure
  - Bleeding
    - Shock
    - Anaemia
    - Melaena
    - Haematemesis
  - Encephalopathy
  - Jaundice

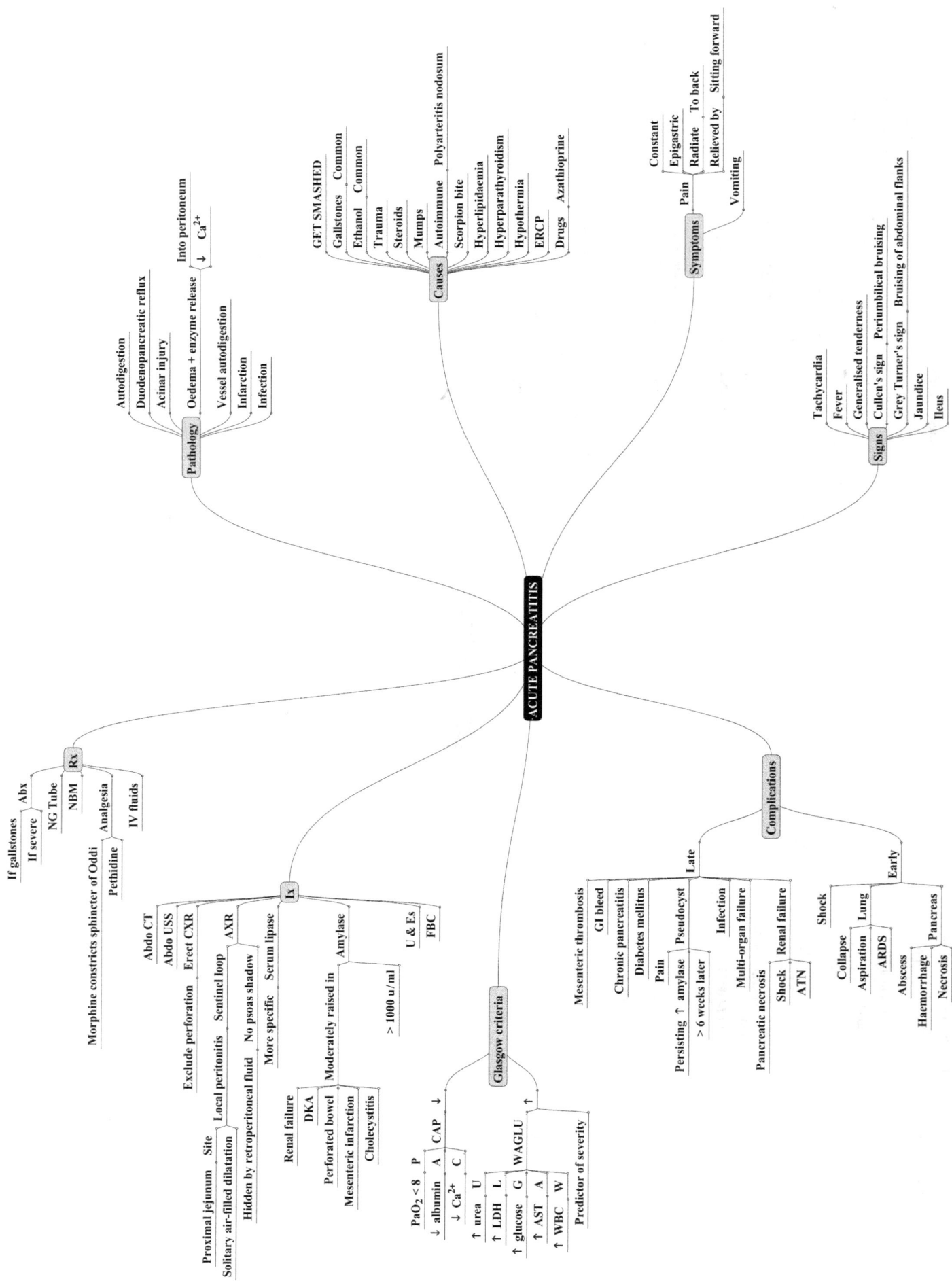

ACUTE PANCREATITIS

Pathology
- Autodigestion
  - Duodenopancreatic reflux
  - Acinar injury
- Oedema + enzyme release
  - Into peritoneum → Ca^{2+} ↓
- Vessel autodigestion
  - Infarction
  - Infection

Causes
GET SMASHED
- Gallstones — Common
- Ethanol — Common
- Trauma
- Steroids
- Mumps
- Autoimmune — Polyarteritis nodosum
- Scorpion bite
- Hyperlipidaemia
- Hyperparathyroidism
- Hypothermia
- ERCP
- Drugs — Azathioprine

Symptoms
- Pain
  - Constant
  - Epigastric
  - Radiate — To back
  - Relieved by — Sitting forward
- Vomiting

Signs
- Tachycardia
- Fever
- Generalised tenderness
- Cullen's sign — Periumbilical bruising
- Grey Turner's sign — Bruising of abdominal flanks
- Jaundice
- Ileus

Rx
- If gallstones — Abx
- If severe — NG Tube
- NBM
  - Morphine constricts sphincter of Oddi
  - Analgesia — Pethidine
  - IV fluids

Ix
- Abdo CT
- Abdo USS
- Erect CXR
  - Exclude perforation
  - Local peritonitis
- AXR
  - Sentinel loop
    - Proximal jejunum
    - Site
  - Solitary air-filled dilatation
  - No psoas shadow
    - Hidden by retroperitoneal fluid
- Serum lipase
  - More specific
- Amylase
  - Moderately raised in
    - Renal failure
    - DKA
    - Perforated bowel
    - Mesenteric infarction
    - Cholecystitis
  - > 1000 u/ml
- U & Es
- FBC

Glasgow criteria
- PaO₂ < 8 — P
- ↓ albumin — A
- ↓ Ca²⁺ — C
- ↑ urea — U
- ↑ LDH — L
- ↓ glucose — G
- ↑ AST — A
- ↑ WBC — W
- PaO$_2$ < 8
- ↓ albumin
- ↓ Ca^{2+}
- ↑ urea
- ↑ LDH
- ↑ glucose
- ↑ AST
- ↑ WBC
- CAP ↓ / WAGLU ↑
- Predictor of severity

Complications
Early
- Shock
- Lung
  - Collapse
  - Aspiration
  - ARDS
- Pancreas
  - Abscess
  - Haemorrhage
  - Necrosis

Late
- Mesenteric thrombosis
- GI bleed
- Chronic pancreatitis
- Diabetes mellitus
- Pseudocyst
  - Pain
  - Persisting ↑ amylase
  - > 6 weeks later
- Infection
  - Multi-organ failure
  - Pancreatic necrosis
- Renal failure
  - Shock
  - ATN

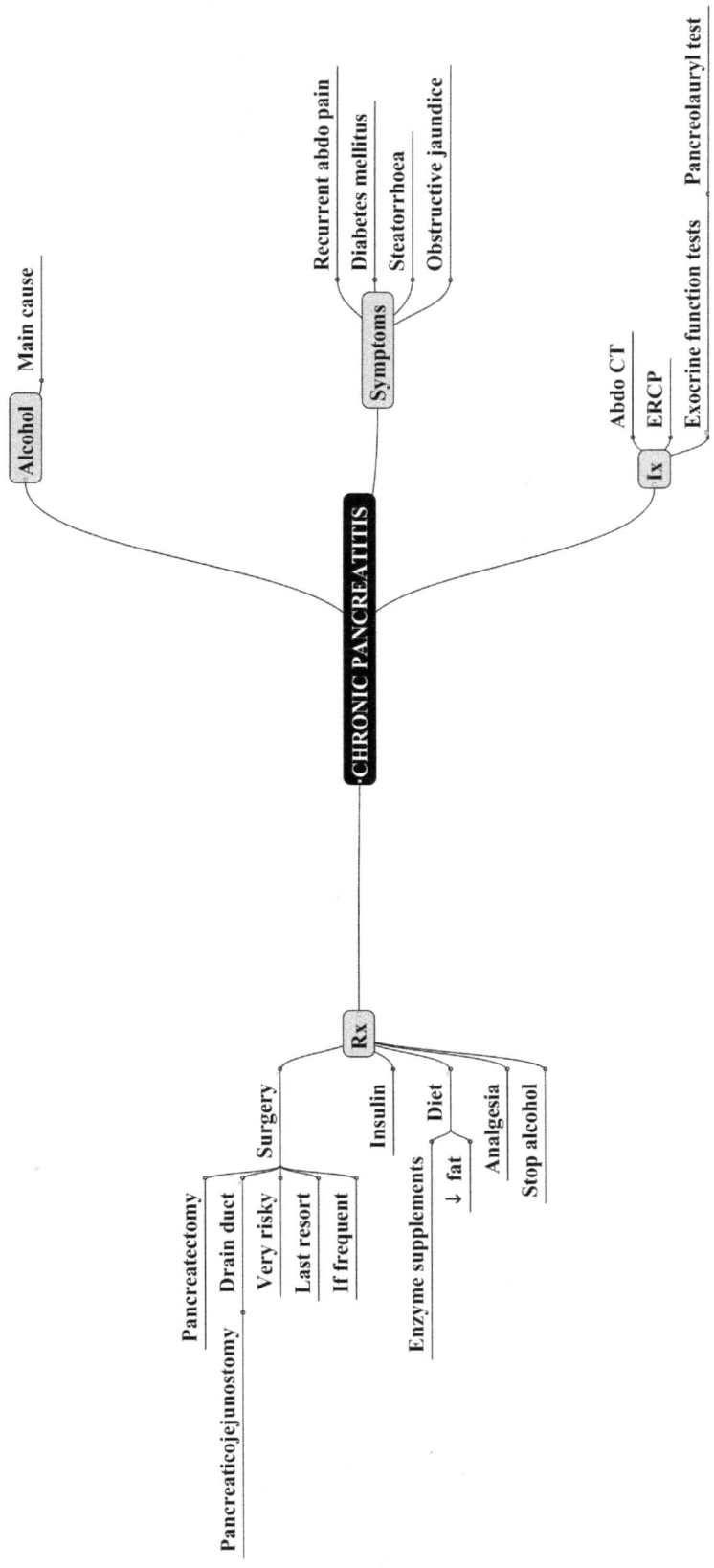

CHRONIC PANCREATITIS

Alcohol
- Main cause

Symptoms
- Recurrent abdo pain
- Diabetes mellitus
- Steatorrhoea
- Obstructive jaundice

Ix
- Abdo CT
- ERCP
- Exocrine function tests
- Pancreolauryl test

Rx
- Surgery
  - Pancreatectomy
  - Pancreaticojejunostomy
  - Drain duct
    - Very risky
    - Last resort
    - If frequent
- Insulin
- Diet
  - Enzyme supplements
  - ↓ fat
- Analgesia
- Stop alcohol

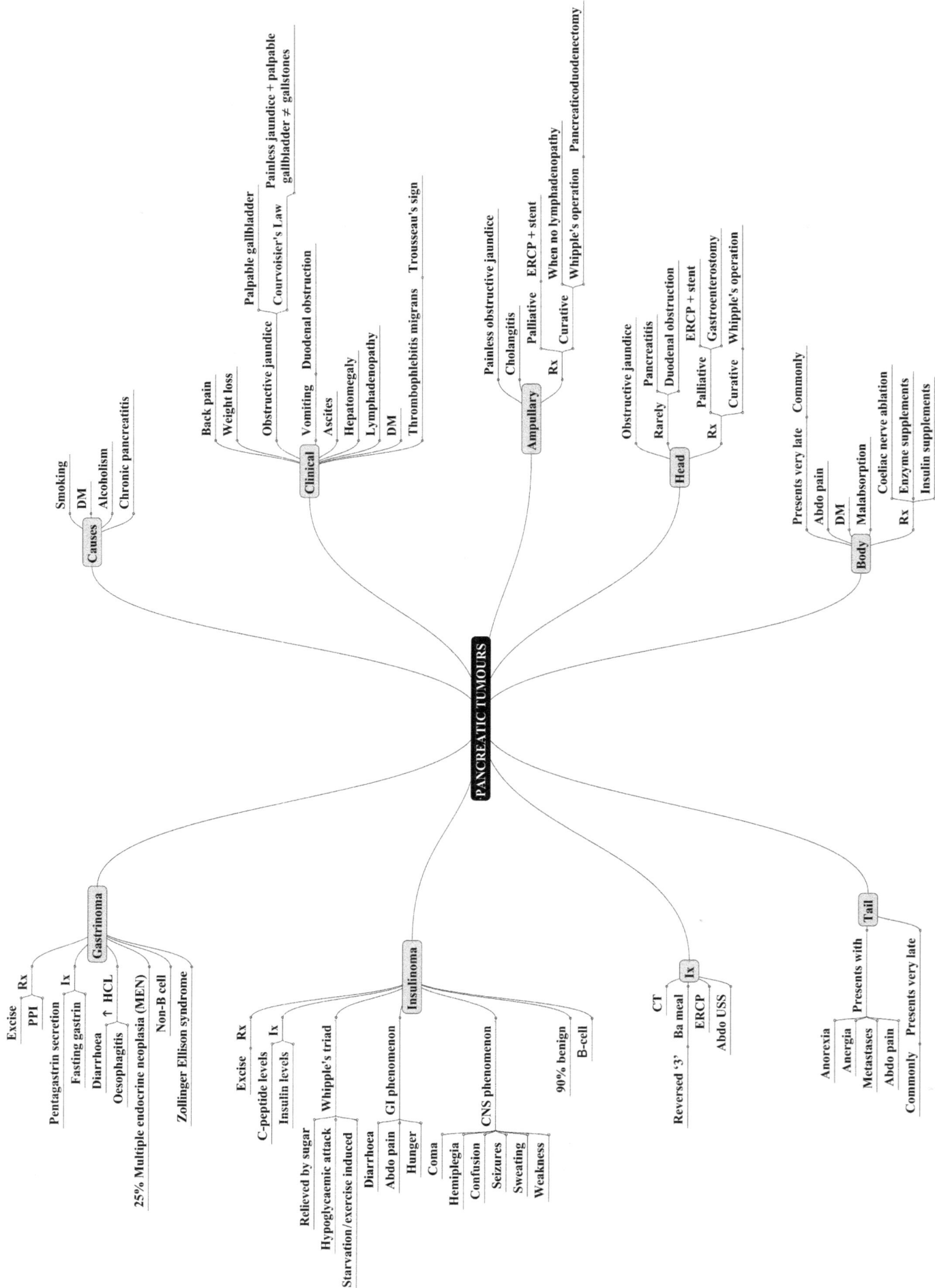

PANCREATIC TUMOURS

Causes
- Smoking
- DM
- Alcoholism
- Chronic pancreatitis

Clinical
- Back pain
- Weight loss
- Obstructive jaundice
  - Palpable gallbladder
  - Courvoisier's Law
    - Painless jaundice + palpable gallbladder ≠ gallstones
- Vomiting
- Duodenal obstruction
- Ascites
- Hepatomegaly
- Lymphadenopathy
- DM
- Thrombophlebitis migrans — Trousseau's sign

Ampullary
- Painless obstructive jaundice
- Cholangitis
- Rx
  - Palliative — ERCP + stent
  - Curative
    - When no lymphadenopathy
    - Whipple's operation — Pancreaticoduodenectomy

Head
- Obstructive jaundice
- Pancreatitis
- Rarely — Duodenal obstruction
- Rx
  - Palliative
    - ERCP + stent
    - Gastroenterostomy
  - Curative — Whipple's operation

Body
- Presents very late — Commonly
- Abdo pain
- DM
- Malabsorption
- Rx
  - Coeliac nerve ablation
  - Enzyme supplements
  - Insulin supplements

Gastrinoma
- Rx
  - Excise
  - PPI
- Ix
  - Pentagastrin secretion
  - Fasting gastrin
- Diarrhoea
- ↑ HCL
- Oesophagitis
- 25% Multiple endocrine neoplasia (MEN)
- Non-B cell
- Zollinger Ellison syndrome

Insulinoma
- Rx
  - Excise
- Ix
  - C-peptide levels
  - Insulin levels
- Whipple's triad
  - Relieved by sugar
  - Hypoglycaemic attack
  - Starvation/exercise induced
- GI phenomenon
  - Diarrhoea
  - Abdo pain
  - Hunger
- CNS phenomenon
  - Coma
  - Hemiplegia
  - Confusion
  - Seizures
  - Sweating
  - Weakness
- 90% benign
- B-cell

Ix
- CT
- Reversed '3' — Ba meal
- ERCP
- Abdo USS

Tail
- Presents with
  - Anorexia
  - Anergia
  - Metastases
  - Abdo pain
- Commonly — Presents very late

Chapter 3

HEAD, NECK AND SKIN

LUMPS IN THE NECK

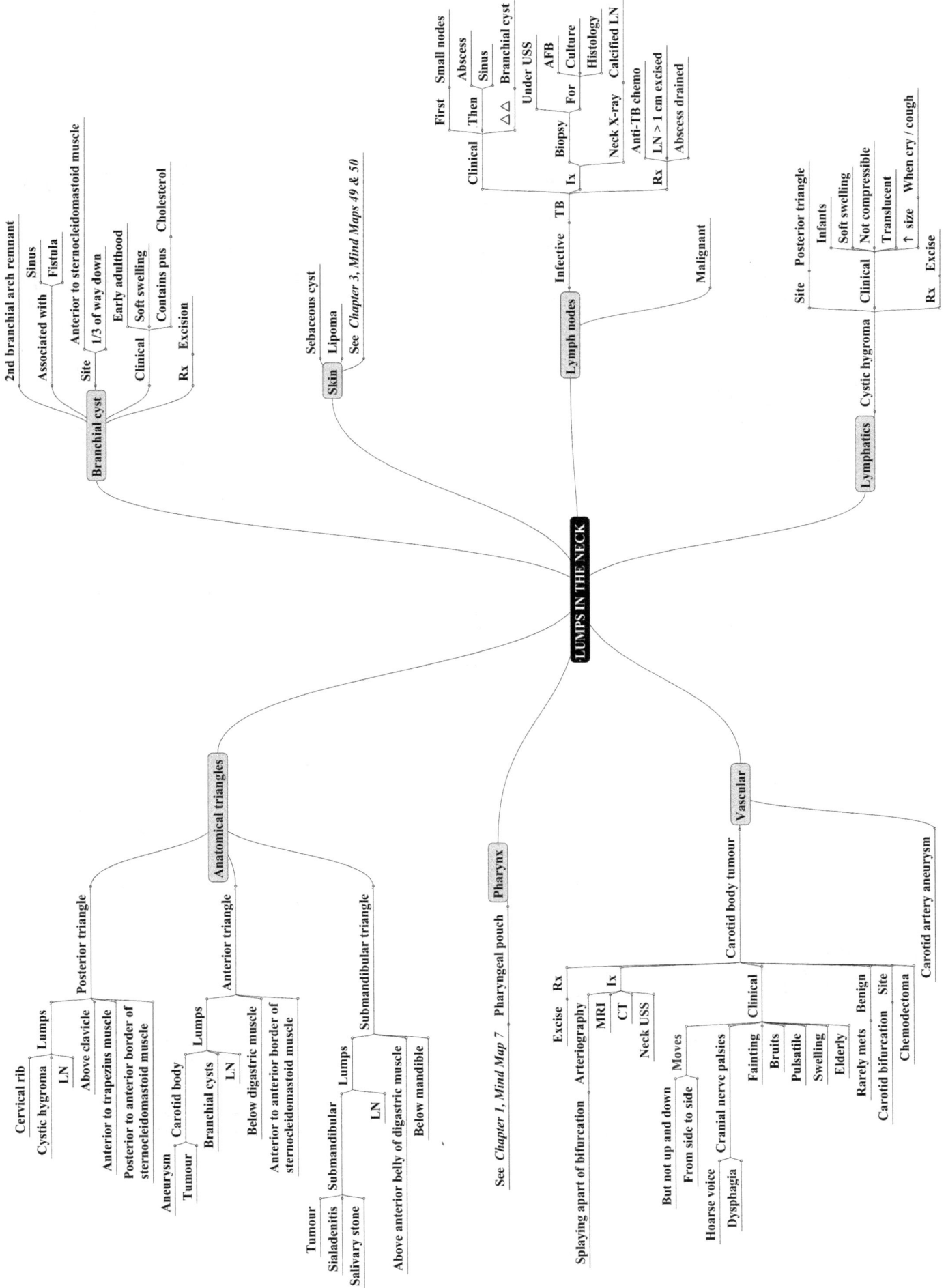

Branchial cyst
- Site
  - 2nd branchial arch remnant
  - Associated with
    - Sinus
    - Fistula
  - Anterior to sternocleidomastoid muscle
  - 1/3 of way down
  - Early adulthood
- Clinical
  - Soft swelling
  - Contains pus
  - Cholesterol
- Rx Excision

Skin
- Sebaceous cyst
- Lipoma
- See *Chapter 3, Mind Maps 49 & 50*

Lymph nodes
- Infective
  - TB
    - Clinical
      - First Small nodes
      - Then
        - Abscess
        - Sinus
        - ΔΔ Branchial cyst
    - Ix
      - Biopsy
        - Under USS
        - For
          - AFB
          - Culture
          - Histology
        - Calcified LN
      - Neck X-ray
    - Rx
      - Anti-TB chemo
      - LN > 1 cm excised
      - Abscess drained
- Malignant

Lymphatics
- Cystic hygroma
  - Site Posterior triangle
  - Clinical
    - Infants
    - Soft swelling
    - Not compressible
    - Translucent
    - ↑ size When cry / cough
  - Rx Excise

Anatomical triangles
- Posterior triangle
  - Cervical rib
  - Cystic hygroma
  - Lumps
  - LN
  - Above clavicle
  - Anterior to trapezius muscle
  - Posterior to anterior border of sternocleidomastoid muscle
- Anterior triangle
  - Aneurysm
  - Carotid body
    - Tumour
  - Branchial cysts
  - Lumps
  - LN
  - Below digastric muscle
  - Anterior to anterior border of sternocleidomastoid muscle
- Submandibular triangle
  - Submandibular
    - Tumour
    - Sialadenitis
    - Salivary stone
  - Lumps
  - LN
  - Above anterior belly of digastric muscle
  - Below mandible

Pharynx
- Pharyngeal pouch
- See *Chapter 1, Mind Map 7*
- Rx Excise

Vascular
- Carotid body tumour
  - Ix
    - Arteriography
    - MRI
    - CT
    - Neck USS
  - Clinical
    - Splaying apart of bifurcation
    - Moves
      - From side to side
      - But not up and down
    - Cranial nerve palsies
      - Hoarse voice
      - Dysphagia
    - Fainting
    - Bruits
    - Pulsatile
    - Swelling
    - Elderly
    - Rarely mets
    - Benign
    - Carotid bifurcation
    - Site
    - Chemodectoma
- Carotid artery aneurysm

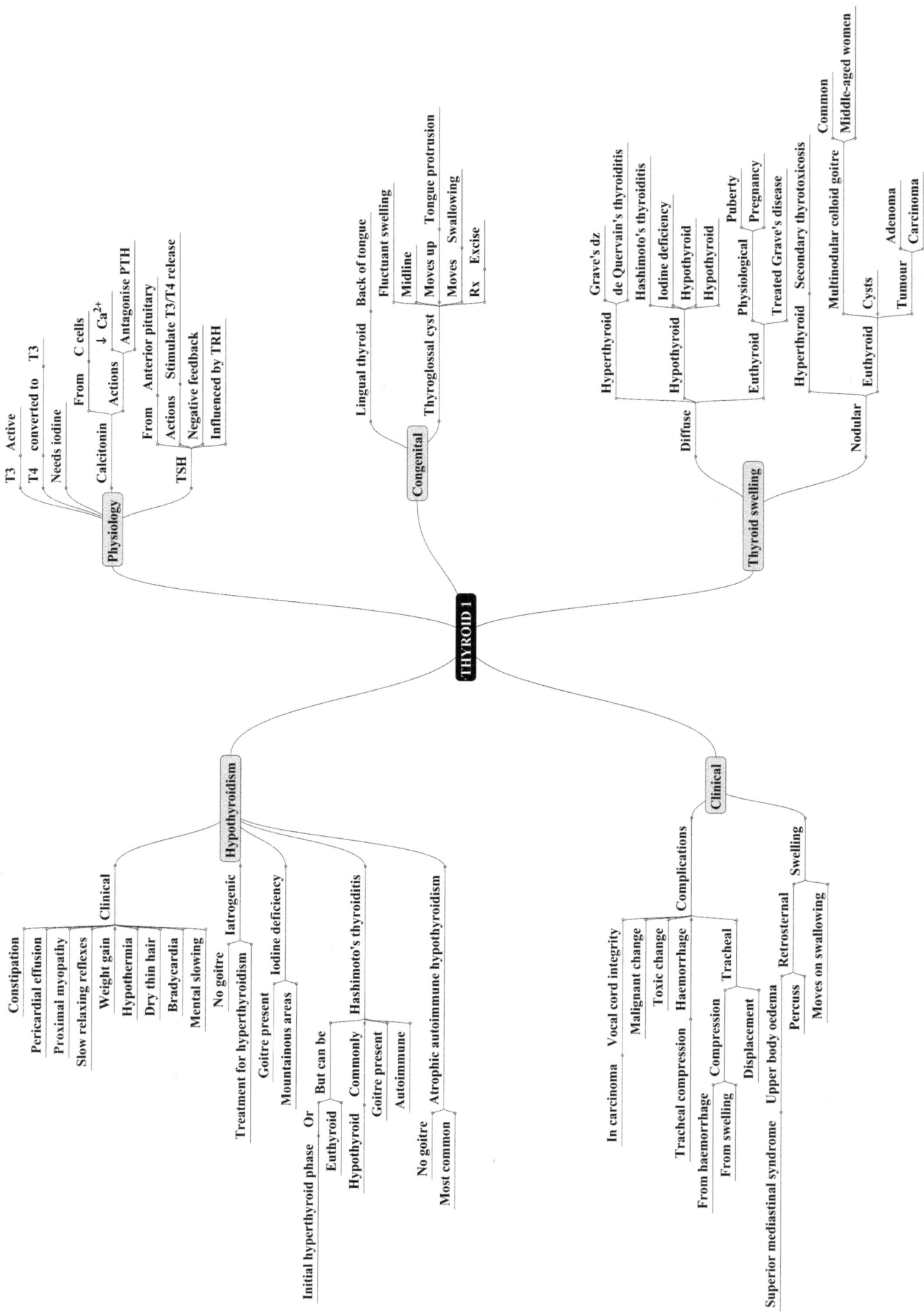

THYROID 1

Physiology

- T3 — Active
- T4 — converted to T3
- Needs iodine
- Calcitonin
  - From C cells
  - Actions
    - ↓ Ca²⁺
    - Antagonise PTH
- TSH
  - From Anterior pituitary
  - Actions — Stimulate T3/T4 release
  - Negative feedback
  - Influenced by TRH

Congenital

- Lingual thyroid — Back of tongue
- Thyroglossal cyst
  - Fluctuant swelling
  - Midline
  - Moves up — Tongue protrusion
  - Moves — Swallowing
  - Rx — Excise

Thyroid swelling

- Diffuse
  - Hyperthyroid
    - Grave's dz
    - de Quervain's thyroiditis
  - Hypothyroid
    - Hashimoto's thyroiditis
    - Iodine deficiency
    - Hypothyroid
    - Hypothyroid
  - Euthyroid
    - Puberty
    - Pregnancy
    - Physiological
    - Treated Grave's disease
- Nodular
  - Hyperthyroid — Secondary thyrotoxicosis
  - Euthyroid — Multinodular colloid goitre
  - Cysts — Common
    - Middle-aged women
  - Tumour
    - Adenoma
    - Carcinoma

Hypothyroidism

- Clinical
  - Constipation
  - Pericardial effusion
  - Proximal myopathy
  - Slow relaxing reflexes
  - Weight gain
  - Hypothermia
  - Dry thin hair
  - Bradycardia
  - Mental slowing
- Iatrogenic
  - No goitre
  - Treatment for hyperthyroidism
- Iodine deficiency
  - Goitre present
  - Mountainous areas
- Hashimoto's thyroiditis
  - Commonly
    - But can be
      - Or
      - Euthyroid
      - Hypothyroid
  - Goitre present
  - Autoimmune
- Atrophic autoimmune hypothyroidism
  - No goitre
  - Most common
- Initial hyperthyroid phase

Clinical

- Complications
  - In carcinoma — Vocal cord integrity
  - Malignant change
  - Toxic change
  - Haemorrhage
    - Tracheal compression
    - From haemorrhage
  - Tracheal
    - Compression
      - From swelling
    - Displacement
- Superior mediastinal syndrome — Upper body oedema
- Swelling
  - Retrosternal
    - Percuss
  - Moves on swallowing

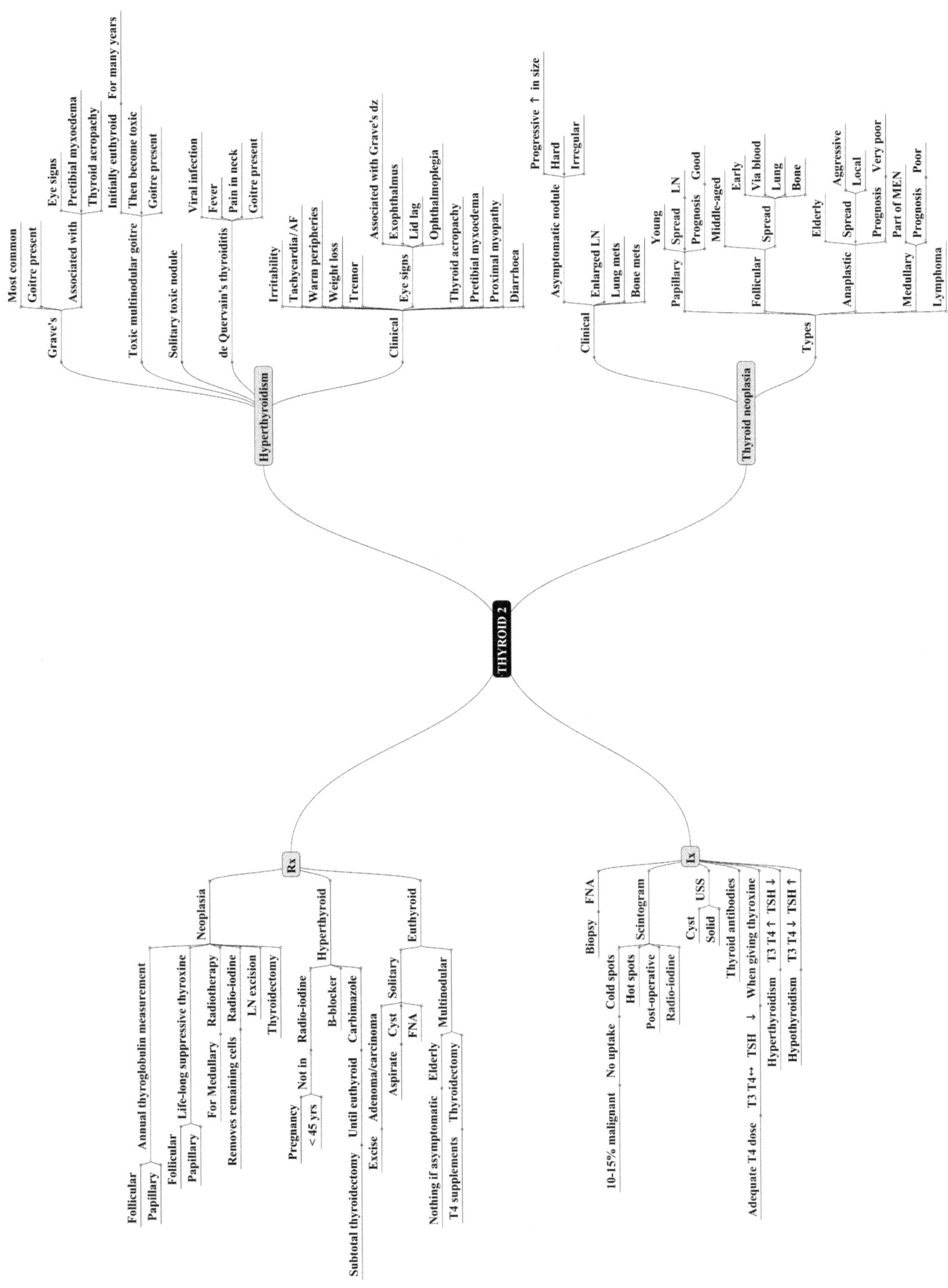

THYROID 2

Hyperthyroidism

- **Grave's**
  - Most common
  - Goitre present
  - Associated with
    - Eye signs
    - Pretibial myxoedema
    - Thyroid acropachy
- **Toxic multinodular goitre**
  - Initially euthyroid — For many years
  - Then become toxic
  - Goitre present
- **Solitary toxic nodule**
- **de Quervain's thyroiditis**
  - Viral infection
  - Fever
  - Pain in neck
  - Goitre present
- **Clinical**
  - Irritability
  - Tachycardia/AF
  - Warm peripheries
  - Weight loss
  - Tremor
  - Eye signs
    - Associated with Grave's dz
    - Exophthalmus
    - Lid lag
    - Ophthalmoplegia
  - Thyroid acropachy
  - Pretibial myxoedema
  - Proximal myopathy
  - Diarrhoea

Thyroid neoplasia

- **Clinical**
  - Asymptomatic nodule
    - Progressive ↑ in size
    - Hard
    - Irregular
  - Enlarged LN
  - Lung mets
  - Bone mets
- **Types**
  - Papillary
    - Young
    - Spread — LN
    - Prognosis — Good
  - Follicular
    - Middle-aged
    - Spread — Via blood
      - Lung
      - Bone
    - Prognosis — Early
  - Anaplastic
    - Elderly
    - Spread — Local
    - Aggressive
    - Prognosis — Very poor
  - Medullary
    - Part of MEN
    - Prognosis — Poor
  - Lymphoma

Rx

- **Neoplasia**
  - Follicular
  - Papillary
    - Annual thyroglobulin measurement
  - Follicular
  - Papillary
    - Life-long suppressive thyroxine
  - Radiotherapy — For Medullary
  - Radio-iodine — Removes remaining cells
  - LN excision
  - Thyroidectomy
- **Hyperthyroid**
  - Radio-iodine
    - Pregnancy — Not in
    - <45 yrs
  - B-blocker
  - Carbimazole — Until euthyroid
  - Subtotal thyroidectomy
- **Euthyroid**
  - Solitary
    - Adenoma/carcinoma — Excise
    - Cyst — Aspirate
    - FNA
  - Multinodular
    - Nothing if asymptomatic
    - Elderly
    - Thyroidectomy
    - T4 supplements

Ix

- **Biopsy**
- **FNA**
  - 10-15% malignant
- **Scintogram**
  - No uptake — Cold spots
  - Hot spots
  - Post-operative
  - Radio-iodine
- **USS**
  - Cyst
  - Solid
- **Thyroid antibodies**
- **When giving thyroxine**
  - Adequate T4 dose — T3 T4↔ TSH →
  - Hyperthyroidism — T3 T4↑ TSH →
  - Hypothyroidism — T3 T4 → TSH ↑

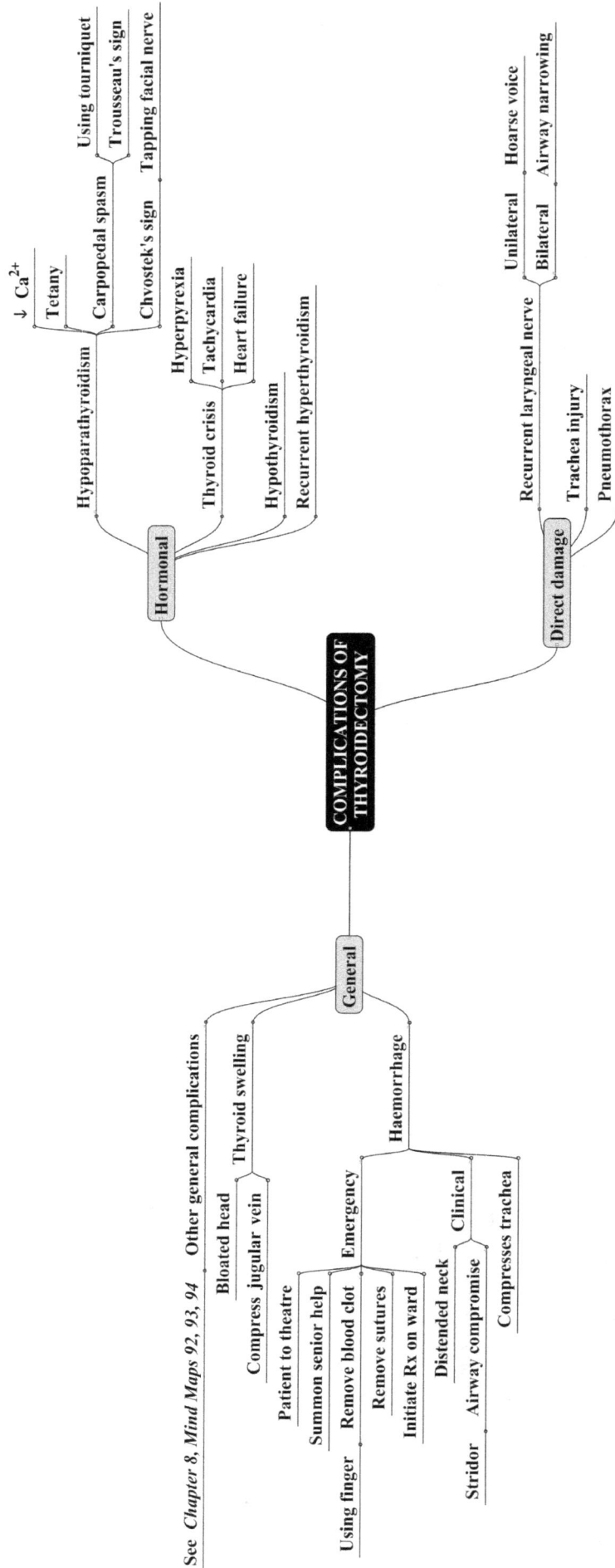

COMPLICATIONS OF THYROIDECTOMY

Hormonal

Hypoparathyroidism
- ↓ Ca²⁺
  - Tetany
  - Carpopedal spasm
    - Using tourniquet
    - Trousseau's sign
  - Chvostek's sign
    - Tapping facial nerve

Thyroid crisis
- Hyperpyrexia
- Tachycardia
- Heart failure

Hypothyroidism

Recurrent hyperthyroidism

Direct damage

Recurrent laryngeal nerve
- Unilateral — Hoarse voice
- Bilateral — Airway narrowing

Trachea injury

Pneumothorax

General

Other general complications
See *Chapter 8, Mind Maps 92, 93, 94*

Thyroid swelling
- Bloated head
- Compress jugular vein

Haemorrhage
- Emergency
  - Patient to theatre
  - Summon senior help
  - Remove blood clot
    - Using finger
  - Remove sutures
  - Initiate Rx on ward
- Clinical
  - Distended neck
  - Airway compromise
    - Stridor
  - Compresses trachea

PARATHYROIDS

Function

↑ Ca²⁺
↓ phosphate

Kidneys
- ↑ Ca²⁺ reabsorption
- ↑ phosphate excretion
- In hypercalcaemia — Exceed resorption capacity — ↑ Ca²⁺ excretion

Bone — Osteoclasts
- ↑ serum Ca²⁺
- ↑ serum phosphate
- ↑ ALP

GIT — ↑ Ca²⁺ absorption

Primary hypoparathyroidism

↓ Ca²⁺

Cause — Thyroidectomy, Bruising

Clinical
- Tetany
- Carpopedal spasm
- Trousseau's sign — Tourniquet around arm — Causes finger spasm
- Chvostek's sign — Tap facial nerve — Causes twitching
- Perioral paraesthesia
- Prolonged Q-T interval

Rx
- Ca²⁺
- Alfacalcidol

Pseudohypoparathyroidism

↓ response to PTH

Signs
- Round face
- Short — Metacarpals, Metatarsals
- ↑ PTH
- ↑ or ↔ ALP

Pseudopseudohypoparathyroidism

- As pseudohypoparathyroidism
- Normal biochemistry

Hyperparathyroidism

Rx — Parathyroidectomy

Ix
- Methylene blue test
- Technetium scan
- MRI
- X-ray bones
- ↑ urine Ca²⁺
- ↑ PTH
- ↑ Ca²⁺

Clinical
- Thirst
- Depression
- Abdo pain — Pancreatitis, Ulcer, Dyspepsia, Constipation
- Renal — Uraemia, Infection, Stones
- Bones — Osteitis fibrosa cystica, Cysts, Fracture, Pain
- Bones, stones, abdo groans, psychic moans

Malignant
- Squamous cell carcinoma
- Ectopic PTH

Tertiary
- Rx — Parathyroidectomy
- Uncontrolled
- Prolonged secondary
- Alfacalcidol

Secondary
- Rx — Commonly Renal failure
- Cause — ↓ Ca²⁺ — ↓ Ca²⁺ absorption, ↓ Vit D activation
- Hyperplasia — All 4 parathyroids

Primary
- Remaining 3 parathyroids suppressed
- Adenoma

SKIN: BENIGN

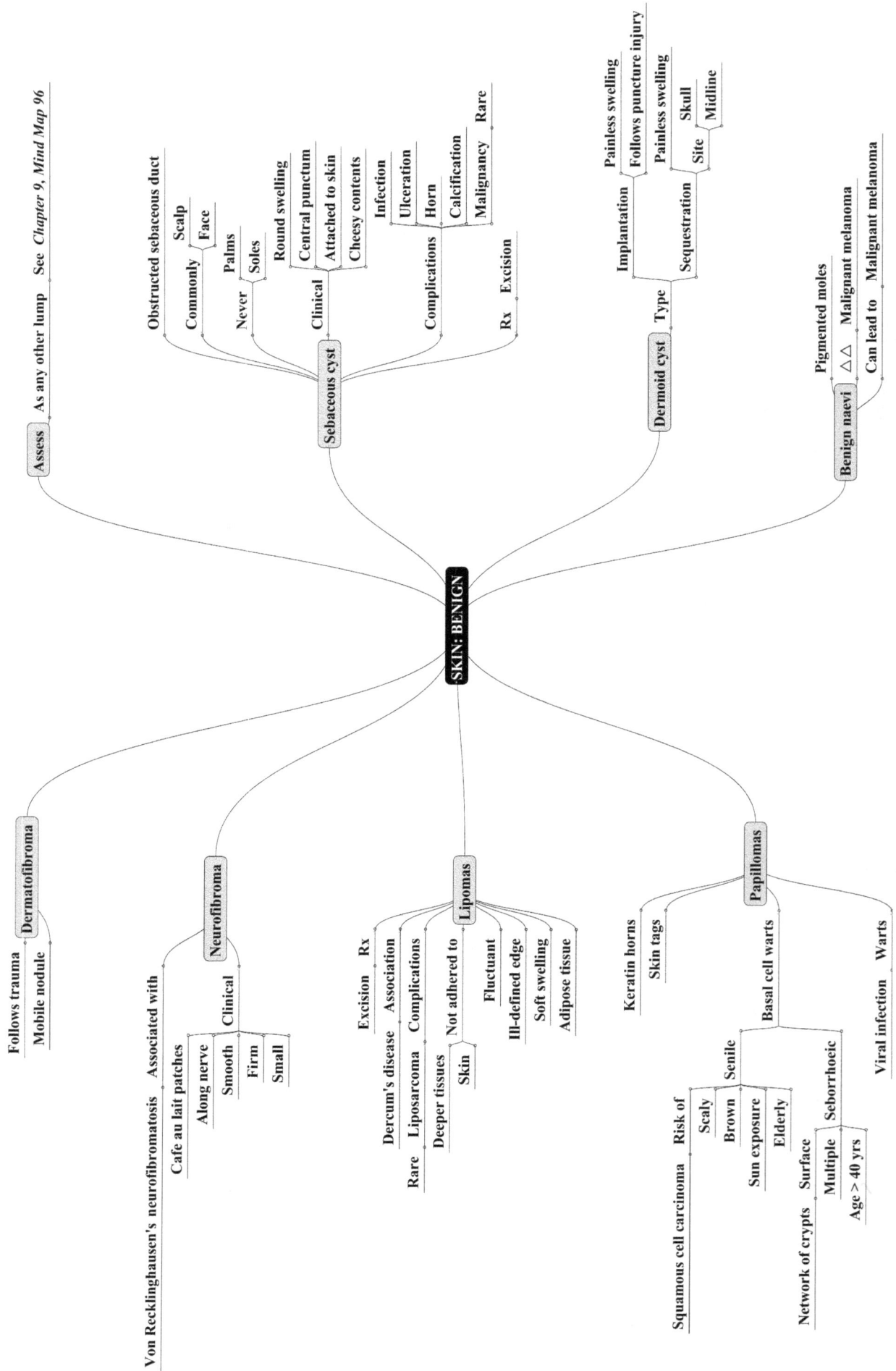

Assess
- As any other lump   *See Chapter 9, Mind Map 96*

Sebaceous cyst
- Obstructed sebaceous duct
- Commonly
  - Scalp
  - Face
- Never
  - Palms
  - Soles
- Clinical
  - Round swelling
  - Central punctum
  - Attached to skin
  - Cheesy contents
- Complications
  - Infection
  - Ulceration
  - Horn
  - Calcification
  - Malignancy   Rare
- Rx   Excision

Dermoid cyst
- Type
  - Implantation
    - Painless swelling
    - Follows puncture injury
  - Sequestration
    - Painless swelling
    - Site
      - Skull
      - Midline

Benign naevi
- Pigmented moles
- △△ Malignant melanoma
- Can lead to   Malignant melanoma

Dermatofibroma
- Follows trauma
- Mobile nodule

Neurofibroma
- Von Recklinghausen's neurofibromatosis   Associated with
  - Cafe au lait patches
- Along nerve
- Clinical
  - Smooth
  - Firm
  - Small

Lipomas
- Excision   Rx
- Dercum's disease   Association
- Rare   Liposarcoma   Complications
- Not adhered to
  - Deeper tissues
  - Skin
- Fluctuant
- Ill-defined edge
- Soft swelling
- Adipose tissue

Papillomas
- Keratin horns
- Skin tags
- Basal cell warts
  - Squamous cell carcinoma   Risk of
  - Senile
    - Scaly
    - Brown
    - Sun exposure
    - Elderly
  - Seborrhoeic
    - Network of crypts   Surface
    - Multiple
    - Age > 40 yrs
- Viral infection   Warts

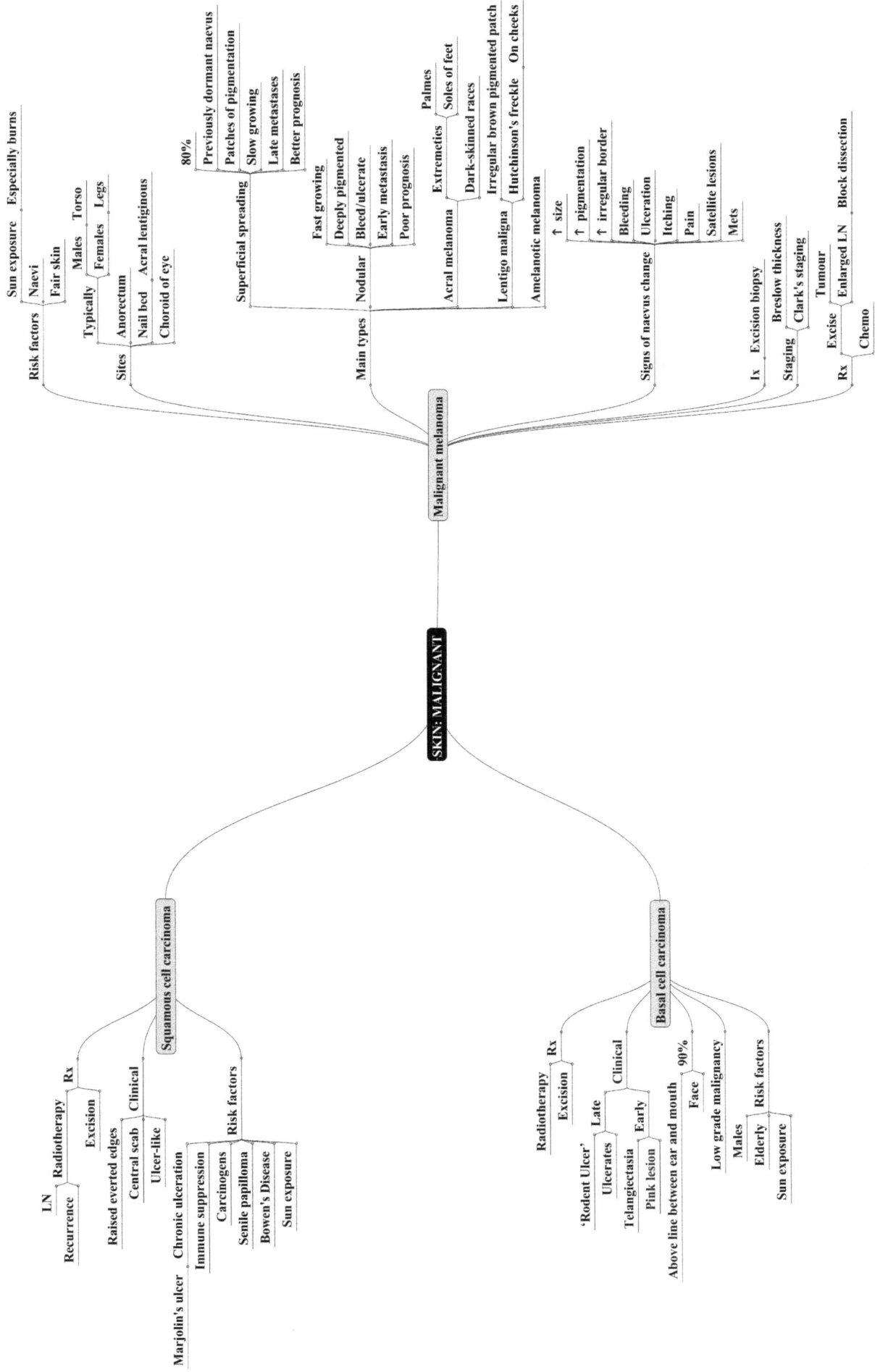

SKIN: MALIGNANT

Malignant melanoma

- **Risk factors**
  - Sun exposure — Especially burns
  - Naevi
  - Fair skin
- **Sites**
  - Typically — Males: Torso; Females: Legs
  - Anorectum
  - Nail bed — Acral lentiginous
  - Choroid of eye
- **Main types**
  - Superficial spreading — 80%; Previously dormant naevus; Patches of pigmentation; Slow growing; Late metastases; Better prognosis
  - Nodular — Fast growing; Deeply pigmented; Bleed/ulcerate; Early metastasis; Poor prognosis
  - Acral melanoma — Extremeties; Palmes, Soles of feet; Dark-skinned races
  - Lentigo maligna — Irregular brown pigmented patch; Hutchinson's freckle; On cheeks
  - Amelanotic melanoma
- **Signs of naevus change**
  - ↑ size
  - ↑ pigmentation
  - irregular border
  - Bleeding
  - Ulceration
  - Itching
  - Pain
  - Satellite lesions
  - Mets
- **Ix** — Excision biopsy
- **Staging** — Breslow thickness; Clark's staging
- **Rx** — Excise: Tumour, Enlarged LN, Block dissection; Chemo

Squamous cell carcinoma

- **Clinical**
  - Raised everted edges
  - Central scab
  - Ulcer-like
- **Risk factors**
  - Marjolin's ulcer — Chronic ulceration
  - Immune suppression
  - Carcinogens
  - Senile papilloma
  - Bowen's Disease
  - Sun exposure
- **Rx**
  - Radiotherapy
  - Excision
  - Recurrence — LN

Basal cell carcinoma

- **Clinical**
  - 'Rodent Ulcer'
  - Late — Ulcerates
  - Telangiectasia
  - Early — Pink lesion
  - Above line between ear and mouth
  - Face — 90%
  - Low grade malignancy
- **Risk factors**
  - Males
  - Elderly
  - Sun exposure
- **Rx**
  - Radiotherapy
  - Excision

Chapter 4

VASCULAR

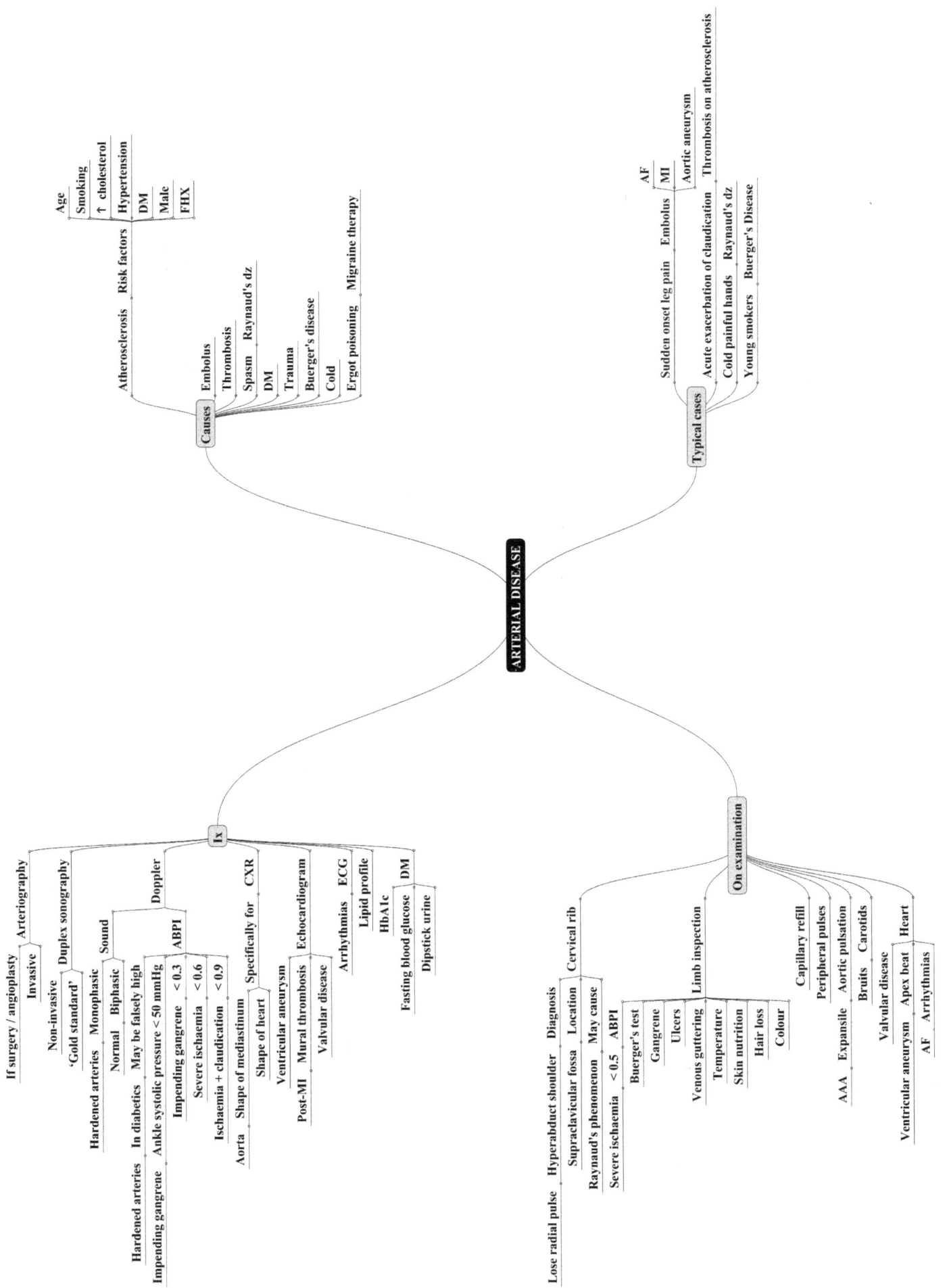

ARTERIAL DISEASE

Causes

Atherosclerosis
Risk factors
- Age
- Smoking
- ↑ cholesterol
- Hypertension
- DM
- Male
- FHX

Causes
- Atherosclerosis
- Embolus
- Thrombosis
- Spasm — Raynaud's dz
- DM
- Trauma
- Buerger's disease
- Cold
- Ergot poisoning — Migraine therapy

Typical cases

- Sudden onset leg pain
  - Embolus — AF, MI, Aortic aneurysm
  - Thrombosis on atherosclerosis
- Acute exacerbation of claudication
- Cold painful hands — Raynaud's dz
- Young smokers — Buerger's Disease

Ix

- Arteriography
  - If surgery / angioplasty
  - Invasive
- Duplex sonography
  - Non-invasive
  - 'Gold standard'
- Doppler
  - Hardened arteries — Monophasic
  - Sound — Normal — Biphasic
  - In diabetics — May be falsely high
  - Ankle systolic pressure <50 mmHg
  - ABPI
    - Impending gangrene — < 0.3
    - Severe ischaemia — < 0.6
    - Ischaemia + claudication — < 0.9
- CXR
  - Specifically for
    - Aorta — Shape of mediastinum
    - Shape of heart
    - Ventricular aneurysm
- Echocardiogram
  - Post-MI — Mural thrombosis
  - Valvular disease
- ECG
  - Arrhythmias
- Lipid profile
- HbA1c
- Fasting blood glucose — DM
- Dipstick urine

On examination

- Cervical rib
  - Lose radial pulse — Hyperabduct shoulder — Diagnosis
  - Supraclavicular fossa — Location
  - Raynaud's phenomenon — May cause
- Limb inspection
  - ABPI
    - Severe ischaemia — < 0.5
  - Buerger's test
  - Gangrene
  - Ulcers
  - Venous guttering
  - Temperature
  - Skin nutrition
  - Hair loss
  - Colour
  - Capillary refill
  - Peripheral pulses
- Aortic pulsation
  - AAA — Expansile
- Bruits — Caroids
- Valvular disease
- Heart
  - Ventricular aneurysm — Apex beat
  - AF — Arrhythmias

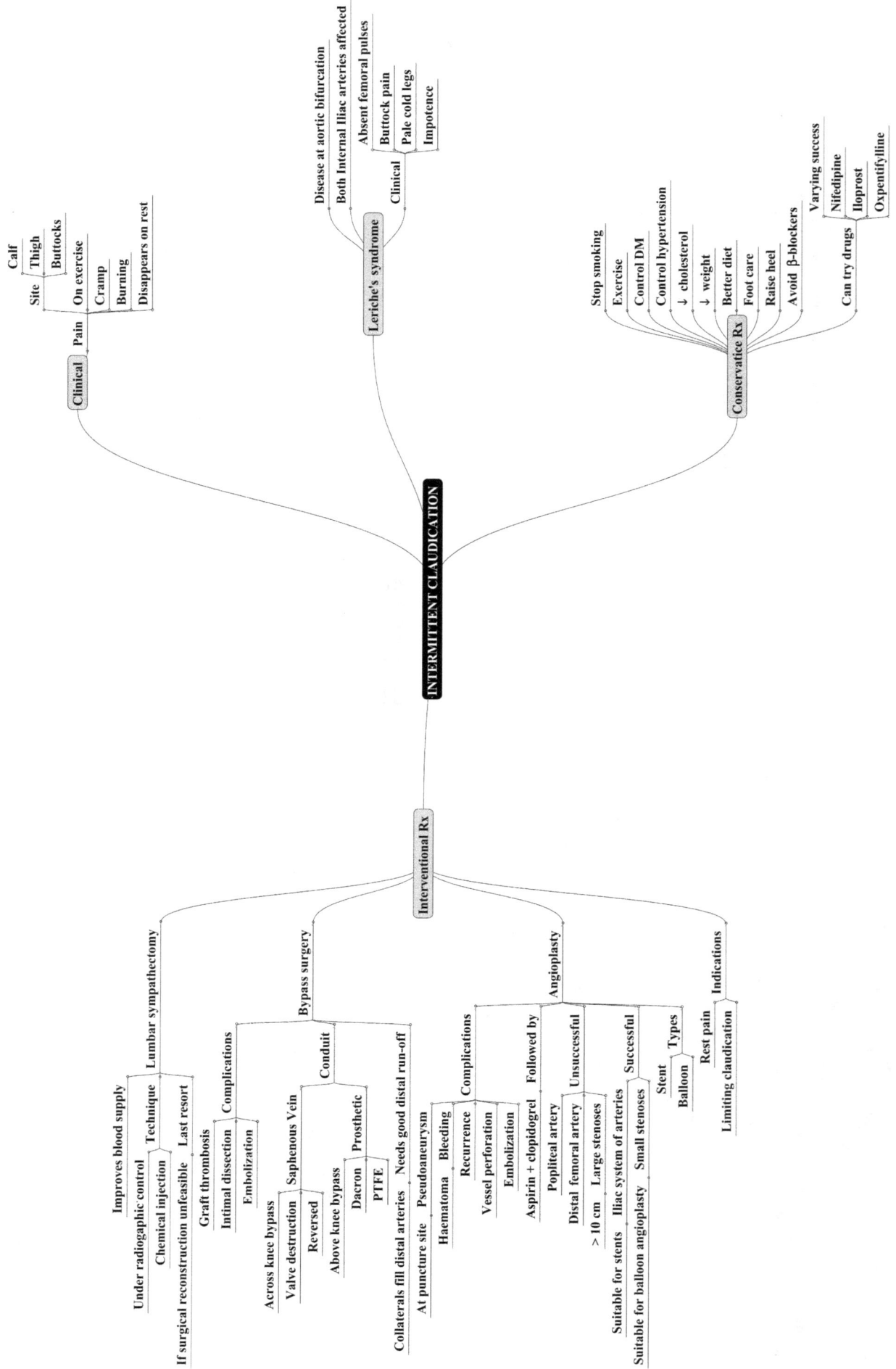

INTERMITTENT CLAUDICATION

Clinical
- Pain
  - Site
    - Calf
    - Thigh
    - Buttocks
  - On exercise
    - Cramp
    - Burning
    - Disappears on rest

Leriche's syndrome
- Disease at aortic bifurcation
- Both Internal Iliac arteries affected
- Clinical
  - Absent femoral pulses
  - Buttock pain
  - Pale cold legs
  - Impotence

Conservative Rx
- Stop smoking
- Exercise
- Control DM
- Control hypertension
- ↓ cholesterol
- ↓ weight
- Better diet
- Foot care
- Raise heel
- Avoid β-blockers
- Can try drugs
  - Varying success
    - Nifedipine
    - Iloprost
    - Oxpentifylline

Interventional Rx

- Lumbar sympathectomy
  - Improves blood supply
  - Technique
    - Under radiographic control
    - Chemical injection
  - Last resort
    - If surgical reconstruction unfeasible

- Bypass surgery
  - Complications
    - Graft thrombosis
    - Intimal dissection
    - Embolization
  - Conduit
    - Saphenous Vein
      - Across knee bypass
      - Valve destruction
      - Reversed
    - Prosthetic
      - Above knee bypass
      - Dacron
      - PTFE
  - Needs good distal run-off
    - Collaterals fill distal arteries

- Angioplasty
  - Complications
    - Pseudoaneurysm
      - At puncture site
    - Haematoma
    - Bleeding
    - Recurrence
    - Vessel perforation
    - Embolization
  - Followed by
    - Aspirin + clopidogrel
  - Unsuccessful
    - Popliteal artery
    - Distal femoral artery
    - >10 cm
    - Large stenoses
  - Successful
    - Iliac system of arteries
    - Small stenoses
  - Types
    - Stent
      - Suitable for stents
    - Balloon
      - Suitable for balloon angioplasty

- Indications
  - Rest pain
  - Limiting claudication

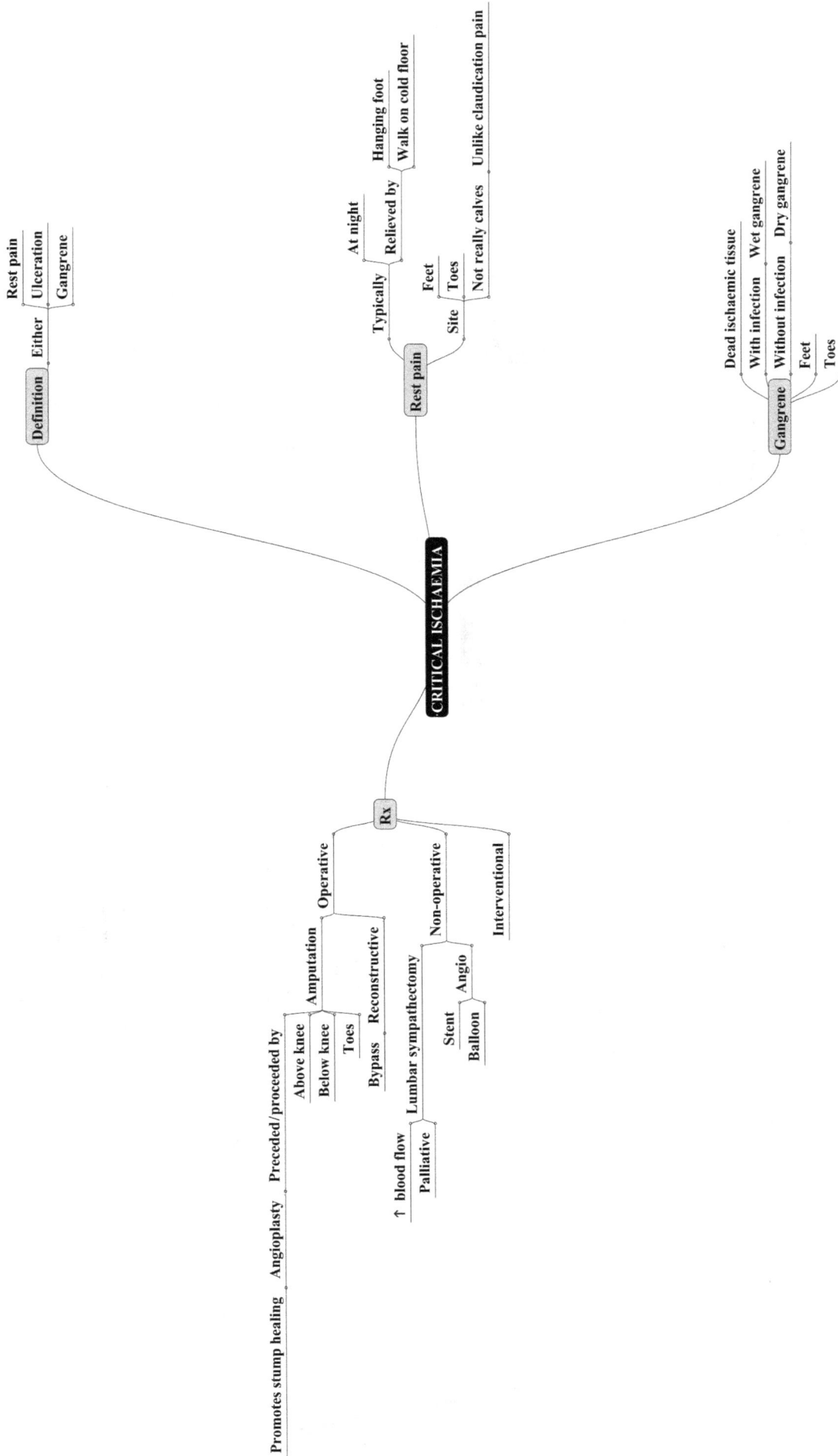

CRITICAL ISCHAEMIA

Definition
- Either
  - **Rest pain**
  - Ulceration
  - Gangrene

Rest pain
- Typically
  - **At night**
- Relieved by
  - **Hanging foot**
  - **Walk on cold floor**
- Site
  - Feet
  - Toes
- Not really calves
- Unlike claudication pain

Gangrene
- Dead ischaemic tissue
- **With infection** → Wet gangrene
- **Without infection** → Dry gangrene
  - Feet
  - Toes

Rx
- **Operative**
  - **Amputation**
    - Preceded/proceeded by
    - Angioplasty
    - Promotes stump healing
    - **Above knee**
    - **Below knee**
    - Toes
  - **Reconstructive**
    - **Bypass**
    - Lumbar sympathectomy
      - ↑ blood flow
      - Palliative
- **Non-operative**
  - **Interventional**
    - Angio
      - Stent
      - **Balloon**

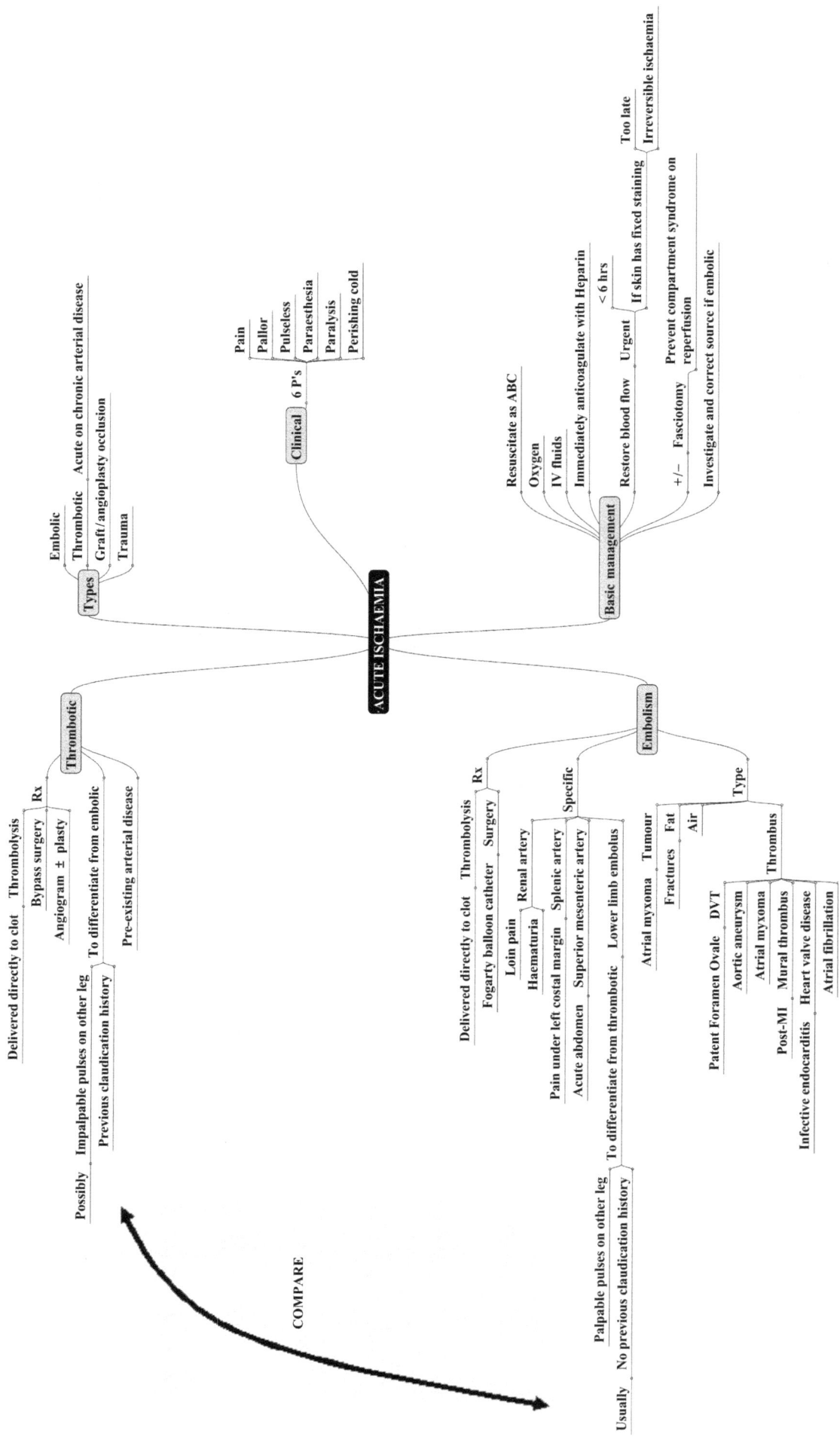

ACUTE ISCHAEMIA

Types

- Embolic
- Thrombotic
  - Acute on chronic arterial disease
  - Graft/angioplasty occlusion
- Trauma

Clinical

- 6 P's
  - Pain
  - Pallor
  - Pulseless
  - Paraesthesia
  - Paralysis
  - Perishing cold

Basic management

- Resuscitate as ABC
  - Oxygen
  - IV fluids
- Immediately anticoagulate with Heparin
- Restore blood flow — Urgent — < 6 hrs
  - If skin has fixed staining — Too late — Irreversible ischaemia
- +/− Fasciotomy — Prevent compartment syndrome on reperfusion
- Investigate and correct source if embolic

Thrombotic

- Rx
  - Thrombolysis — Delivered directly to clot
  - Bypass surgery
  - Angiogram ± plasty
- To differentiate from embolic
  - Pre-existing arterial disease
  - Possibly — Impalpable pulses on other leg
  - Previous claudication history

Embolism

- Rx
  - Thrombolysis — Delivered directly to clot
  - Surgery — Fogarty balloon catheter
- Specific
  - Renal artery — Loin pain — Haematuria
  - Splenic artery — Pain under left costal margin
  - Superior mesenteric artery — Acute abdomen
  - Lower limb embolus
- To differentiate from thrombotic
  - Usually — Palpable pulses on other leg — No previous claudication history
- Type
  - Tumour — Atrial myxoma
  - Fat — Fractures
  - Air
  - Thrombus
    - Patent Foramen Ovale — DVT
    - Aortic aneurysm
    - Atrial myxoma
    - Mural thrombus — Post-MI
    - Heart valve disease — Infective endocarditis
    - Atrial fibrillation

COMPARE

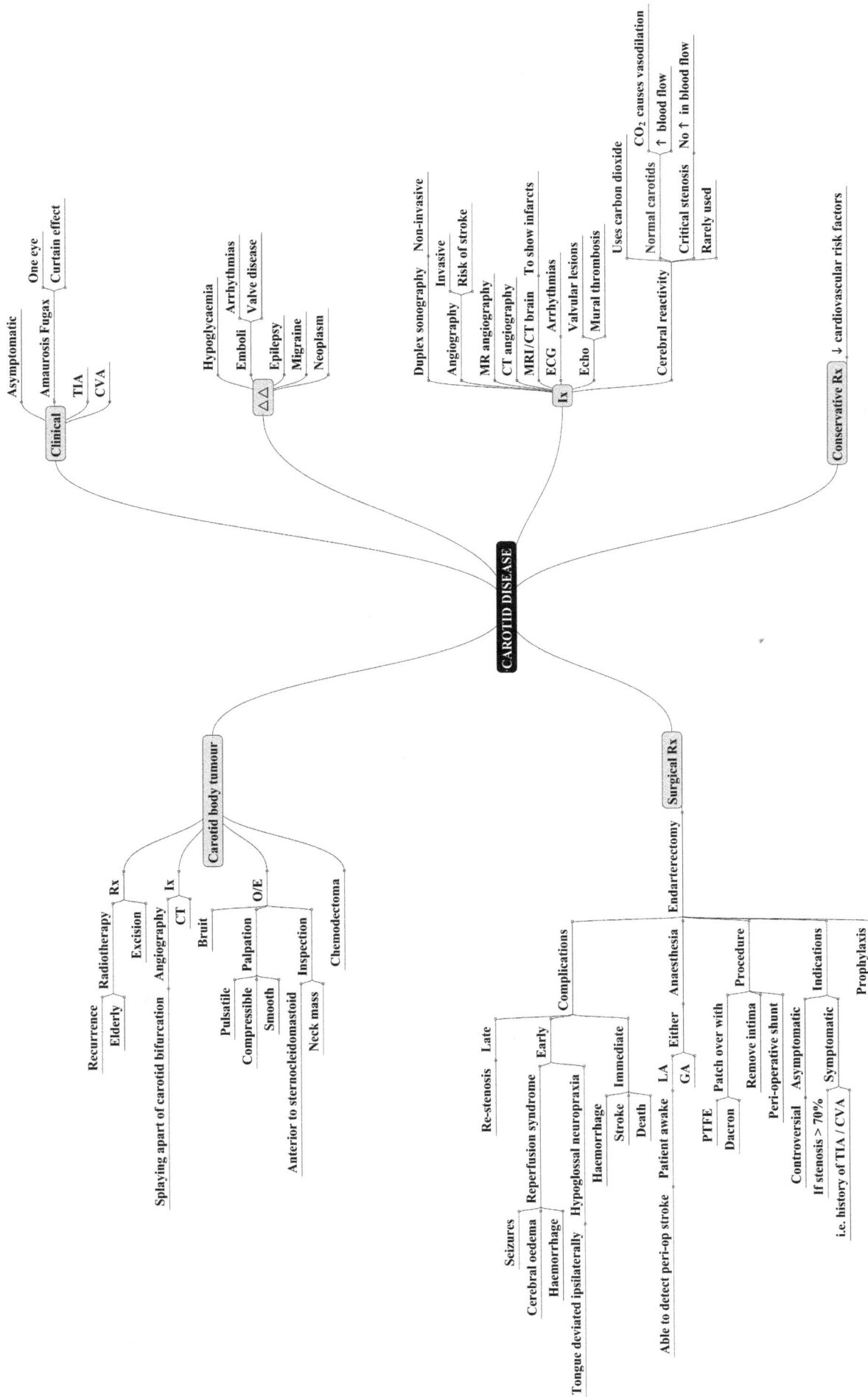

CAROTID DISEASE

Clinical
- Asymptomatic
- Amaurosis Fugax
  - One eye
  - Curtain effect
- TIA
- CVA

ΔΔ
- Hypoglycaemia
- Emboli
  - Arrhythmias
  - Valve disease
- Epilepsy
- Migraine
- Neoplasm

Ix
- Duplex sonography — Non-invasive
- Angiography — Invasive — Risk of stroke
- MR angiography
- CT angiography
- MRI/CT brain — To show infarcts
- ECG — Arrhythmias
- Echo — Valvular lesions / Mural thrombosis
- Cerebral reactivity — Uses carbon dioxide
  - CO_2 causes vasodilation
  - Normal carotids — ↑ blood flow
  - Critical stenosis — No ↑ in blood flow
  - Rarely used

Conservative Rx
- ↓ cardiovascular risk factors

Carotid body tumour
- Rx
  - Radiotherapy — Recurrence / Elderly
  - Excision
- Ix
  - Angiography — Splaying apart of carotid bifurcation
  - CT
- O/E
  - Bruit — Pulsatile
  - Palpation — Compressible / Smooth
  - Inspection — Anterior to sternocleidomastoid
  - Neck mass
- Chemodectoma

Surgical Rx
- Endarterectomy
- Complications
  - Late — Re-stenosis
  - Early
    - Seizures
    - Reperfusion syndrome — Cerebral oedema / Haemorrhage
    - Hypoglossal neuropraxia — Tongue deviated ipsilaterally
    - Immediate — Haemorrhage / Stroke / Death
- Anaesthesia
  - LA — Patient awake — Able to detect peri-op stroke
  - GA
  - Either
- Procedure
  - Patch over with — PTFE / Dacron
  - Remove intima
  - Peri-operative shunt
- Indications
  - Asymptomatic — Controversial
  - Symptomatic — If stenosis > 70% — i.e. history of TIA / CVA
- Prophylaxis

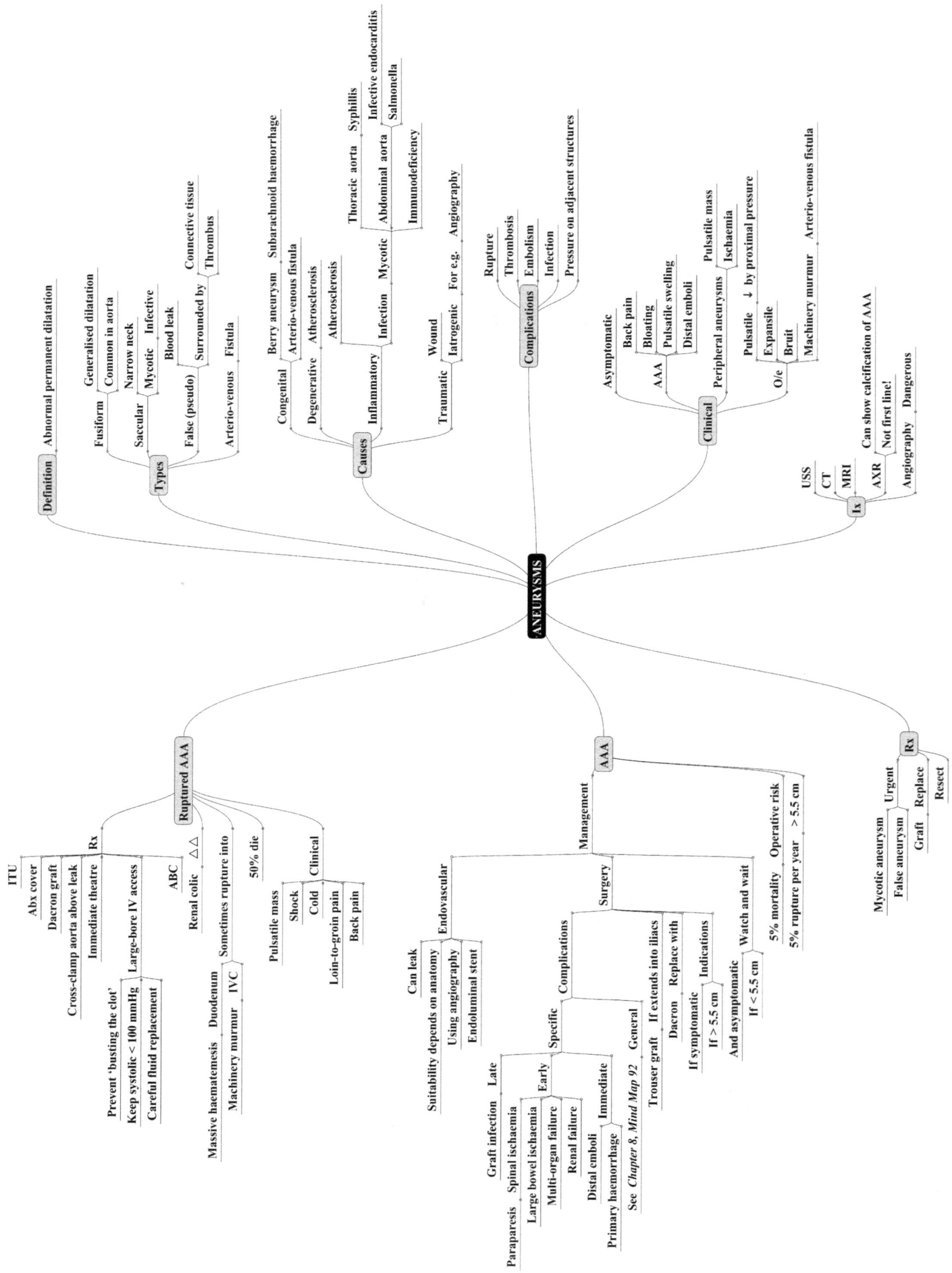

ANEURYSMS

Definition
- Abnormal permanent dilatation

Types
- Fusiform — Generalised dilatation
- Saccular
  - Common in aorta
  - Narrow neck
  - Mycotic — Infective
- False (pseudo)
  - Blood leak
  - Surrounded by — Connective tissue / Thrombus
- Arterio-venous — Fistula

Causes
- Congenital
  - Berry aneurysm
  - Arterio-venous fistula
  - Subarachnoid haemorrhage
- Degenerative — Atherosclerosis
- Inflammatory — Atherosclerosis
- Infection — Mycotic
- Traumatic
  - Wound
  - Iatrogenic — For e.g. Angiography
- Thoracic aorta — Syphilis
- Abdominal aorta
  - Infective endocarditis
  - Salmonella
- Immunodeficiency

Complications
- Rupture
- Thrombosis
- Embolism
- Infection
- Pressure on adjacent structures

Clinical
- Asymptomatic
- AAA
  - Back pain
  - Bloating
  - Pulsatile swelling
  - Distal emboli
- Peripheral aneurysm
  - Pulsatile mass
  - Ischaemia
- O/e
  - Pulsatile — ↓ by proximal pressure
  - Expansile
  - Bruit
  - Machinery murmur — Arterio-venous fistula

Ix
- USS
- CT
- MRI
- AXR
  - Can show calcification of AAA
  - Not first line!
- Angiography — Dangerous

Ruptured AAA
- Rx
  - ITU
  - Abx cover
  - Dacron graft
  - Cross-clamp aorta above leak
  - Immediate theatre
  - Large-bore IV access
    - Prevent 'busting the clot'
    - Keep systolic < 100 mmHg
    - Careful fluid replacement
- ABC
- Renal colic ΔΔ
- Sometimes rupture into — Duodenum / IVC
  - Massive haematemesis
  - Machinery murmur
- 50% die
- Clinical
  - Pulsatile mass
  - Shock
  - Cold
  - Loin-to-groin pain
  - Back pain

AAA
- Management
  - Endovascular
    - Can leak
    - Suitability depends on anatomy
    - Using angiography
    - Endoluminal stent
  - Surgery
    - Complications
      - Specific
        - Late — Graft infection
        - Early
          - Spinal ischaemia
          - Large bowel ischaemia
          - Multi-organ failure
          - Renal failure
        - Immediate
          - Distal emboli
          - Primary haemorrhage
      - General — See Chapter 8, Mind Map 92
      - Paraparesis
    - Trouser graft — If extends into iliacs
    - Replace with — Dacron
    - Indications
      - If > 5.5 cm
      - If symptomatic
      - And asymptomatic
      - If < 5.5 cm — Watch and wait
    - Operative risk
      - 5% mortality
      - 5% rupture per year — > 5.5 cm

Rx
- Mycotic aneurysm
- False aneurysm
- Urgent
  - Graft
  - Replace
  - Resect

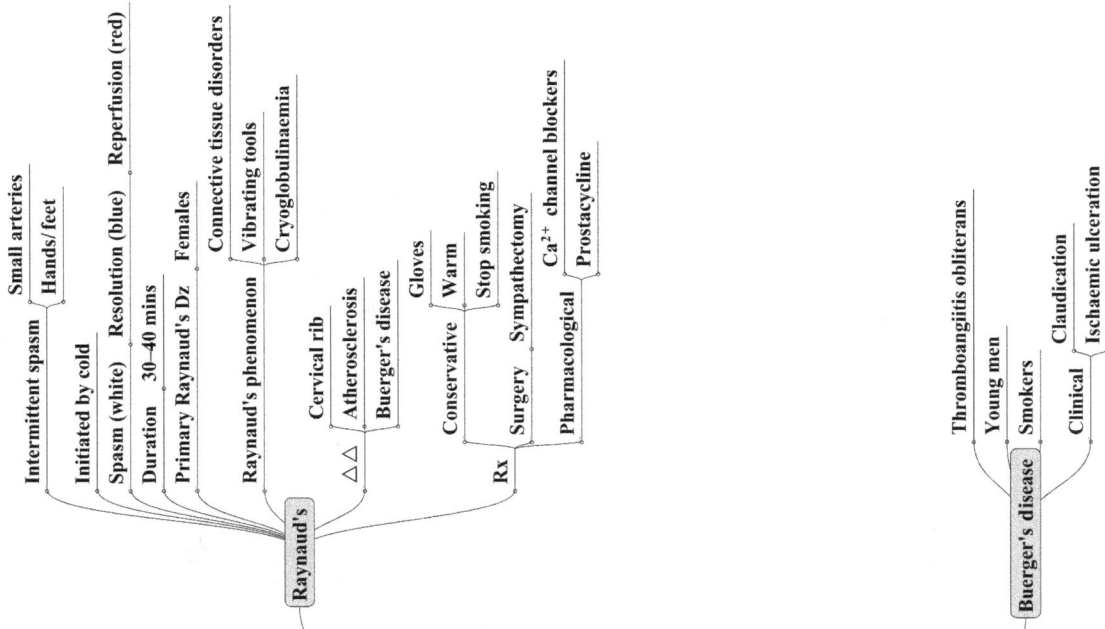

MISCELLANEOUS ARTERIAL DISEASE

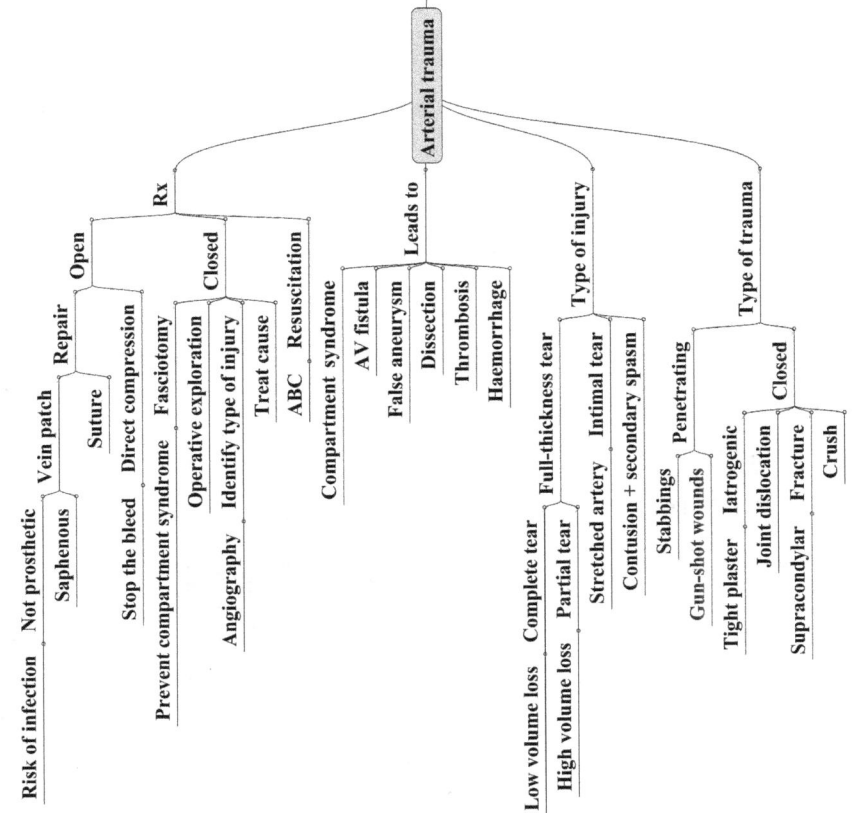

Raynaud's

- Intermittent spasm
  - Small arteries
    - Hands/feet
- Initiated by cold
- Spasm (white)
  - Resolution (blue)
    - Reperfusion (red)
- Duration 30–40 mins
- Primary Raynaud's Dz — Females
- Raynaud's phenomenon
  - Connective tissue disorders
  - Vibrating tools
  - Cryoglobulinaemia
- ΔΔ
  - Cervical rib
  - Atherosclerosis
  - Buerger's disease
- Rx
  - Conservative
    - Gloves
    - Warm
    - Stop smoking
  - Surgery — Sympathectomy
  - Pharmacological
    - Ca²⁺ channel blockers
    - Prostacycline

Ca^{2+} channel blockers

Buerger's disease

- Thromboangiitis obliterans
- Young men
- Smokers
- Clinical
  - Claudication
  - Ischaemic ulceration

Arterial trauma

- Rx
  - Open
    - Repair
      - Vein patch
        - Saphenous
        - Not prosthetic — Risk of infection
      - Suture
    - Direct compression — Stop the bleed
  - Fasciotomy — Prevent compartment syndrome
  - Operative exploration
  - Closed
    - Identify type of injury
    - Treat cause
    - Resuscitation — ABC
    - Angiography
- Leads to
  - Compartment syndrome
  - AV fistula
  - False aneurysm
  - Dissection
  - Thrombosis
  - Haemorrhage
- Type of injury
  - Complete tear — Low volume loss
  - Partial tear — High volume loss
  - Full-thickness tear — Stretched artery
  - Intimal tear — Contusion + secondary spasm
- Type of trauma
  - Penetrating
    - Stabbings
    - Gun-shot wounds
  - Closed
    - Iatrogenic — Tight plaster
    - Joint dislocation
    - Fracture — Supracondylar
    - Crush

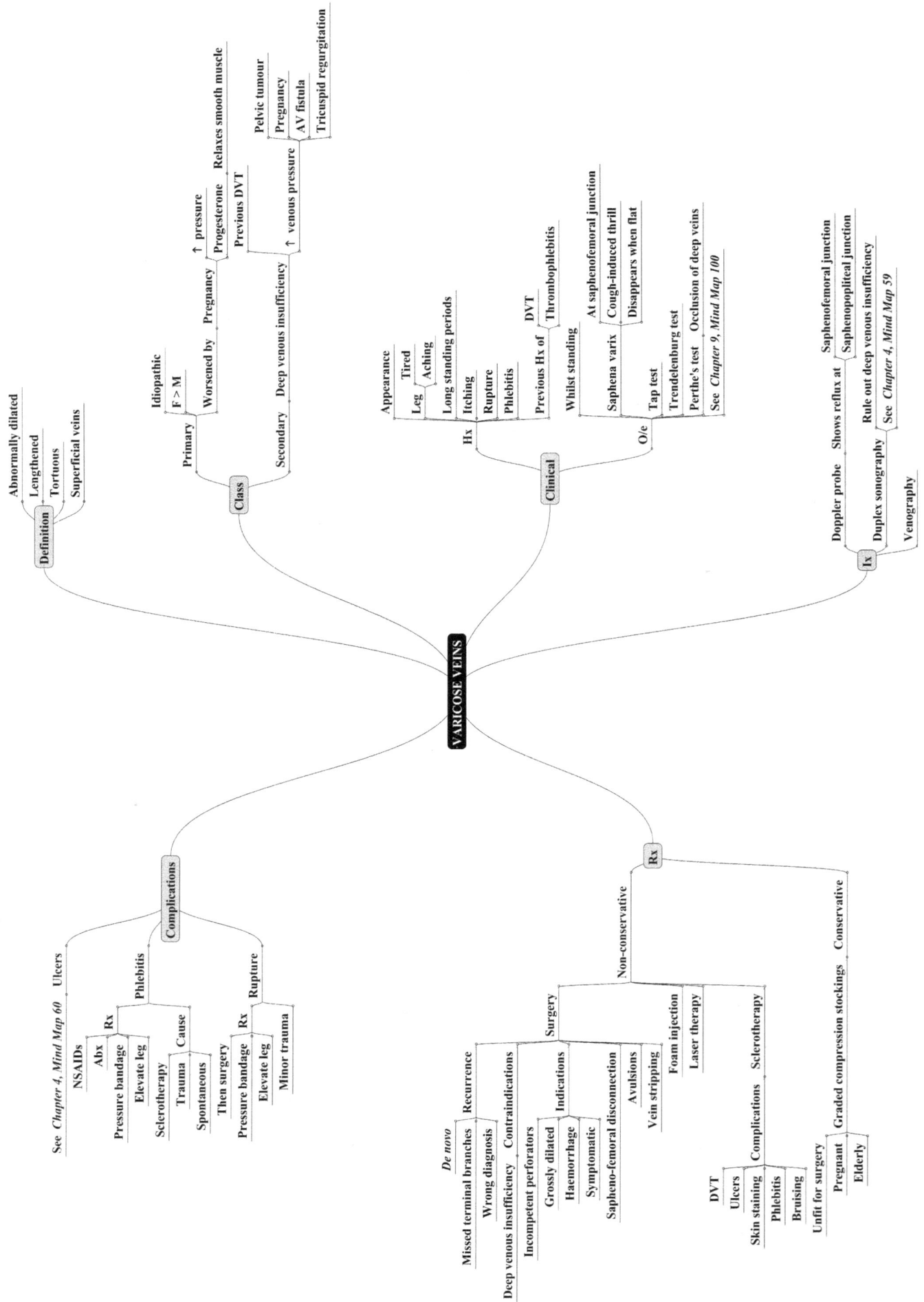

VARICOSE VEINS

Definition
- Abnormally dilated
- Lengthened
- Tortuous
- Superficial veins

Class
- Primary
  - Idiopathic
  - F > M
  - Worsened by
    - Pregnancy
      - ↑ pressure
      - Progesterone → Relaxes smooth muscle
    - Previous DVT
- Secondary → Deep venous insufficiency → ↑ venous pressure
  - Pelvic tumour
  - Pregnancy
  - AV fistula
  - Tricuspid regurgitation

Clinical
- Hx
  - Appearance
  - Leg
    - Tired
    - Aching
  - Long standing periods
  - Itching
  - Rupture
  - Phlebitis
  - Previous Hx of
    - DVT
    - Thrombophlebitis
- O/e
  - Whilst standing
  - Saphena varix
    - At saphenofemoral junction
    - Cough-induced thrill
    - Disappears when flat
  - Tap test
  - Trendelenburg test
  - Perthe's test → Occlusion of deep veins
  - See *Chapter 9, Mind Map 100*

Ix
- Doppler probe → Shows reflux at
  - Saphenofemoral junction
  - Saphenopopliteal junction
- Duplex sonography → Rule out deep venous insufficiency → See *Chapter 4, Mind Map 59*
- Venography

Complications
- See *Chapter 4, Mind Map 60* Ulcers
- Phlebitis
  - Rx
    - NSAIDs
    - Abx
    - Pressure bandage
    - Elevate leg
    - Sclerotherapy
  - Cause
    - Trauma
    - Spontaneous
    - Then surgery
- Rupture
  - Rx
    - Pressure bandage
    - Elevate leg
  - Minor trauma

Rx
- Non-conservative
  - Surgery
    - Recurrence
      - *De novo*
      - Missed terminal branches
      - Wrong diagnosis
      - Deep venous insufficiency
      - Incompetent perforators
    - Contraindications
    - Indications
      - Grossly dilated
      - Haemorrhage
      - Symptomatic
    - Saphmeno-femoral disconnection
    - Avulsions
    - Vein stripping
    - Complications
      - DVT
      - Ulcers
      - Skin staining
      - Phlebitis
      - Bruising
  - Foam injection
  - Laser therapy
  - Sclerotherapy
- Conservative
  - Unfit for surgery
    - Pregnant
    - Elderly
  - Graded compression stockings

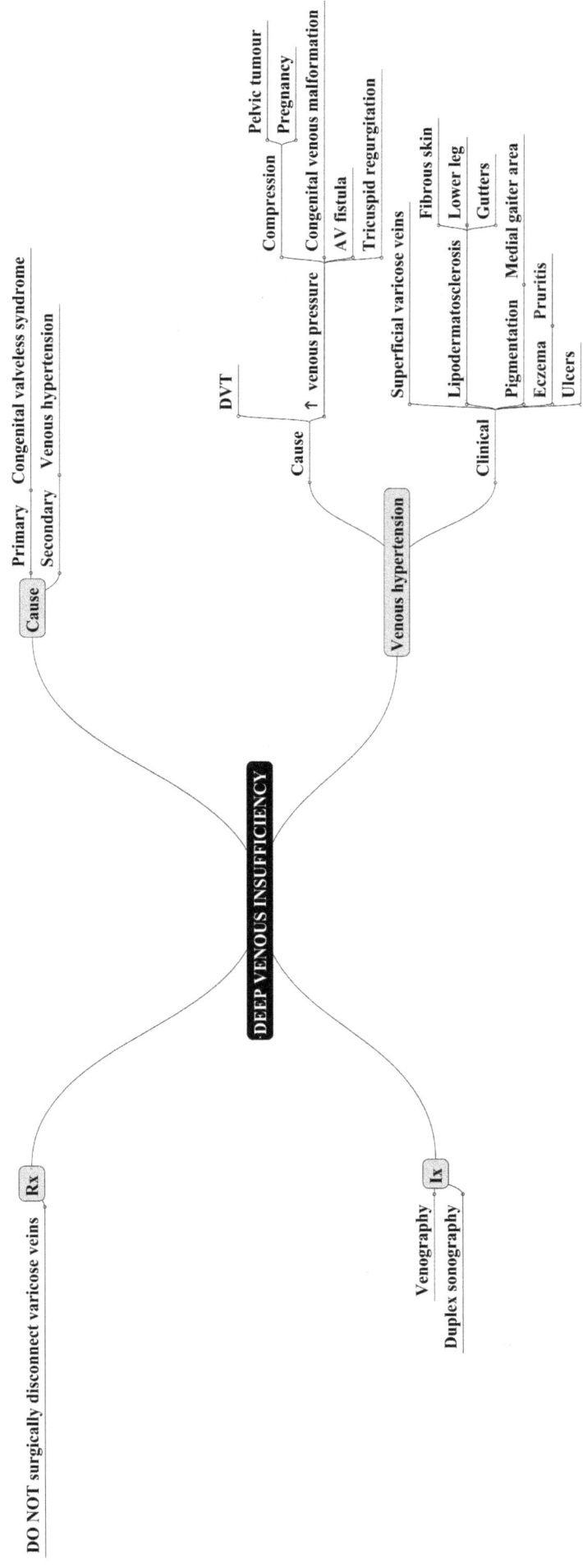

DEEP VENOUS INSUFFICIENCY

Cause

Primary
- Congenital valveless syndrome

Secondary
- Venous hypertension

Venous hypertension

Cause
- DVT
- ↑ venous pressure
  - Compression
    - Pelvic tumour
    - Pregnancy
  - Congenital venous malformation
  - AV fistula
  - Tricuspid regurgitation

Clinical
- Superficial varicose veins
- Lipodermatosclerosis
  - Fibrous skin
  - Lower leg
  - Gutters
  - Medial gaiter area
- Pigmentation
- Eczema
- Pruritis
- Ulcers

Rx
- DO NOT surgically disconnect varicose veins

Ix
- Venography
- Duplex sonography

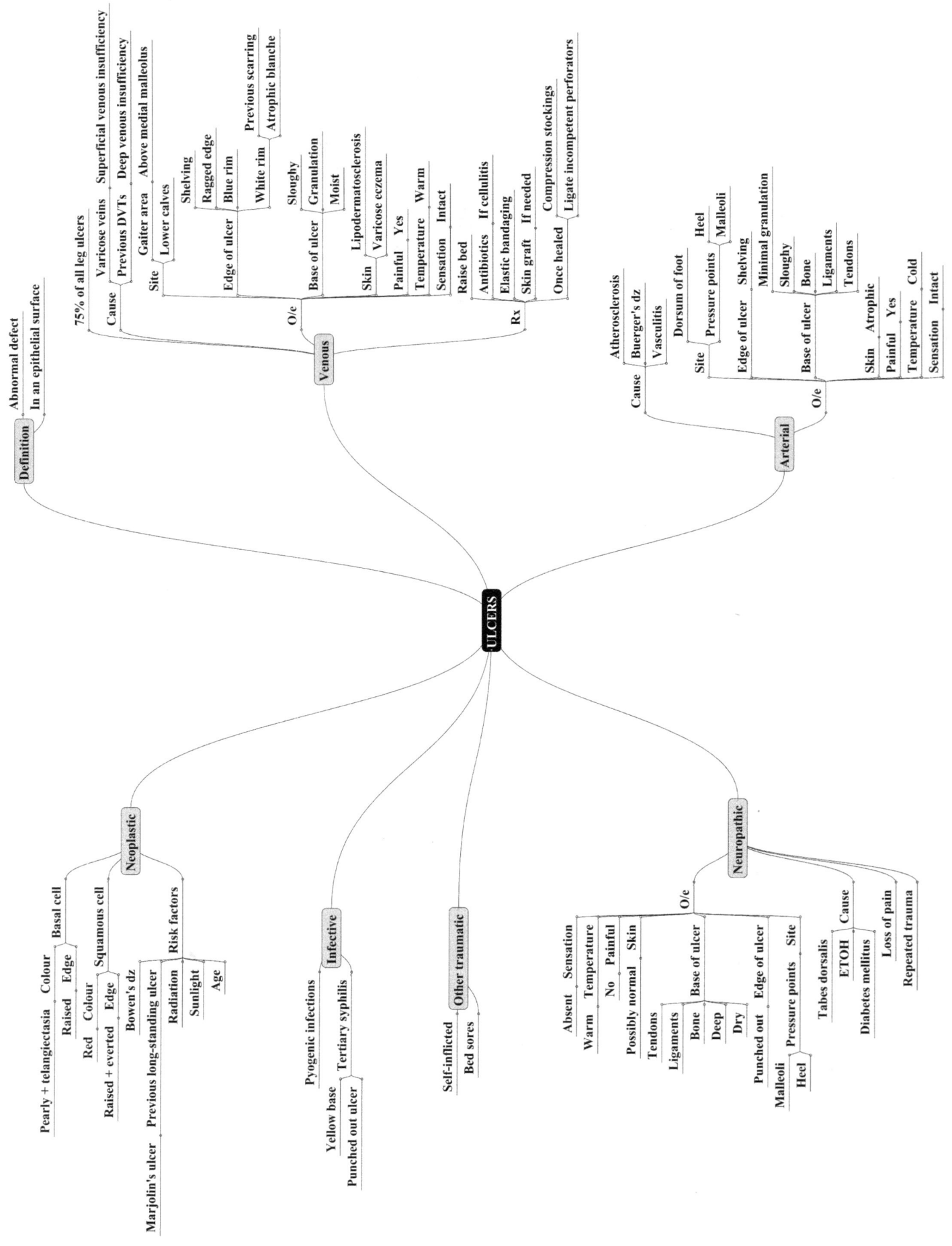

ULCERS

Definition
- Abnormal defect
- In an epithelial surface

Venous
- 75% of all leg ulcers
- **Cause**
  - Varicose veins — Superficial venous insufficiency
  - Previous DVTs — Deep venous insufficiency
- **Site**
  - Gaiter area — Above medial malleolus
  - Lower calves
- **O/e**
  - Edge of ulcer
    - Shelving
    - Ragged edge
    - Blue rim
    - White rim — Previous scarring
    - Atrophic blanche
  - Base of ulcer
    - Sloughy
    - Granulation
    - Moist
  - Skin
    - Lipodermatosclerosis
    - Varicose eczema
  - Painful — Yes
  - Temperature — Warm
  - Sensation — Intact
- **Rx**
  - Raise bed
  - Antibiotics — If cellulitis
  - Elastic bandaging
  - Skin graft — If needed
  - Compression stockings
  - Once healed
  - Ligate incompetent perforators

Arterial
- **Cause**
  - Atherosclerosis
  - Buerger's dz
  - Vasculitis
- **Site**
  - Dorsum of foot
  - Pressure points
    - Heel
    - Malleoli
- **O/e**
  - Edge of ulcer
    - Shelving
    - Minimal granulation
  - Base of ulcer
    - Sloughy
    - Bone
    - Ligaments
    - Tendons
  - Skin — Atrophic
  - Painful — Yes
  - Temperature — Cold
  - Sensation — Intact

Neoplastic
- Basal cell
  - Pearly + telangiectasia
  - Colour
  - Edge — Raised
- Squamous cell
  - Colour — Red
  - Edge — Raised + everted
  - Bowen's dz
- Marjolin's ulcer
  - Previous long-standing ulcer
- Risk factors
  - Radiation
  - Sunlight
  - Age

Infective
- Pyogenic infections
- Tertiary syphilis — Punched out ulcer
  - Yellow base

Other traumatic
- Self-inflicted
- Bed sores

Neuropathic
- **O/e**
  - Sensation — Absent
  - Temperature — Warm
  - Painful — No
  - Skin — Possibly normal
  - Base of ulcer
    - Tendons
    - Ligaments
    - Bone
    - Deep
    - Dry
  - Edge of ulcer — Punched out
  - Site — Pressure points
    - Malleoli
    - Heel
- **Cause**
  - Tabes dorsalis
  - ETOH
  - Diabetes mellitus
  - Loss of pain
  - Repeated trauma

Chapter 5

BREAST

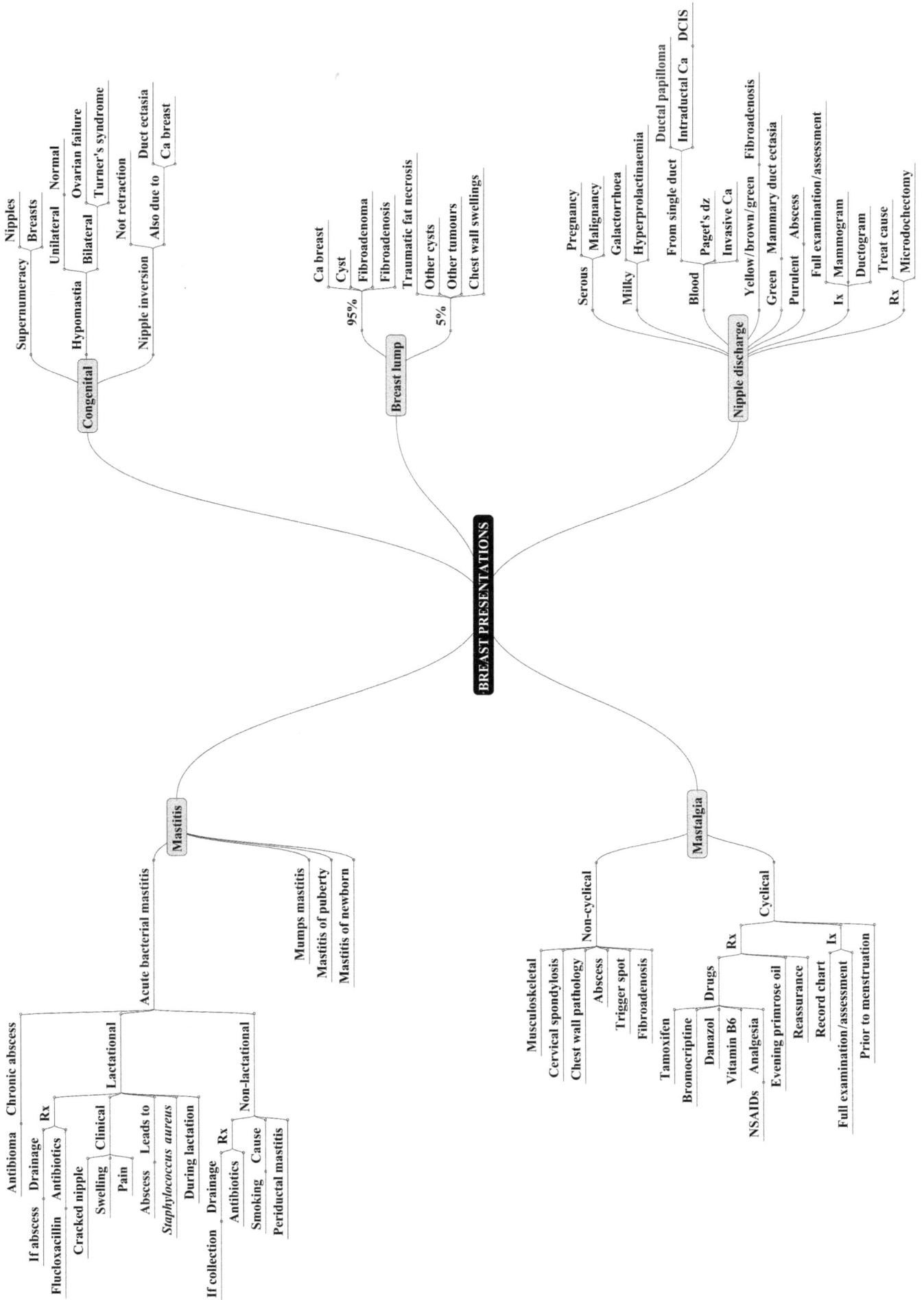

BREAST PRESENTATIONS

Congenital

- Supernumeracy
  - Nipples
  - Breasts
- Hypomastia
  - Unilateral
  - Bilateral
    - Normal
    - Ovarian failure
    - Turner's syndrome
- Nipple inversion
  - Not retraction
  - Also due to
    - Duct ectasia
    - Ca breast

Breast lump

- 95%
  - Ca breast
  - Cyst
  - Fibroadenoma
  - Fibroadenosis
- 5%
  - Traumatic fat necrosis
  - Other cysts
  - Other tumours
  - Chest wall swellings

Nipple discharge

- Serous
  - Pregnancy
  - Malignancy
- Milky
  - Galactorrhoea
  - Hyperprolactinaemia
- Blood
  - From single duct
    - Ductal papilloma
    - Intraductal Ca   DCIS
  - Paget's dz
  - Invasive Ca
- Yellow/brown/green
  - Fibroadenosis
- Green
  - Mammary duct ectasia
- Purulent
  - Abscess
- Ix
  - Full examination/assessment
  - Mammogram
  - Ductogram
- Rx
  - Treat cause
  - Microdochectomy

Mastitis

- Acute bacterial mastitis
  - Lactational
    - Cracked nipple
    - Clinical
      - Swelling
      - Pain
    - Leads to
      - Abscess
    - *Staphylococcus aureus*
    - During lactation
    - Rx
      - Antibiotics
        - Flucloxacillin
      - Drainage
        - If abscess
    - Chronic abscess
      - Antibioma
  - Non-lactational
    - Rx
      - Antibiotics
      - Drainage
        - If collection
    - Cause
      - Smoking
    - Periductal mastitis
- Mumps mastitis
- Mastitis of puberty
- Mastitis of newborn

Mastalgia

- Non-cyclical
  - Musculoskeletal
  - Cervical spondylosis
  - Chest wall pathology
  - Abscess
  - Trigger spot
  - Fibroadenosis
- Cyclical
  - Rx
    - Drugs
      - Tamoxifen
      - Bromocriptine
      - Danazol
      - Vitamin B6
    - Analgesia
      - NSAIDs
    - Evening primrose oil
    - Reassurance
    - Record chart
  - Ix
    - Full examination/assessment
    - Prior to menstruation

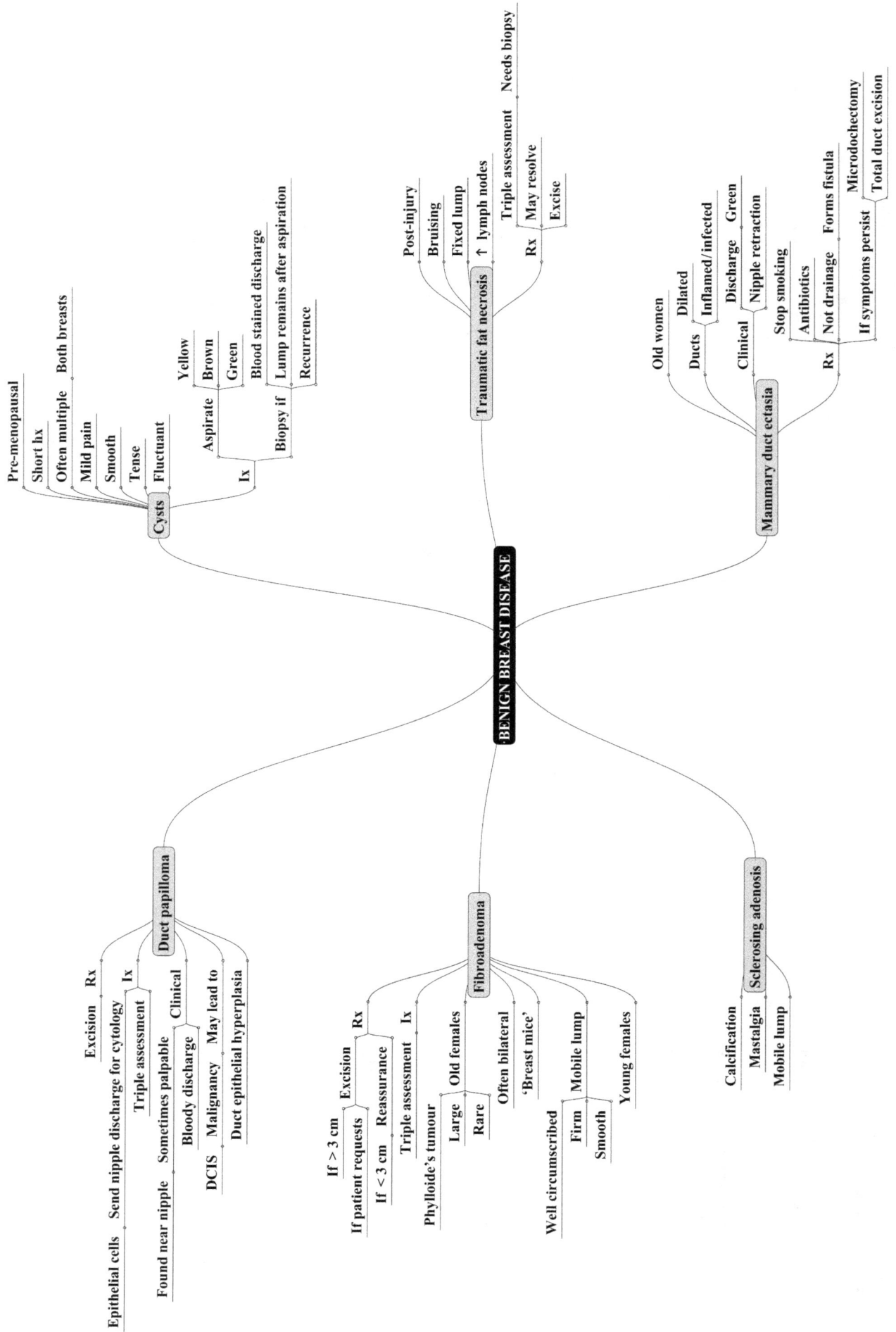

BENIGN BREAST DISEASE

Cysts
- Pre-menopausal
- Short hx
- Often multiple
- Both breasts
- Mild pain
- Smooth
- Tense
- Fluctuant
- Ix
  - Aspirate
    - Yellow
    - Brown
    - Green
    - Blood stained discharge
  - Biopsy if
    - Lump remains after aspiration
    - Recurrence

Traumatic fat necrosis
- Post-injury
- Bruising
- Fixed lump
- ↑ lymph nodes
- Triple assessment
  - Needs biopsy
- Rx
  - May resolve
  - Excise

Mammary duct ectasia
- Old women
- Ducts
  - Dilated
  - Inflamed / infected
- Clinical
  - Discharge — Green
  - Nipple retraction
- Rx
  - Stop smoking
  - Antibiotics
  - Not drainage
    - Forms fistula
  - If symptoms persist
    - Microdochectomy
    - Total duct excision

Duct papilloma
- Epithelial cells
- Found near nipple
- Sometimes palpable
- Ix
  - Send nipple discharge for cytology
  - Triple assessment
  - Clinical
    - Bloody discharge
    - Malignancy
      - DCIS
    - May lead to
      - Duct epithelial hyperplasia
- Rx
  - Excision

Fibroadenoma
- Young females
- Mobile lump
  - Firm
  - Smooth
- Well circumscribed
- 'Breast mice'
- Often bilateral
- Rare
- Large — Old females
- Phylloide's tumour
- Ix
  - Triple assessment
- Rx
  - If > 3 cm — Excision
  - If patient requests — Excision
  - If < 3 cm — Reassurance

Sclerosing adenosis
- Mobile lump
- Mastalgia
- Calcification

BREAST CANCER 1

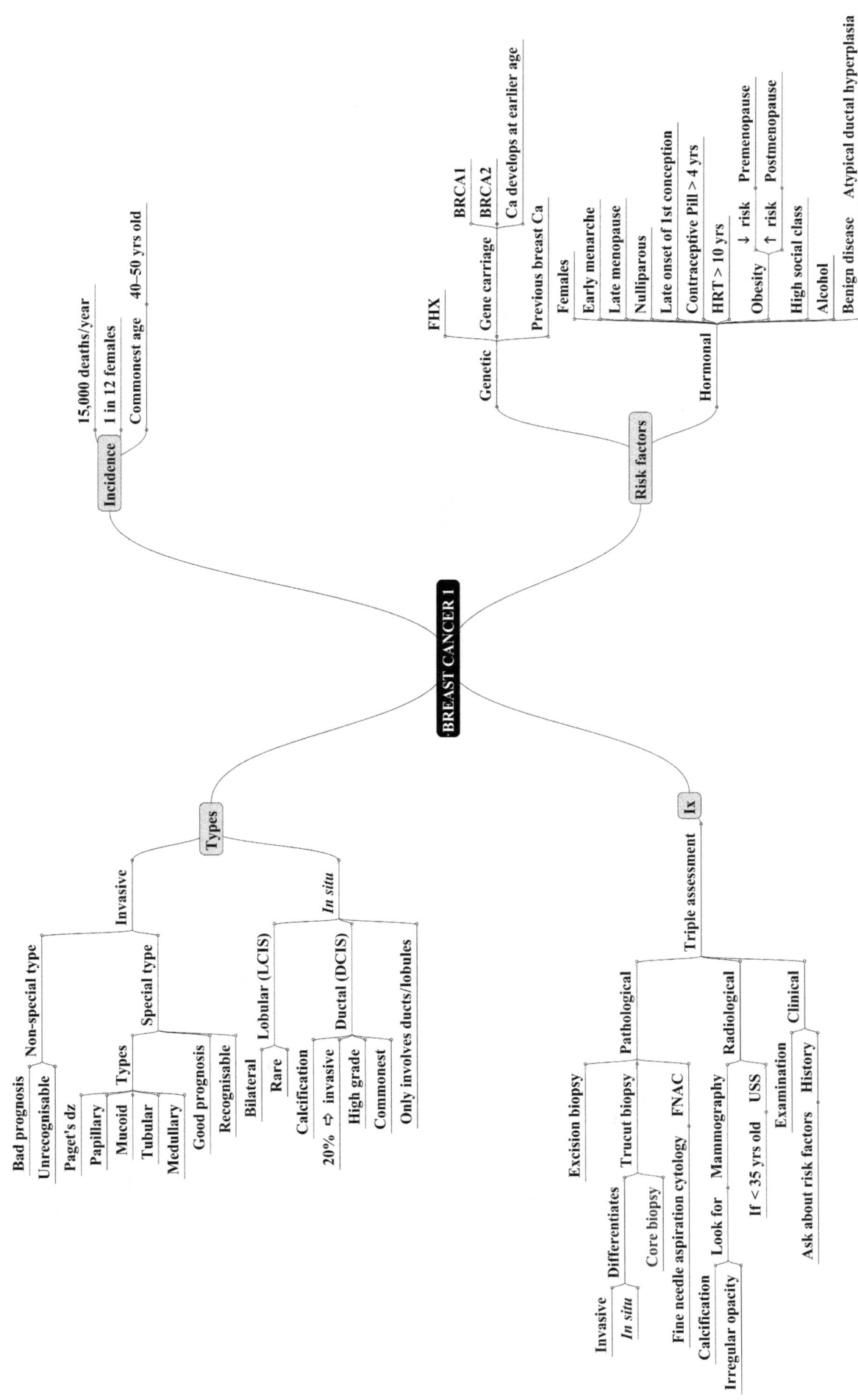

Incidence
- 15,000 deaths/year
- 1 in 12 females
- Commonest age
  - 40–50 yrs old

Risk factors

Genetic
- FHX
- Gene carriage
  - BRCA1
  - BRCA2
    - Ca develops at earlier age
- Previous breast Ca

Hormonal
- Females
- Early menarche
- Late menopause
- Nulliparous
- Late onset of 1st conception
- Contraceptive Pill > 4 yrs
- HRT > 10 yrs
- Obesity
  - ↓ risk — Premenopause
  - ↑ risk — Postmenopause
- High social class
- Alcohol
- Benign disease — Atypical ductal hyperplasia

Types

Invasive
- Non-special type
  - Bad prognosis
  - Unrecognisable
  - Paget's dz
- Special type
  - Types
    - Papillary
    - Mucoid
    - Tubular
    - Medullary
  - Good prognosis
  - Recognisable

In situ
- Lobular (LCIS)
  - Bilateral
  - Rare
- Ductal (DCIS)
  - Calcification
  - 20% ⇔ invasive
  - High grade
  - Commonest
  - Only involves ducts/lobules

Ix

Triple assessment

Pathological
- Excision biopsy
- Trucut biopsy
  - Differentiates
    - Invasive
    - *In situ*
  - Core biopsy
- Fine needle aspiration cytology (FNAC)

Radiological
- Mammography
  - Look for
    - Calcification
    - Irregular opacity
  - If <35 yrs old — USS

Clinical
- Examination
- History
  - Ask about risk factors

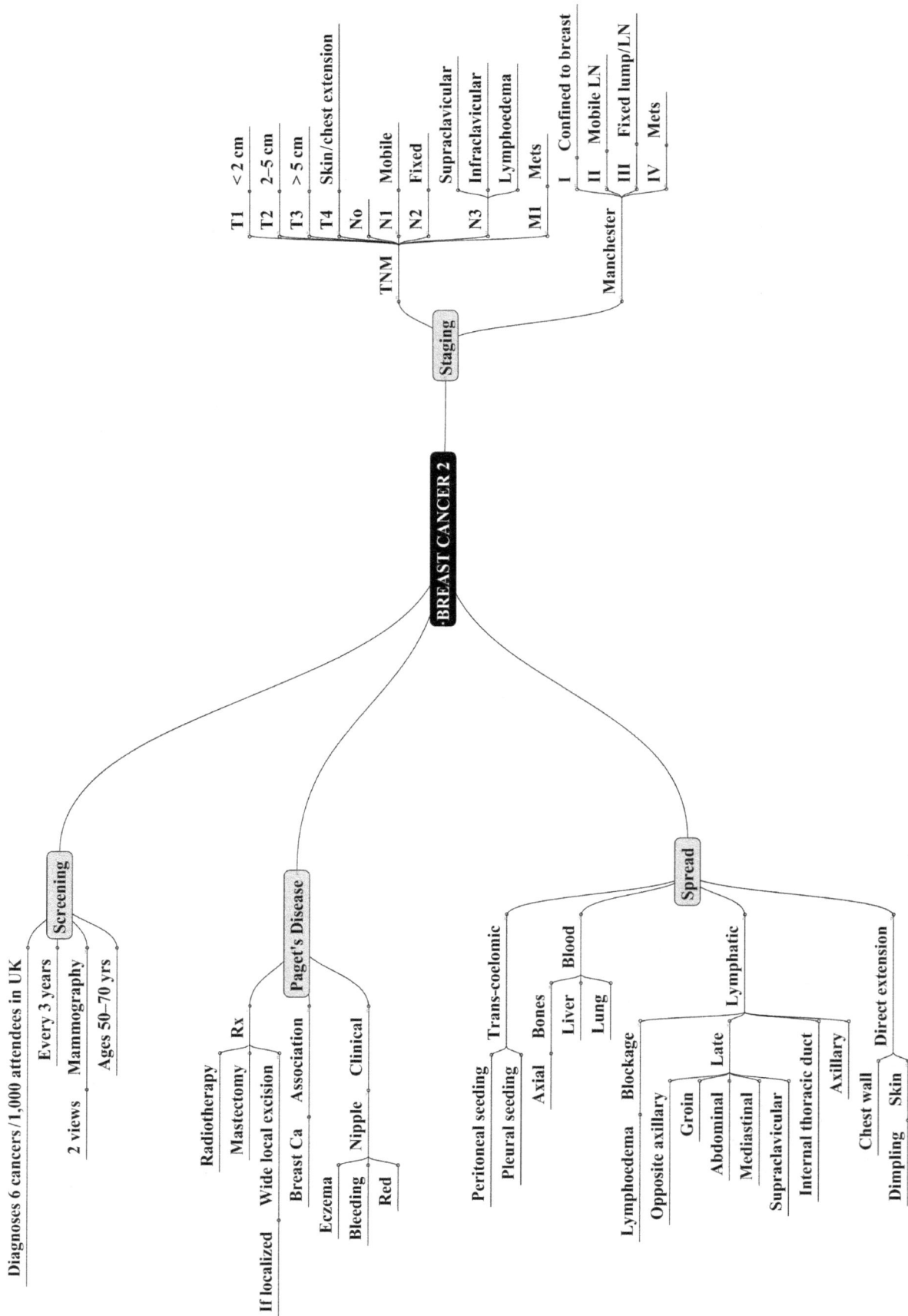

BREAST CANCER 2

Staging

TNM

- T1   < 2 cm
- T2   2–5 cm
- T3   > 5 cm
- T4   Skin/chest extension
- N0   Mobile
- N1   Mobile
- N2   Fixed
- N3   Supraclavicular
       Infraclavicular
       Lymphoedema
- M1   Mets

Manchester
- I   Confined to breast
- II   Mobile LN
- III   Fixed lump/LN
- IV   Mets

Screening
- Diagnoses 6 cancers/1,000 attendees in UK
- Every 3 years
- Mammography
  - 2 views
- Ages 50–70 yrs

Paget's Disease
- Rx
  - Radiotherapy
  - Mastectomy
  - Wide local excision (If localized)
- Association
  - Breast Ca
- Clinical
  - Eczema
  - Nipple
    - Bleeding
    - Red

Spread
- Trans-coelomic
  - Peritoneal seeding
  - Pleural seeding
- Bones
  - Axial
- Blood
  - Liver
  - Lung
- Lymphatic
  - Blockage
    - Lymphoedema
    - Opposite axillary
  - Late
    - Groin
    - Abdominal
    - Mediastinal
    - Supraclavicular
    - Internal thoracic duct
    - Axillary
- Direct extension
  - Chest wall
    - Dimpling
    - Skin

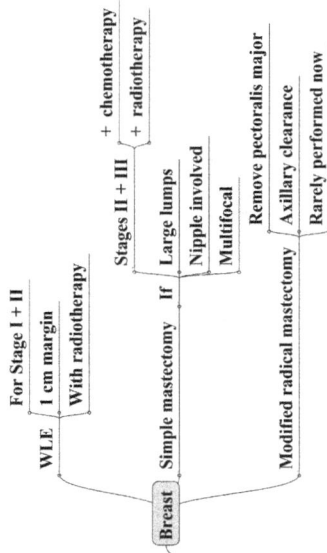

BREAST CANCER TREATMENT 1

Breast

WLE — For Stage I + II
- 1 cm margin
- With radiotherapy

Simple mastectomy
- If
  - Large lumps
  - Nipple involved
  - Multifocal
- Stages II + III
  - + chemotherapy
  - + radiotherapy

Modified radical mastectomy
- Remove pectoralis major
- Axillary clearance
- Rarely performed now

Axilla

Contains 28+ nodes
- Level 1 — Lateral to pec minor
- Level 2 — Behind pec minor
- Level 3 — Medial to pec minor

Options
- Sampling
  - 4 nodes
  - At level 1
  - If +ve — Axillary clearance
- Sentinel node biopsy
  - Sentinel node — 1st node to drain tumour
  - Aim → needless axillary clearance
    - In LN −ve patients
  - Technique
    - Blue dye or radiocolloid
    - Injected into tumour area
    - Axillary incision
    - Either
      - Visual inspection
      - Gamma probe
    - Sentinel node identified
    - Sentinel node sent for histology
    - If +ve — Axillary clearance
- Clearance
  - No survival effect
  - Useful for
    - Staging
    - Preventing recurrence

Adjuvant therapy

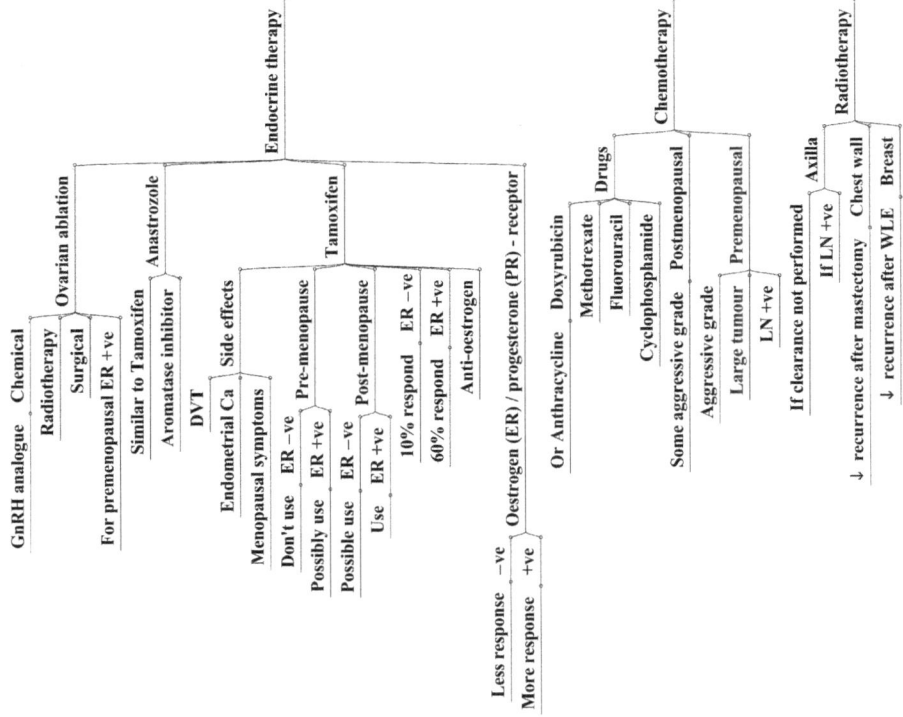

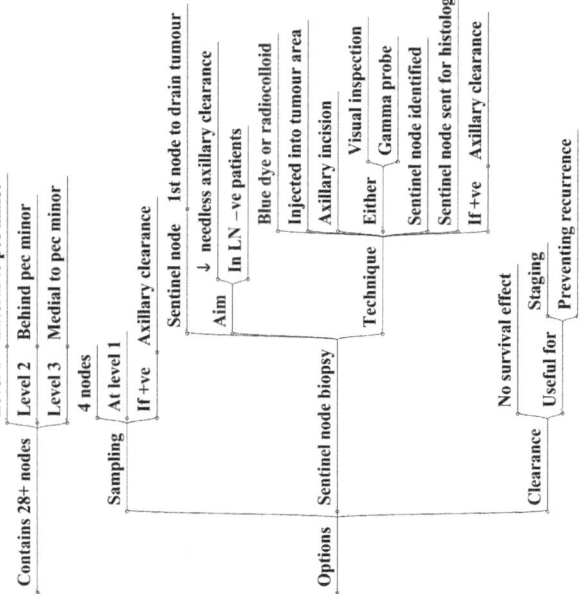

Endocrine therapy

Ovarian ablation
- GnRH analogue
- Chemical
- Radiotherapy
- Surgical
- For premenopausal ER +ve

Anastrozole
- Similar to Tamoxifen
- Aromatase inhibitor

Tamoxifen
- Side effects
  - DVT
  - Endometrial Ca
  - Menopausal symptoms
- Pre-menopause
  - Don't use — ER −ve
  - Possibly use — ER +ve
- Post-menopause
  - Possible use — ER −ve
  - Use — ER +ve
- ER −ve — 10% respond
- ER +ve — 60% respond
- Anti-oestrogen

Oestrogen (ER) / progesterone (PR) - receptor
- Less response — −ve
- More response — +ve

Chemotherapy

Drugs
- Doxyrubicin — Or Anthracycline
- Methotrexate
- Fluorouracil
- Cyclophosphamide

- Postmenopausal — Some aggressive grade
- Premenopausal
  - Aggressive grade
  - Large tumour
  - LN +ve

Radiotherapy

Axilla — If clearance not performed
- If LN +ve → recurrence after mastectomy

Chest wall — → recurrence after WLE

Breast

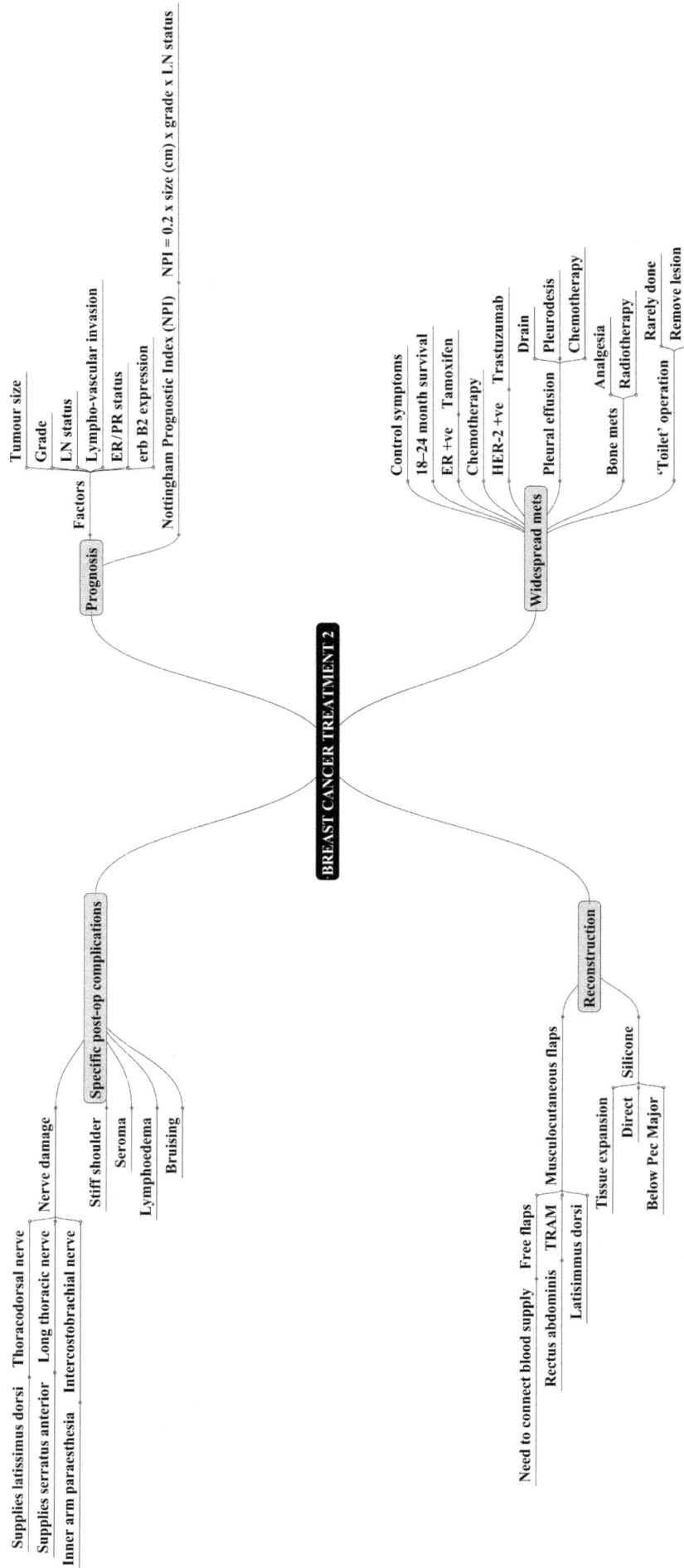

BREAST CANCER TREATMENT 2

Prognosis

Factors
- Tumour size
- Grade
- LN status
- Lympho-vascular invasion
- ER/PR status
- erb B2 expression
- Nottingham Prognostic Index (NPI)

NPI = 0.2 x size (cm) x grade x LN status

Widespread mets

- Control symptoms
- 18–24 month survival
- ER +ve — Tamoxifen
- Chemotherapy
- HER-2 +ve — Trastuzumab
- Pleural effusion
  - Drain
  - Pleurodesis
  - Chemotherapy
- Bone mets
  - Analgesia
  - Radiotherapy
- 'Toilet' operation
  - Rarely done
  - Remove lesion

Specific post-op complications

- Nerve damage
  - Supplies latissimus dorsi — Thoracodorsal nerve
  - Supplies serratus anterior — Long thoracic nerve
  - Inner arm paraesthesia — Intercostobrachial nerve
- Stiff shoulder
- Seroma
- Lymphoedema
- Bruising

Reconstruction

- Need to connect blood supply — Free flaps
- Musculocutaneous flaps
  - TRAM — Rectus abdominis
  - Latissimus dorsi
- Tissue expansion
  - Direct — Silicone
  - Below Pec Major

Chapter 6

UROLOGY

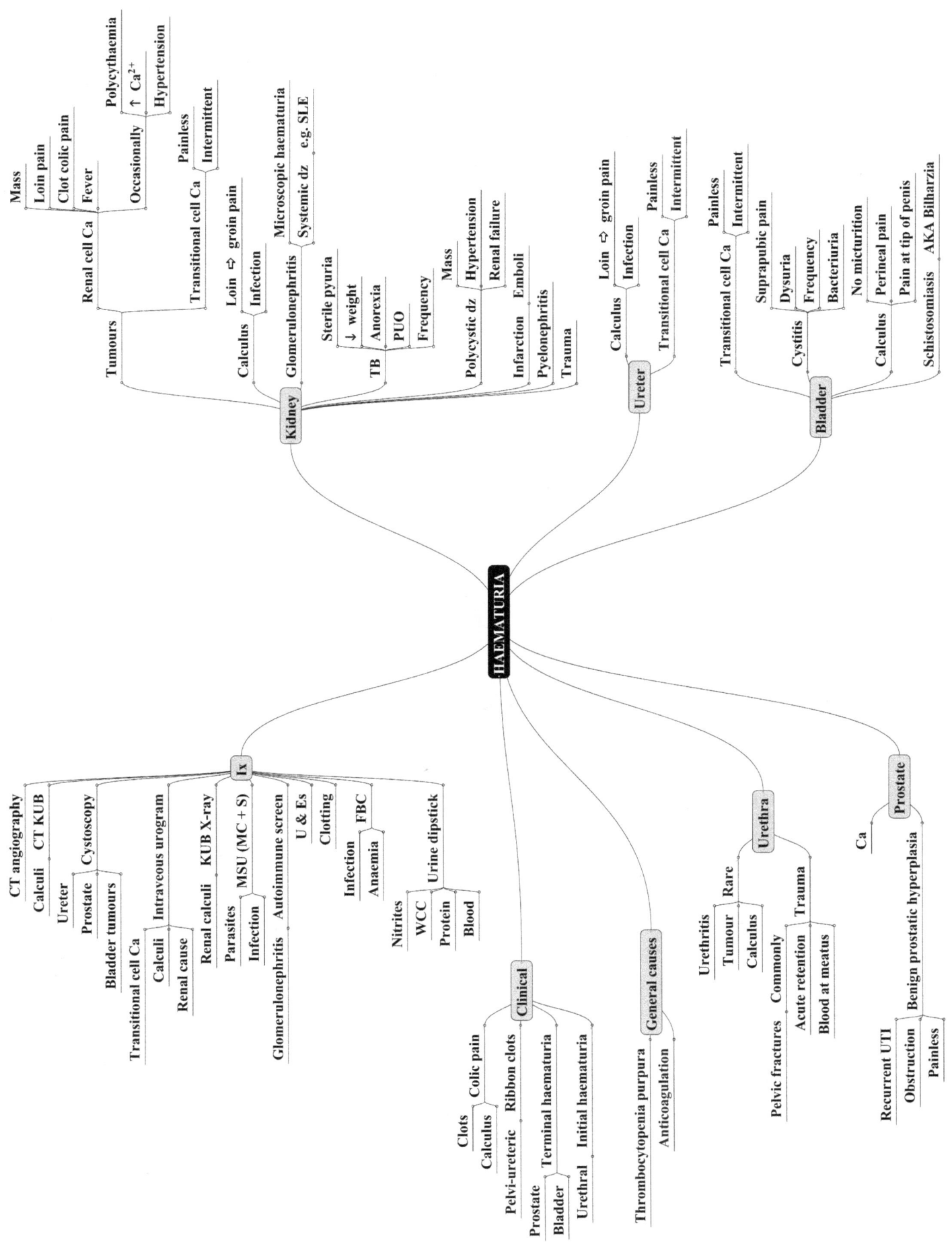

HAEMATURIA

Kidney

- Tumours
  - Renal cell Ca
    - Mass
    - Loin pain
    - Clot colic pain
    - Fever
    - Occasionally
      - Polycythaemia
      - ↑ Ca^{2+}
      - Hypertension
  - Transitional cell Ca
    - Painless
    - Intermittent
- Calculus
  - Loin ⇌ groin pain
  - Infection
- Glomerulonephritis
  - Microscopic haematuria
  - Systemic dz e.g. SLE
- TB
  - Sterile pyuria
  - ↓ weight
  - Anorexia
  - PUO
  - Frequency
- Polycystic dz
  - Mass
  - Hypertension
  - Renal failure
- Infarction
  - Emboli
- Pyelonephritis
- Trauma

Ureter

- Calculus
  - Loin ⇌ groin pain
  - Infection
- Transitional cell Ca
  - Painless
  - Intermittent

Bladder

- Transitional cell Ca
  - Painless
  - Intermittent
- Cystitis
  - Suprapubic pain
  - Dysuria
  - Frequency
  - Bacteriuria
- Calculus
  - No micturition
  - Perineal pain
  - Pain at tip of penis
- Schistosomiasis AKA Bilharzia

Ix

- CT angiography
- Calculi CT KUB
  - Ureter
  - Prostate
  - Bladder tumours
- Cystoscopy
  - Transitional cell Ca
  - Calculi
  - Renal cause
- Intraveous urogram
  - Renal calculi
- KUB X-ray
  - Renal calculi
- MSU (MC + S)
  - Parasites
  - Infection
    - Glomerulonephritis
  - Autoimmune screen
- U & Es
- Clotting
- FBC
  - Infection
  - Anaemia
- Urine dipstick
  - Nitrites
  - WCC
  - Protein
  - Blood

Clinical

- Clots
  - Colic pain
  - Calculus
- Ribbon clots
  - Pelvi-ureteric
- Terminal haematuria
  - Prostate
  - Bladder
- Initial haematuria
  - Urethral

General causes

- Thrombocytopenia purpura
- Anticoagulation

Urethra

- Urethritis
- Tumour
  - Rare
- Calculus
- Trauma
  - Commonly
    - Pelvic fractures
  - Acute retention
  - Blood at meatus

Prostate

- Ca
- Benign prostatic hyperplasia
  - Recurrent UTI
  - Obstruction
  - Painless

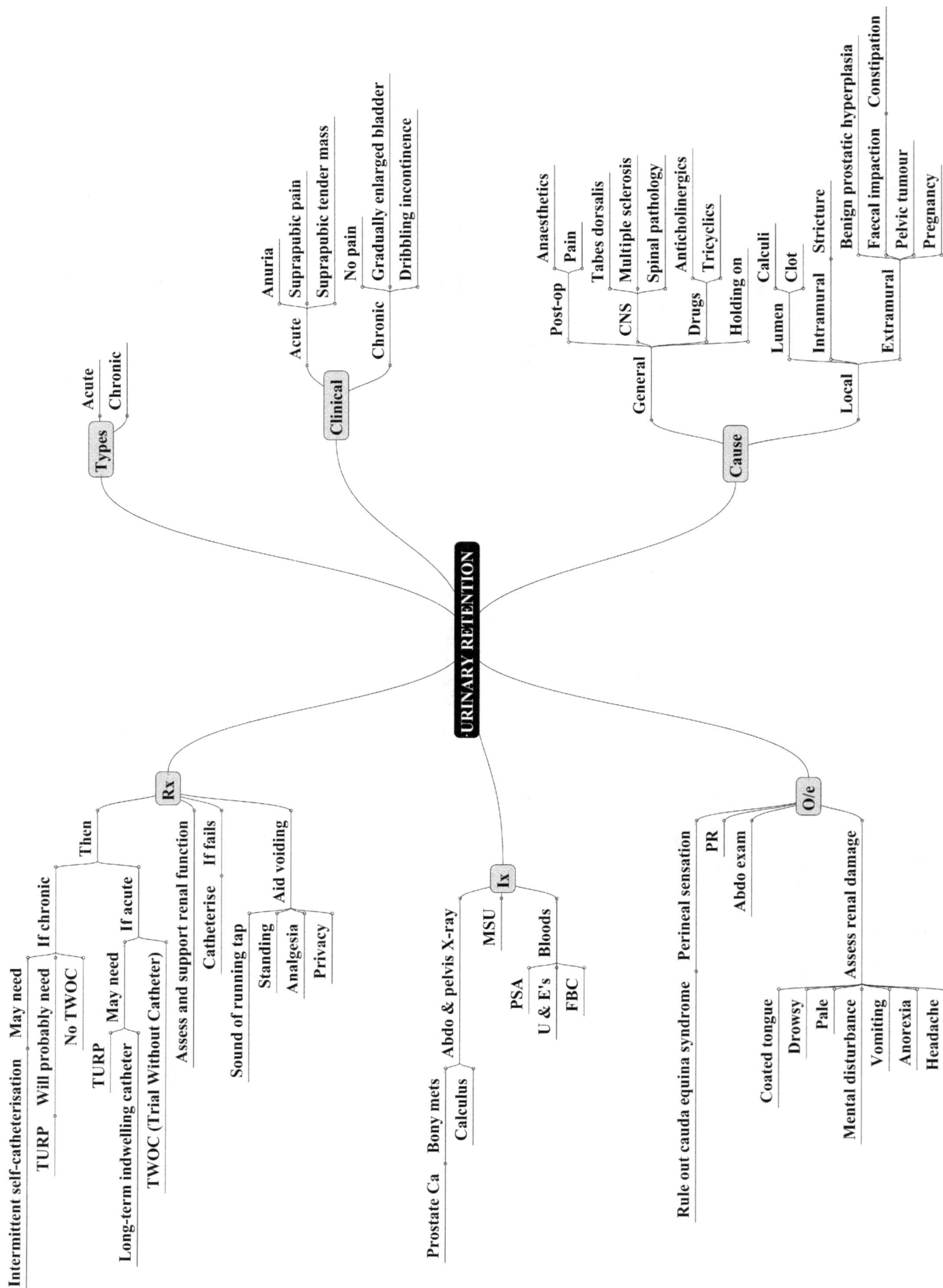

URINARY RETENTION

Types
- Acute
- Chronic

Clinical
- Acute
  - Anuria
  - Suprapubic pain
  - Suprapubic tender mass
- Chronic
  - No pain
  - Gradually enlarged bladder
  - Dribbling incontinence

Cause
- General
  - Post-op
    - Anaesthetics
    - Pain
  - CNS
    - Tabes dorsalis
    - Multiple sclerosis
    - Spinal pathology
  - Drugs
    - Anticholinergics
    - Tricyclics
  - Holding on
- Local
  - Lumen
    - Calculi
    - Clot
  - Intramural
    - Stricture
    - Benign prostatic hyperplasia
  - Extramural
    - Faecal impaction
    - Pelvic tumour
    - Pregnancy
    - Constipation

Rx
- If chronic
  - Intermittent self-catheterisation
  - May need
  - TURP
  - Will probably need
  - No TWOC
- Then
  - TURP
  - May need
  - TURP
  - Long-term indwelling catheter
  - TWOC (Trial Without Catheter)
- If acute
- Assess and support renal function
- Catheterise   If fails
  - Aid voiding
    - Sound of running tap
    - Standing
    - Analgesia
    - Privacy

Ix
- Abdo & pelvis X-ray
  - Prostate Ca
  - Bony mets
  - Calculus
- MSU
- Bloods
  - PSA
  - U & E's
  - FBC

O/e
- Perineal sensation
  - Rule out cauda equina syndrome
- PR
- Abdo exam
- Assess renal damage
  - Coated tongue
  - Drowsy
  - Pale
  - Mental disturbance
  - Vomiting
  - Anorexia
  - Headache

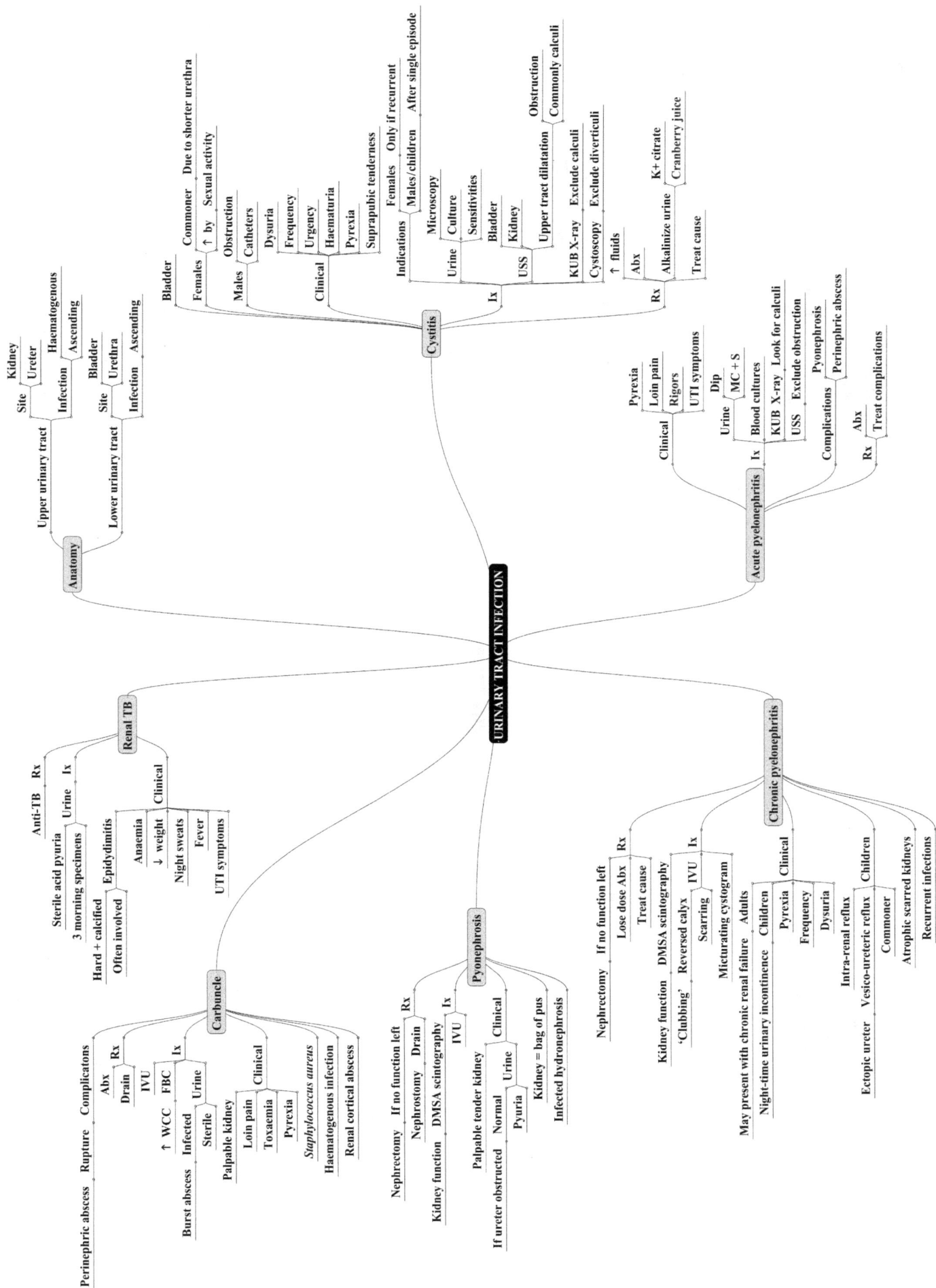

URINARY TRACT INFECTION

Anatomy

- **Upper urinary tract**
  - Site
    - Kidney
    - Ureter
  - Infection
    - Haematogenous
    - Ascending
- **Lower urinary tract**
  - Site
    - Bladder
    - Urethra
  - Infection
    - Ascending

Cystitis

- **Females** — Commoner / Due to shorter urethra
  - ↑ by — Sexual activity
  - Obstruction
- **Males** — Catheters / Obstruction
- **Clinical**
  - Dysuria
  - Frequency
  - Urgency
  - Haematuria
  - Pyrexia
  - Suprapubic tenderness
- **Ix**
  - Indications — Females (Only if recurrent) / Males/children (After single episode)
  - Urine — Microscopy / Culture / Sensitivities
  - USS — Bladder / Kidney — Upper tract dilatation
  - KUB X-ray — Exclude calculi (Obstruction — Commonly calculi)
  - Cystoscopy — Exclude diverticuli
- **Rx**
  - ↑ fluids
  - Abx
  - Alkalinize urine — K+ citrate / Cranberry juice
  - Treat cause

Acute pyelonephritis

- **Clinical**
  - Pyrexia
  - Loin pain
  - Rigors
  - UTI symptoms
- **Ix**
  - Urine — Dip / MC + S
  - Blood cultures
  - KUB X-ray — Look for calculi
  - USS — Exclude obstruction
- **Complications** — Pyonephrosis / Perinephric abscess
- **Rx** — Abx / Treat complications

Renal TB

- **Clinical**
  - Anaemia
  - ↓ weight
  - Night sweats
  - Fever
  - UTI symptoms
- **Ix**
  - Urine — Sterile acid pyuria / 3 morning specimens
  - Epididimitis — Hard + calcified / Often involved
- **Rx** — Anti-TB

Carbuncle

- **Clinical**
  - Palpable kidney
  - Loin pain
  - Toxaemia
  - Pyrexia
  - *Staphylococcus aureus*
  - Haematogenous infection
  - Renal cortical abscess
- **Ix**
  - Urine — Infected / Sterile
  - FBC — ↑ WCC
  - IVU
- **Rx** — Abx / Drain
- **Complications** — Burst abscess / Perinephric abscess / Rupture

Pyonephrosis

- **Clinical**
  - Palpable tender kidney
  - Urine — Normal / Pyuria
  - Kidney = bag of pus
  - If ureter obstructed — Infected hydronephrosis
- **Ix** — IVU / DMSA scintography
- **Rx** — Nephrostomy / Drain / Nephrectomy (If no function left)
  - Kidney function

Chronic pyelonephritis

- **Clinical**
  - Pyrexia
  - Frequency
  - Dysuria
  - Children — Vesico-ureteric reflux — Intra-renal reflux
    - Ectopic ureter
  - Adults — Commoner
  - Atrophic scarred kidneys
  - Recurrent infections
  - May present with chronic renal failure
  - Night-time urinary incontinence
- **Ix**
  - IVU — Scarring / Reversed calyx / 'Clubbing'
  - Micturating cystogram
  - DMSA scintography — Kidney function
- **Rx** — Treat cause / Lose dose Abx / Nephrectomy (If no function left)

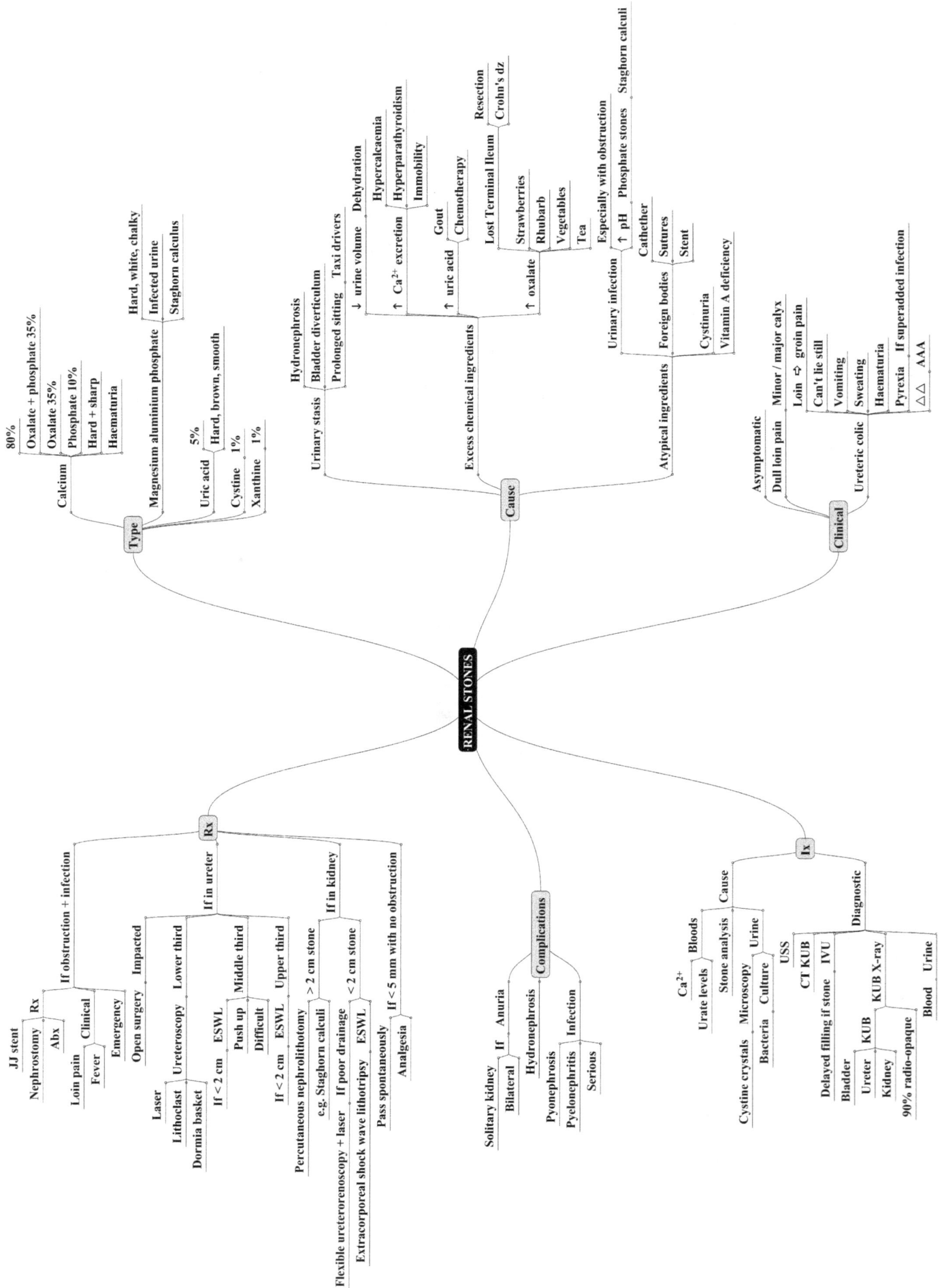

RENAL STONES

Type

- **Calcium (80%)**
  - Oxalate + phosphate 35%
  - Oxalate 35%
  - Phosphate 10%
  - Hard + sharp
  - Haematuria
- **Magnesium aluminium phosphate**
  - Hard, white, chalky
  - Infected urine
  - Staghorn calculus
- **Uric acid (5%)**
  - Hard, brown, smooth
- **Cystine 1%**
- **Xanthine 1%**

Cause

- **Urinary stasis**
  - Hydronephrosis
  - Bladder diverticulum
  - Prolonged sitting — Taxi drivers
- **Excess chemical ingredients**
  - ↓ urine volume — Dehydration
  - ↑ Ca²⁺ excretion
    - Hypercalcaemia
    - Hyperparathyroidism
    - Immobility
  - ↑ uric acid
    - Gout
    - Chemotherapy
  - ↑ oxalate
    - Lost Terminal Ileum — Resection — Crohn's dz
    - Strawberries
    - Rhubarb
    - Vegetables
    - Tea
- **Atypical ingredients**
  - Urinary infection
    - ↑ pH — Phosphate stones — Staghorn calculi
    - Especially with obstruction
  - Foreign bodies
    - Cathether
    - Sutures
    - Stent
  - Cystinuria
  - Vitamin A deficiency

Clinical

- **Asymptomatic**
- **Dull loin pain** — Minor / major calyx
- **Ureteric colic**
  - Loin ⇄ groin pain
  - Can't lie still
  - Vomiting
  - Sweating
  - Haematuria
  - Pyrexia — If superadded infection
  - ΔΔ — AAA

Rx

- **If obstruction + infection**
  - JJ stent
  - Nephrostomy
  - Rx — Abx
  - Loin pain
  - Clinical — Fever
  - Emergency
- **If in ureter**
  - Impacted — Open surgery
  - Lower third — Ureteroscopy
    - Laser
    - Lithoclast
    - Dormia basket
  - Middle third
    - If < 2 cm — ESWL
    - Push up — Difficult
  - Upper third
    - If < 2 cm — ESWL
- **If in kidney**
  - > 2 cm stone — Percutaneous nephrolithotomy
    - e.g. Staghorn calculi — Flexible ureterorenoscopy + laser
    - If poor drainage — Extracorporeal shock wave lithotripsy
  - < 2 cm stone — ESWL
  - If < 5 mm with no obstruction
    - Pass spontaneously
    - Analgesia

Complications

- Solitary kidney — If — Anuria
- Bilateral
- Hydronephrosis
- Infection
  - Pyonephrosis
  - Pyelonephritis
  - Serious

Ix

- **Cause**
  - Bloods
    - Ca²⁺
    - Urate levels
  - Stone analysis
  - Urine — Microscopy
    - Cystine crystals
    - Bacteria
    - Culture
- **Diagnostic**
  - USS
  - CT KUB
  - IVU — Delayed filling if stone
  - KUB X-ray
    - KUB
      - Bladder
      - Ureter
      - Kidney
    - 90% radio-opaque
  - Urine
    - Blood
    - Urine

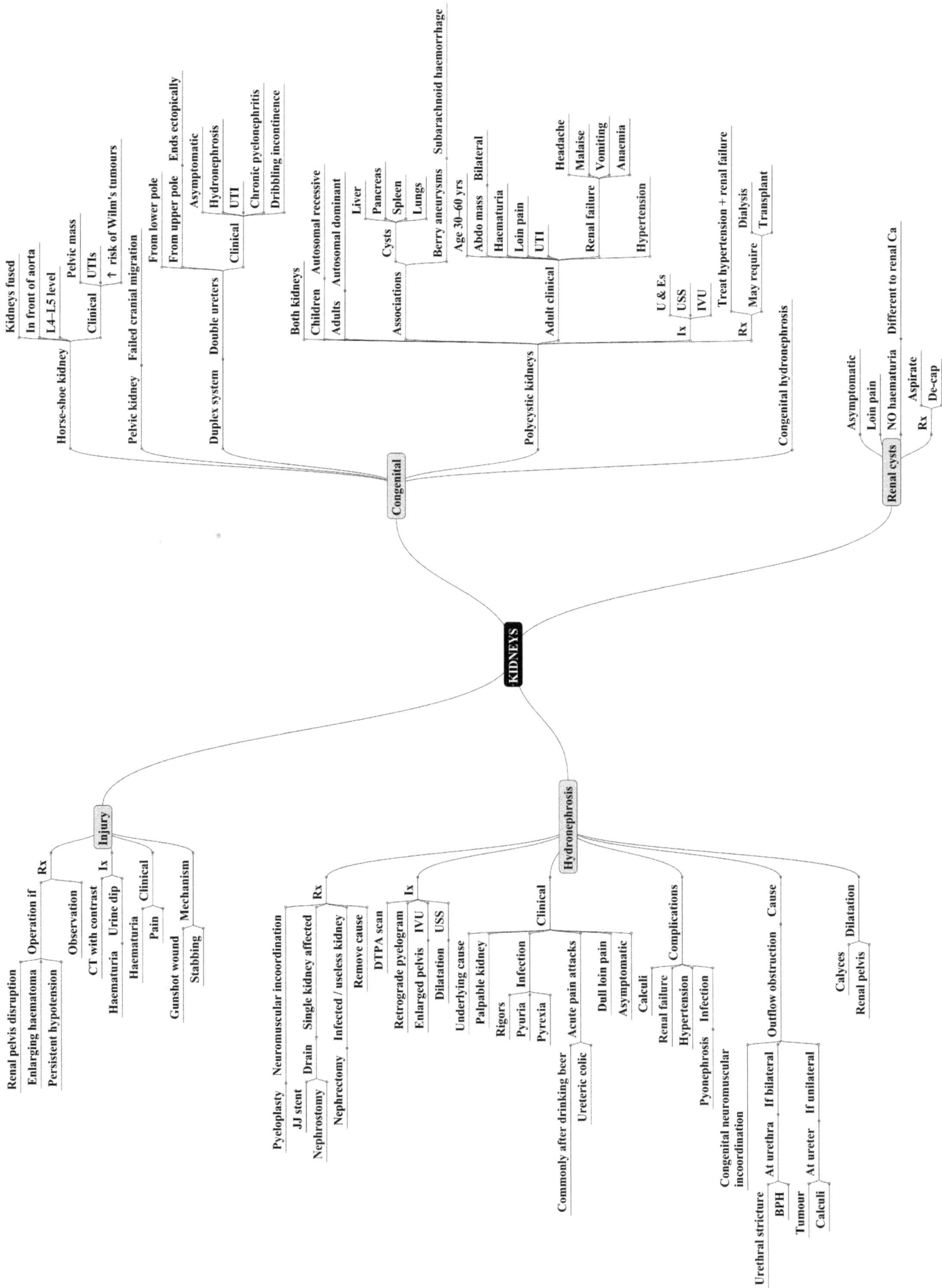

KIDNEYS

Congenital

Horse-shoe kidney
- Kidneys fused
- In front of aorta
- L4–L5 level
- Clinical
  - Pelvic mass
  - UTIs
  - ↑ risk of Wilm's tumours

Pelvic kidney
- Failed cranial migration

Duplex system
- Double ureters
  - From lower pole
  - From upper pole — Ends ectopically
  - Clinical
    - Asymptomatic
    - Hydronephrosis
    - UTI
    - Chronic pyelonephritis
    - Dribbling incontinence

Polycystic kidneys
- Both kidneys
- Children — Autosomal recessive
- Adults — Autosomal dominant
- Associations
  - Cysts
    - Liver
    - Pancreas
    - Spleen
    - Lungs
  - Berry aneurysms — Subarachnoid haemorrhage
- Adult clinical
  - Age 30–60 yrs
  - Abdo mass — Bilateral
  - Haematuria
  - Loin pain
  - UTI
  - Renal failure
    - Headache
    - Malaise
    - Vomiting
    - Anaemia
  - Hypertension
- Ix
  - U & Es
  - USS
  - IVU
- Rx
  - Treat hypertension + renal failure
  - May require
    - Dialysis
    - Transplant

Congenital hydronephrosis

Renal cysts
- Asymptomatic
- Loin pain
- NO haematuria — Different to renal Ca
- Rx
  - Aspirate
  - De-cap

Injury
- Mechanism
  - Gunshot wound
  - Stabbing
- Clinical
  - Pain
  - Haematuria
- Ix
  - Urine dip — Haematuria
  - CT with contrast
- Rx
  - Observation
  - Operation if
    - Enlarging haematoma
    - Persistent hypotension
    - Renal pelvis disruption

Hydronephrosis
- Dilatation
  - Calyces
  - Renal pelvis
- Cause
  - Outflow obstruction
    - If bilateral — At urethra
      - BPH
      - Tumour
      - Urethral stricture
    - If unilateral — At ureter
      - Calculi
      - Congenital neuromuscular incoordination
  - Complications
    - Renal failure
    - Hypertension
    - Infection — Pyonephrosis
- Clinical
  - Asymptomatic
  - Dull loin pain
  - Acute pain attacks — Ureteric colic
    - Commonly after drinking beer
  - Underlying cause
    - Palpable kidney
    - Infection
      - Pyrexia
      - Pyuria
      - Rigors
- Ix
  - USS — Dilatation
  - IVU — Enlarged pelvis
  - Retrograde pyelogram
  - DTPA scan
- Rx
  - Remove cause
    - Infected / useless kidney — Nephrectomy
    - Single kidney affected — Drain
      - Nephrostomy
      - JJ stent
    - Neuromuscular incoordination — Pyeloplasty
  - Calculi

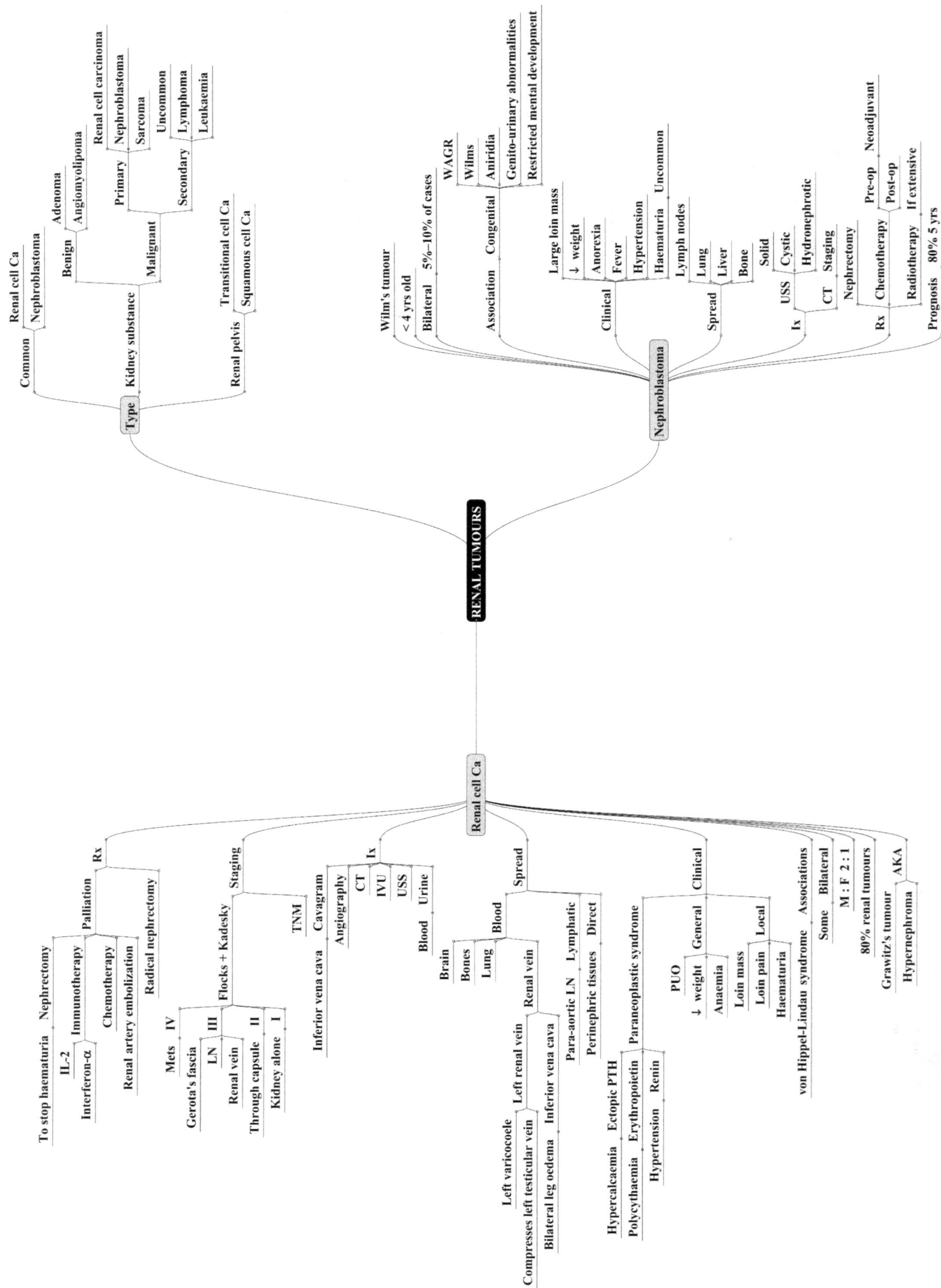

RENAL TUMOURS

Type

- **Common**
  - Renal cell Ca
  - Nephroblastoma
- **Kidney substance**
  - Benign
    - Adenoma
    - Angiomyolipoma
  - Malignant
    - Primary
      - Renal cell carcinoma
      - Nephroblastoma
      - Sarcoma
    - Secondary / Uncommon
      - Lymphoma
      - Leukaemia
- **Renal pelvis**
  - Transitional cell Ca
  - Squamous cell Ca

Nephroblastoma

- **Wilm's tumour**
- **<4 yrs old**
- **Bilateral** 5%–10% of cases
- **Association**
  - Congenital
    - WAGR
      - Wilms
      - Aniridia
      - Genito-urinary abnormalities
      - Restricted mental development
- **Clinical**
  - Large loin mass
  - ↓ weight
  - Anorexia
  - Fever
  - Hypertension
  - Haematuria Uncommon
- **Spread**
  - Lymph nodes
  - Lung
  - Liver
  - Bone
- **Ix**
  - USS
    - Solid
    - Cystic
    - Hydronephrotic
  - CT Staging
- **Rx**
  - Nephrectomy
  - Chemotherapy
    - Pre-op Neoadjuvant
    - Post-op
  - Radiotherapy If extensive
- **Prognosis** 80% 5 yrs

Renal cell Ca

- **Rx**
  - Palliation
    - To stop haematuria Nephrectomy
    - Immunotherapy
      - IL-2
      - Interferon-α
    - Chemotherapy
    - Renal artery embolization
  - Radical nephrectomy
- **Staging**
  - Flocks + Kadesky
    - IV Mets
    - III LN / Gerota's fascia
    - II Renal vein / Through capsule
    - I Kidney alone
  - TNM
- **Ix**
  - Cavagram Inferior vena cava
  - Angiography
  - CT
  - IVU
  - USS
  - Urine
  - Blood
- **Spread**
  - Blood
    - Brain
    - Bones
    - Lung
    - Renal vein
      - Left renal vein
        - Left varicocele Compresses left testicular vein
        - Inferior vena cava Bilateral leg oedema
  - Lymphatic
    - Para-aortic LN
  - Direct
    - Perinephric tissues
- **Paraneoplastic syndrome**
  - Hypercalcaemia Ectopic PTH
  - Polycythaemia Erythropoietin
  - Hypertension Renin
- **Clinical**
  - General
    - PUO
    - ↓ weight
    - Anaemia
  - Local
    - Loin mass
    - Loin pain
    - Haematuria
- **Associations**
  - von Hippel-Lindau syndrome
  - Some Bilateral
  - 80% renal tumours
- M : F 2 : 1
- **AKA**
  - Grawitz's tumour
  - Hypernephroma

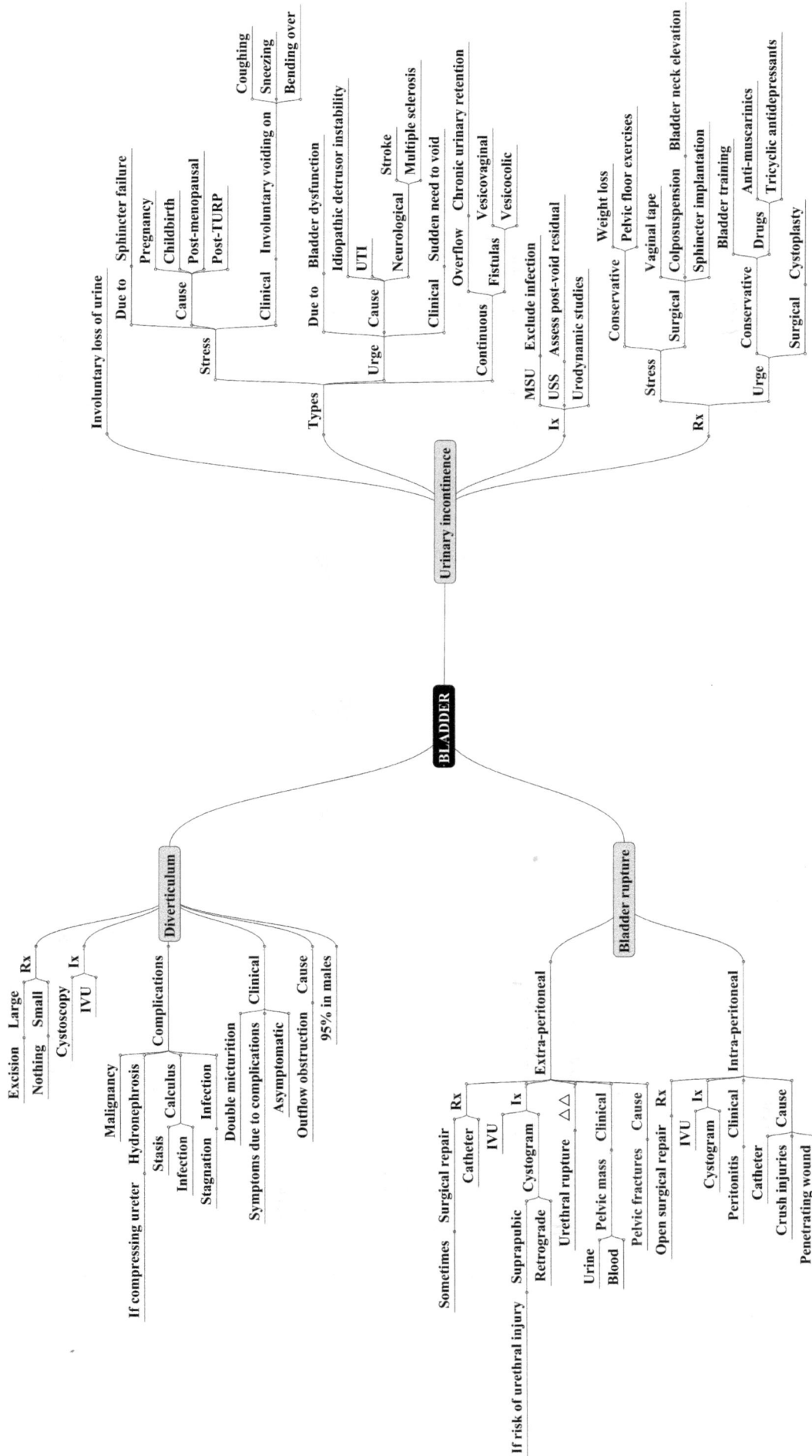

Urinary incontinence

Types

Involuntary loss of urine
- Stress — Due to Sphincter failure
  - Cause
    - Pregnancy
    - Childbirth
    - Post-menopausal
    - Post-TURP
  - Clinical — Involuntary voiding on
    - Coughing
    - Sneezing
    - Bending over
- Urge — Due to Bladder dysfunction
  - Idiopathic detrusor instability
  - Cause
    - UTI
    - Neurological
      - Stroke
      - Multiple sclerosis
  - Clinical — Sudden need to void
- Overflow — Chronic urinary retention
- Continuous — Fistulas
  - Vesicovaginal
  - Vesicocolic

Ix
- MSU — Exclude infection
- USS — Assess post-void residual
- Urodynamic studies

Rx
- Stress
  - Conservative
    - Weight loss
    - Pelvic floor exercises
  - Surgical
    - Vaginal tape
    - Colposuspension
    - Sphincter implantation
    - Bladder neck elevation
- Urge
  - Conservative
    - Bladder training
    - Drugs
      - Anti-muscarinics
      - Tricyclic antidepressants
  - Surgical — Cystoplasty

BLADDER

Diverticulum
- Cause — 95% in males — Outflow obstruction
- Clinical
  - Asymptomatic
  - Symptoms due to complications
  - Double micturition
- Complications
  - Infection — Stagnation
  - Calculus — Stasis
  - Hydronephrosis — If compressing ureter
  - Malignancy
- Ix
  - IVU
  - Cystoscopy
- Rx
  - Small — Nothing
  - Large — Excision

Bladder rupture
- Extra-peritoneal
  - Cause
    - Pelvic fractures
    - Urethral rupture ΔΔ
  - Clinical
    - Blood
    - Urine
    - Pelvic mass
  - Ix
    - IVU
    - Cystogram
  - Rx
    - Catheter
      - Retrograde
      - Suprapubic — If risk of urethral injury
    - Surgical repair — Sometimes
    - Open surgical repair
- Intra-peritoneal
  - Cause
    - Penetrating wound
    - Crush injuries
  - Clinical
    - Catheter
    - Peritonitis
  - Ix
    - IVU
    - Cystogram

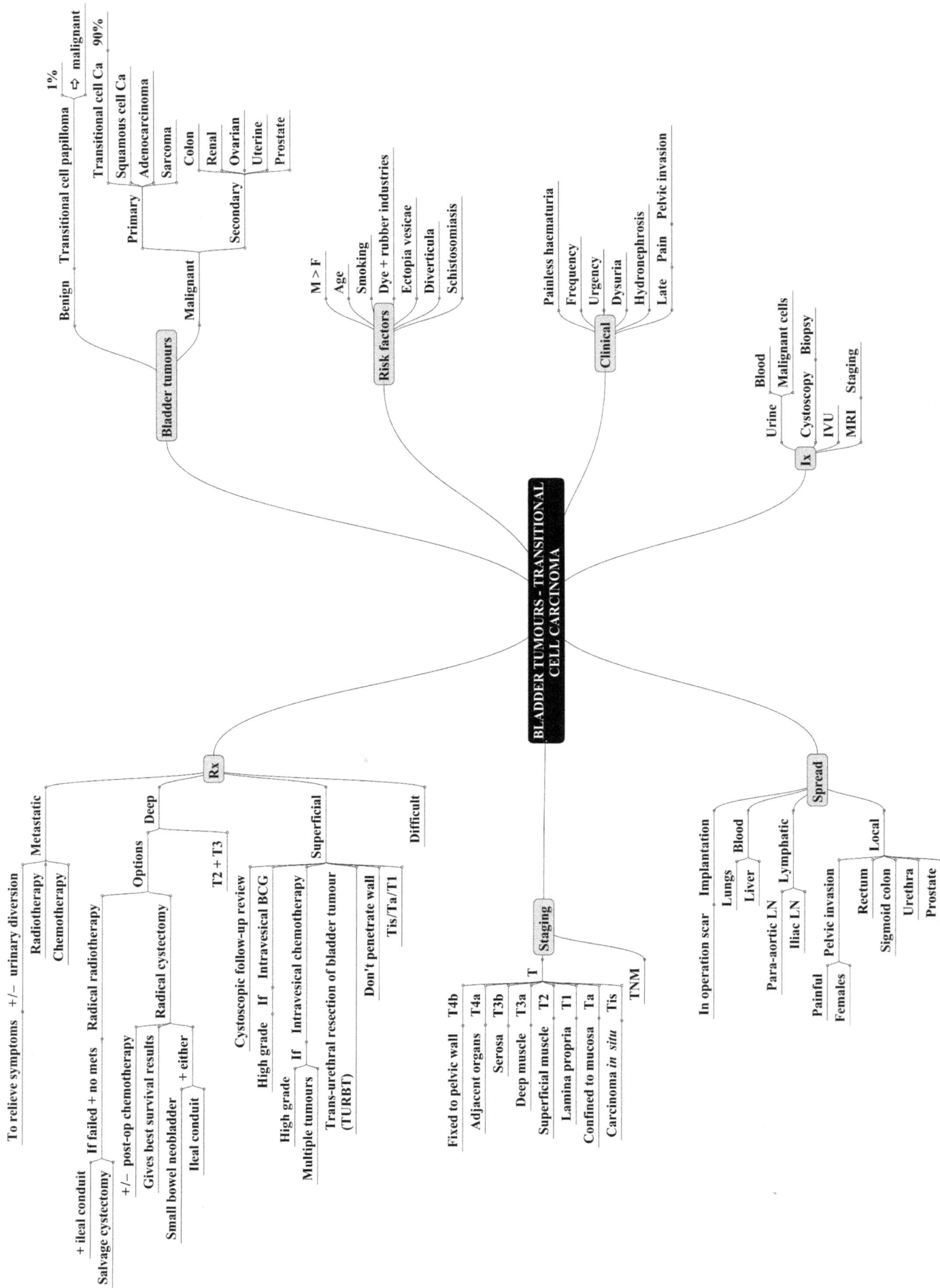

BLADDER TUMOURS – TRANSITIONAL CELL CARCINOMA

Bladder tumours

- Benign — Transitional cell papilloma — 1% ⇨ malignant
- Malignant
  - Transitional cell Ca — 90% malignant
  - Squamous cell Ca
  - Adenocarcinoma
  - Primary
    - Sarcoma
  - Secondary
    - Colon
    - Renal
    - Ovarian
    - Uterine
    - Prostate

Risk factors
- M > F
- Age
- Smoking
- Dye + rubber industries
- Ectopia vesicae
- Diverticula
- Schistosomiasis

Clinical
- Painless haematuria
- Frequency
- Urgency
- Dysuria
- Hydronephrosis
- Late — Pain — Pelvic invasion

Ix
- Urine — Blood — Malignant cells
- Cystoscopy — Biopsy
- IVU
- MRI — Staging

Rx
- Metastatic
  - To relieve symptoms +/− urinary diversion
  - Radiotherapy
  - Chemotherapy
- Deep — T2 + T3
  - Options
  - Radical radiotherapy
    - + ileal conduit
    - Salvage cystectomy
    - If failed + no mets
  - Radical cystectomy
    - +/− post-op chemotherapy
    - Gives best survival results
    - Small bowel neobladder
    - Ileal conduit
    - + either
- Superficial — Tis/Ta/T1
  - Cystoscopic follow-up review
  - Intravesical BCG — If — High grade
  - Intravesical chemotherapy — If — High grade, Multiple tumours
  - Trans-urethral resection of bladder tumour (TURBT)
  - Don't penetrate wall
- Difficult

Staging
- T
  - T4b — Fixed to pelvic wall
  - T4a — Adjacent organs
  - T3b — Serosa
  - T3a — Deep muscle
  - T2 — Superficial muscle
  - T1 — Lamina propria
  - Ta — Confined to mucosa
  - Tis — Carcinoma *in situ*
- TNM

Spread
- Implantation — In operation scar
- Blood
  - Lungs
  - Liver
- Lymphatic
  - Para-aortic LN
  - Iliac LN
- Local
  - Pelvic invasion — Painful — Females
  - Rectum
  - Sigmoid colon
  - Urethra
  - Prostate

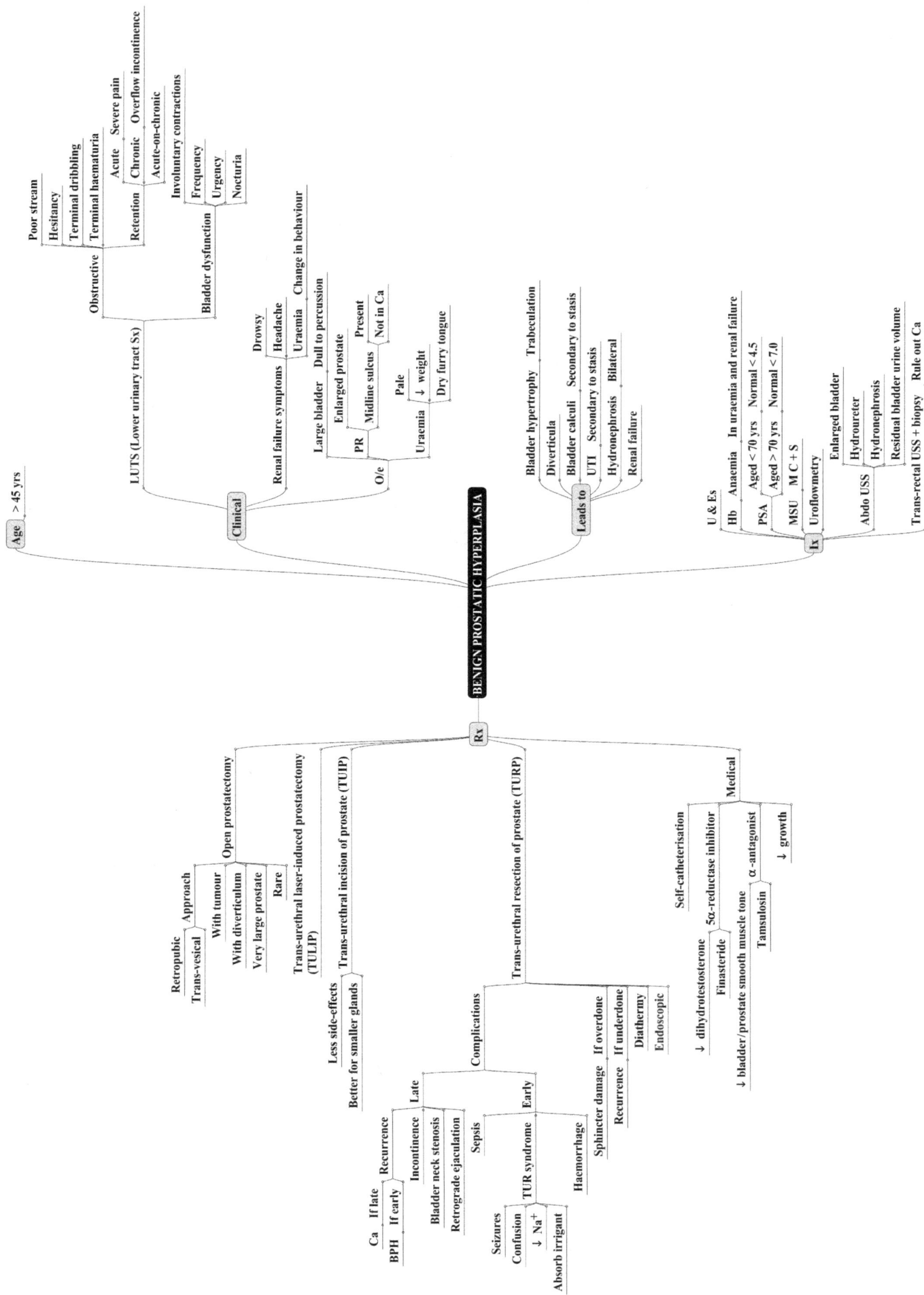

BENIGN PROSTATIC HYPERPLASIA

Age
- >45 yrs

Clinical
- LUTS (Lower urinary tract Sx)
  - Obstructive
    - Poor stream
    - Hesitancy
    - Terminal dribbling
    - Terminal haematuria
    - Retention
      - Acute — Severe pain
      - Chronic — Overflow incontinence
      - Acute-on-chronic
  - Bladder dysfunction
    - Involuntary contractions
      - Frequency
      - Urgency
      - Nocturia
- Renal failure symptoms
  - Drowsy
  - Headache
  - Uraemia
  - Change in behaviour
- O/e
  - Large bladder — Dull to percussion
  - PR
    - Enlarged prostate
    - Midline sulcus
      - Present
      - Not in Ca
  - Uraemia
    - Pale
    - ↓ weight
    - Dry furry tongue

Leads to
- Bladder hypertrophy — Trabeculation
- Diverticula
- Bladder calculi — Secondary to stasis
- UTI — Secondary to stasis
- Hydronephrosis — Bilateral
- Renal failure

Ix
- U & Es
  - Hb — Anaemia — In uraemia and renal failure
  - PSA
    - Aged <70 yrs — Normal <4.5
    - Aged >70 yrs — Normal <7.0
  - MSU — M C + S
  - Uroflowmetry
- Abdo USS
  - Enlarged bladder
  - Hydroureter
  - Hydronephrosis
  - Residual bladder urine volume
- Trans-rectal USS + biopsy — Rule out Ca

Rx
- Open prostatectomy
  - Approach
    - Retropubic
    - Trans-vesical
  - With tumour
  - With diverticulum
  - Very large prostate
  - Rare
- Trans-urethral laser-induced prostatectomy (TULIP)
- Trans-urethral incision of prostate (TUIP)
  - Less side-effects
  - Better for smaller glands
- Trans-urethral resection of prostate (TURP)
  - Complications
    - Late
      - Recurrence
        - Ca — If late
        - BPH — If early
      - Incontinence
      - Bladder neck stenosis
      - Retrograde ejaculation
    - Early
      - Sepsis
      - TUR syndrome
        - Seizures
        - Confusion
        - ↓ Na⁺
        - Absorb irrigant
      - Haemorrhage
    - Sphincter damage
      - If overdone
      - If underdone
    - Recurrence
    - Diathermy
    - Endoscopic
- Medical
  - Self-catheterisation
  - 5α-reductase inhibitor
    - Finasteride
      - ↓ dihydrotestosterone
      - ↓ growth
  - α-antagonist
    - Tamsulosin
      - ↓ bladder/prostate smooth muscle tone

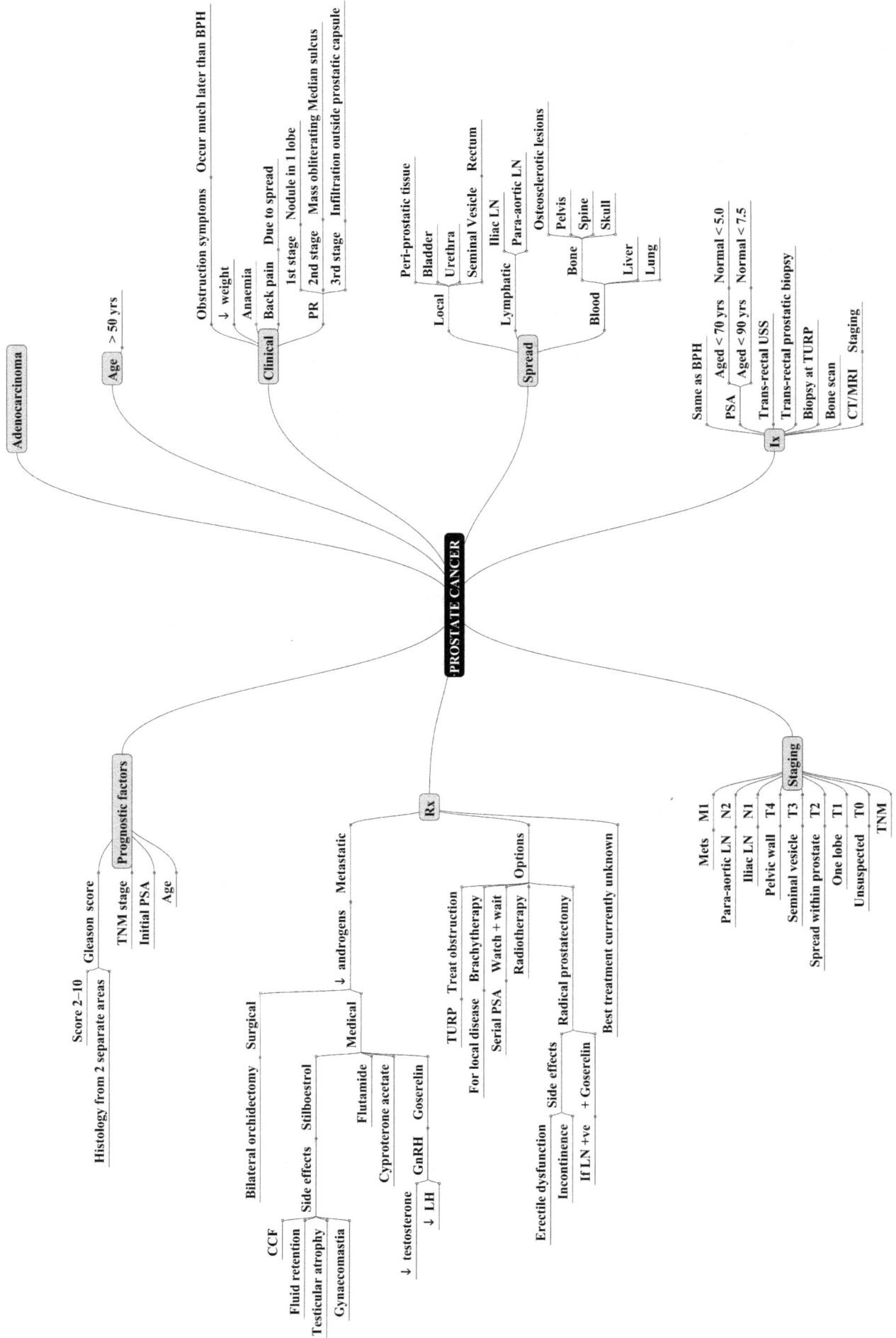

PROSTATE CANCER

Adenocarcinoma

Age
- > 50 yrs

Clinical
- Obstruction symptoms — Occur much later than BPH
- ↓ weight
- Anaemia
- Back pain — Due to spread
- PR
  - 1st stage — Nodule in 1 lobe
  - 2nd stage — Mass obliterating Median sulcus
  - 3rd stage — Infiltration outside prostatic capsule

Spread
- Local
  - Peri-prostatic tissue
  - Bladder
  - Urethra
  - Seminal Vesicle
  - Rectum
- Lymphatic
  - Iliac LN
  - Para-aortic LN
- Blood
  - Osteosclerotic lesions
  - Bone
    - Pelvis
    - Spine
    - Skull
  - Liver
  - Lung

Ix
- Same as BPH
- PSA
  - Aged < 70 yrs — Normal < 5.0
  - Aged < 90 yrs — Normal < 7.5
- Trans-rectal USS
- Trans-rectal prostatic biopsy
- Biopsy at TURP
- Bone scan
- CT/MRI — Staging

Prognostic factors
- Gleason score
  - Score 2–10
  - Histology from 2 separate areas
- TNM stage
- Initial PSA
- Age

Rx
- ↓ androgens
  - Surgical
    - Bilateral orchidectomy
  - Medical
    - Stilboestrol
      - Side effects
        - CCF
        - Fluid retention
        - Testicular atrophy
        - Gynaecomastia
    - Flutamide
    - Cyproterone acetate
    - Goserelin
      - GnRH — ↓ testosterone — ↓ LH
- Metastatic
  - Treat obstruction
    - TURP
- For local disease
  - Brachytherapy
  - Watch + wait
    - Serial PSA
  - Radiotherapy
  - Radical prostatectomy
    - Options
      - Side effects
        - Erectile dysfunction
        - Incontinence
      - If LN +ve — + Goserelin
  - Best treatment currently unknown

Staging
- Mets — M1
- Para-aortic LN — N2
- Iliac LN — N1
- Pelvic wall — T4
- Seminal vesicle — T3
- Spread within prostate — T2
- One lobe — T1
- Unsuspected — T0
- TNM

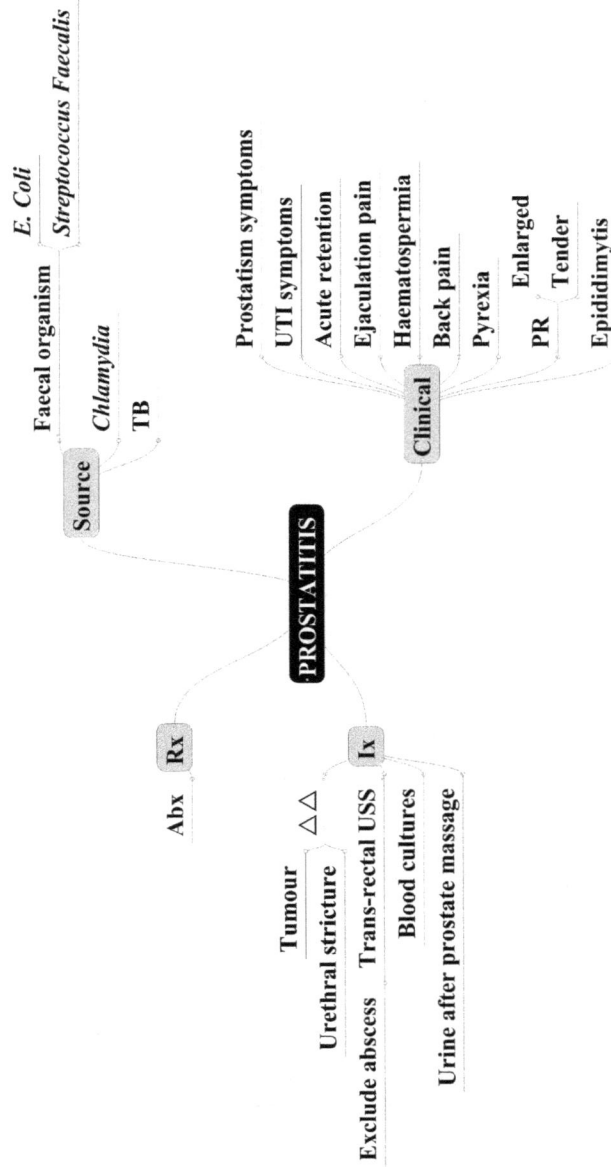

PROSTATITIS

Source
- Faecal organism
  - *E. Coli*
  - *Streptococcus Faecalis*
- *Chlamydia*
- TB

Clinical
- Prostatism symptoms
- UTI symptoms
- Acute retention
- Ejaculation pain
- Haematospermia
- Back pain
- Pyrexia
- PR
  - Enlarged
  - Tender
- Epididimytis

Rx
- Abx

Ix
- ΔΔ
  - Tumour
  - Urethral stricture
- Exclude abscess
- Trans-rectal USS
- Blood cultures
- Urine after prostate massage

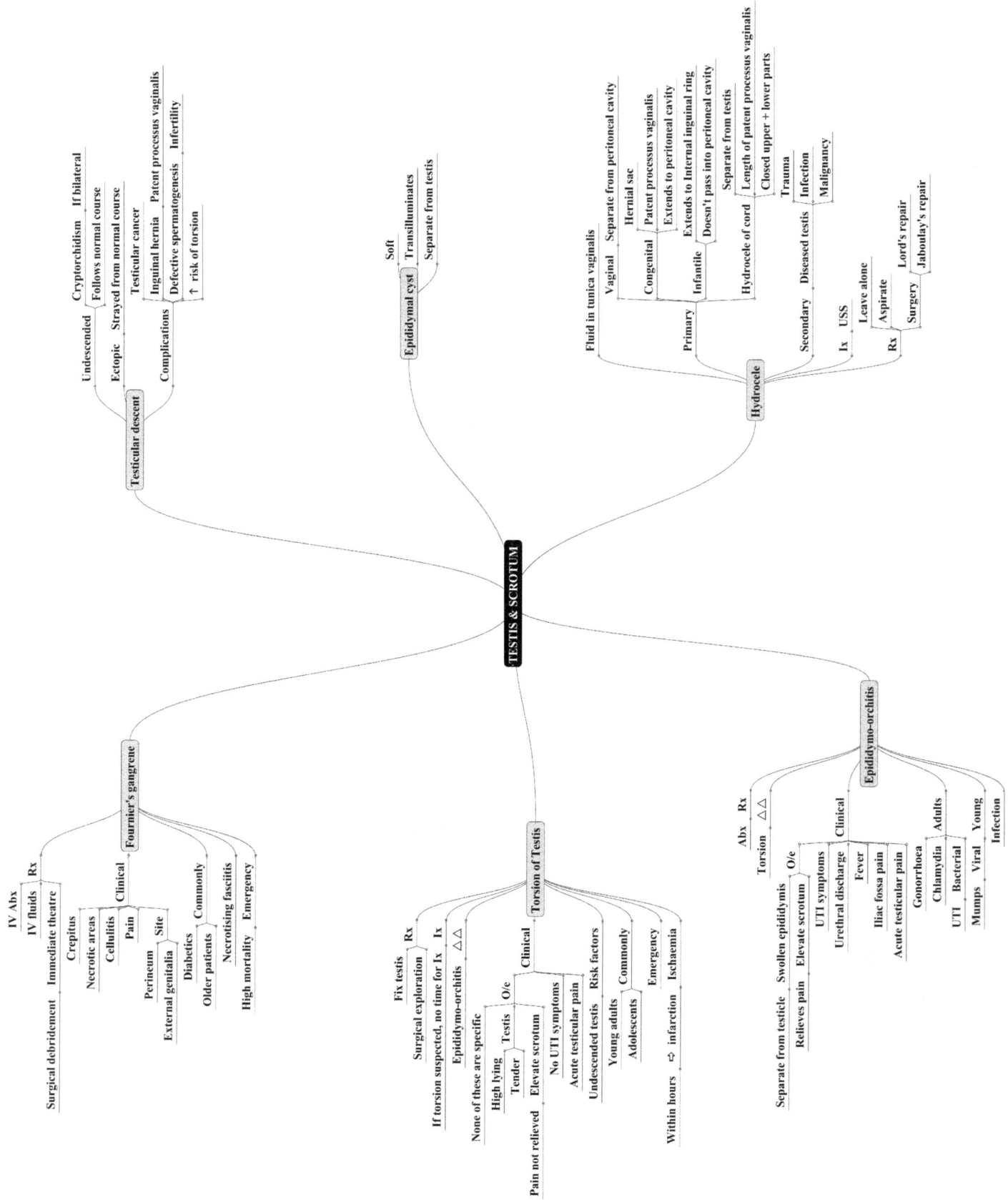

TESTIS & SCROTUM

Testicular descent

- Undescended
  - Cryptorchidism — If bilateral
  - Follows normal course
- Ectopic — Strayed from normal course
- Complications
  - Testicular cancer
  - Inguinal hernia — Patent processus vaginalis
  - Defective spermatogenesis — Infertility
  - ↑ risk of torsion

Epididymal cyst

- Soft
- Transilluminates
- Separate from testis

Hydrocele

- Fluid in tunica vaginalis
- Primary
  - Vaginal — Separate from peritoneal cavity
  - Hernial sac
  - Congenital — Patent processus vaginalis — Extends to peritoneal cavity
  - Infantile — Doesn't pass into peritoneal cavity — Extends to Internal inguinal ring
  - Hydrocele of cord — Separate from testis — Length of patent processus vaginalis — Closed upper + lower parts
- Secondary
  - Trauma
  - Infection
  - Malignancy
  - Diseased testis
- Ix — USS
- Rx
  - Leave alone
  - Aspirate
  - Surgery
    - Lord's repair
    - Jaboulay's repair

Fournier's gangrene

- Rx
  - IV Abx
  - IV fluids
  - Surgical debridement — Immediate theatre
- Clinical
  - Crepitus
  - Necrotic areas
  - Cellulitis
  - Pain
  - Site
    - Perineum
    - External genitalia
- Commonly
  - Diabetics
  - Older patients
- Necrotising fasciitis
- High mortality — Emergency

Torsion of Testis

- Rx
  - Fix testis
  - Surgical exploration
- Ix — If torsion suspected, no time for Ix — ΔΔ
  - Epididymo-orchitis
- Clinical — None of these are specific
  - O/e
    - High lying
    - Testis — Tender
    - Elevate scrotum — Pain not relieved
  - No UTI symptoms
  - Acute testicular pain
  - Risk factors — Undescended testis
- Commonly
  - Young adults
  - Adolescents
- Emergency — Within hours ⇨ infarction — Ischaemia

Epididymo-orchitis

- Abx — Rx
- Torsion — ΔΔ
- Clinical
  - O/e
    - Separate from testicle
    - Swollen epididymis
    - Elevate scrotum — Relieves pain
  - UTI symptoms
  - Urethral discharge
  - Fever
  - Iliac fossa pain
  - Acute testicular pain
- Adults
  - Gonorrhoea
  - Chlamydia
- Young
  - Bacterial — UTI
  - Viral — Mumps
- Infection

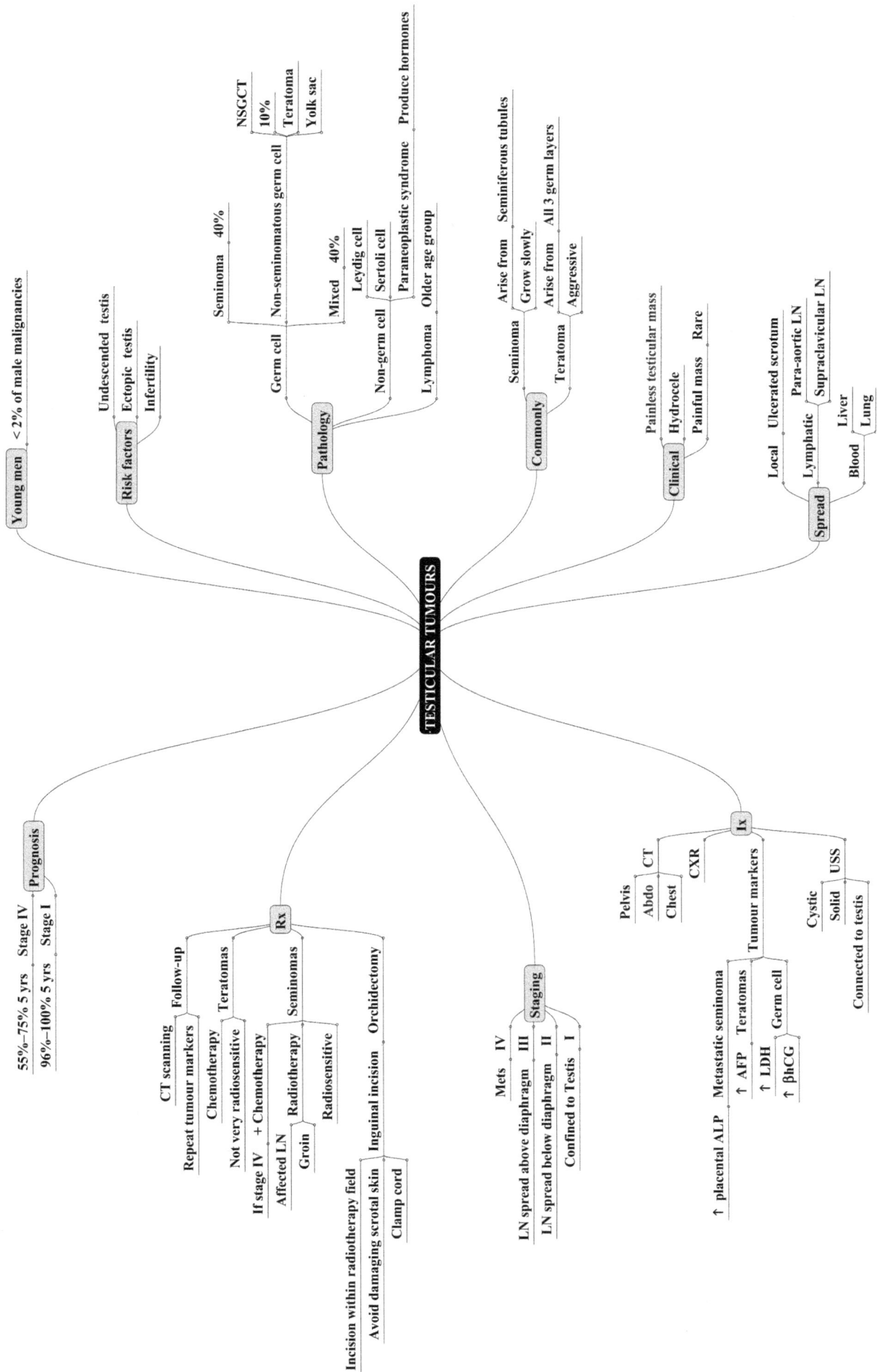

TESTICULAR TUMOURS

Young men — <2% of male malignancies

Risk factors
- Undescended testis
- Ectopic testis
- Infertility

Pathology
- Germ cell
  - Seminoma 40%
  - Non-seminomatous germ cell
    - NSGCT 10%
    - Teratoma
    - Yolk sac
  - Mixed 40%
- Non-germ cell
  - Leydig cell
  - Sertoli cell
  - Paraneoplastic syndrome — Produce hormones
- Lymphoma — Older age group

Commonly
- Seminoma
  - Arise from Seminiferous tubules
  - Grow slowly
- Teratoma
  - Arise from All 3 germ layers
  - Aggressive

Clinical
- Painless testicular mass
- Hydrocele
- Painful mass — Rare

Spread
- Local — Ulcerated scrotum
- Lymphatic — Para-aortic LN, Supraclavicular LN
- Blood — Liver, Lung

Ix
- CT — Pelvis, Abdo, Chest
- CXR
- Tumour markers
  - ↑ placental ALP — Metastatic seminoma
  - ↑ AFP — Teratomas
  - ↑ LDH — Germ cell
  - ↑ βhCG
- USS — Cystic, Solid, Connected to testis

Staging
- Mets — IV
- LN spread above diaphragm — III
- LN spread below diaphragm — II
- Confined to Testis — I

Rx
- Follow-up
  - CT scanning
  - Repeat tumour markers
- Teratomas
  - Chemotherapy
  - Not very radiosensitive
- Seminomas
  - If stage IV + Chemotherapy
  - Affected LN, Groin — Radiotherapy
  - Radiosensitive
- Orchidectomy
  - Inguinal incision
  - Incision within radiotherapy field
  - Avoid damaging scrotal skin
  - Clamp cord

Prognosis
- Stage IV — 55%–75% 5 yrs
- Stage I — 96%–100% 5 yrs

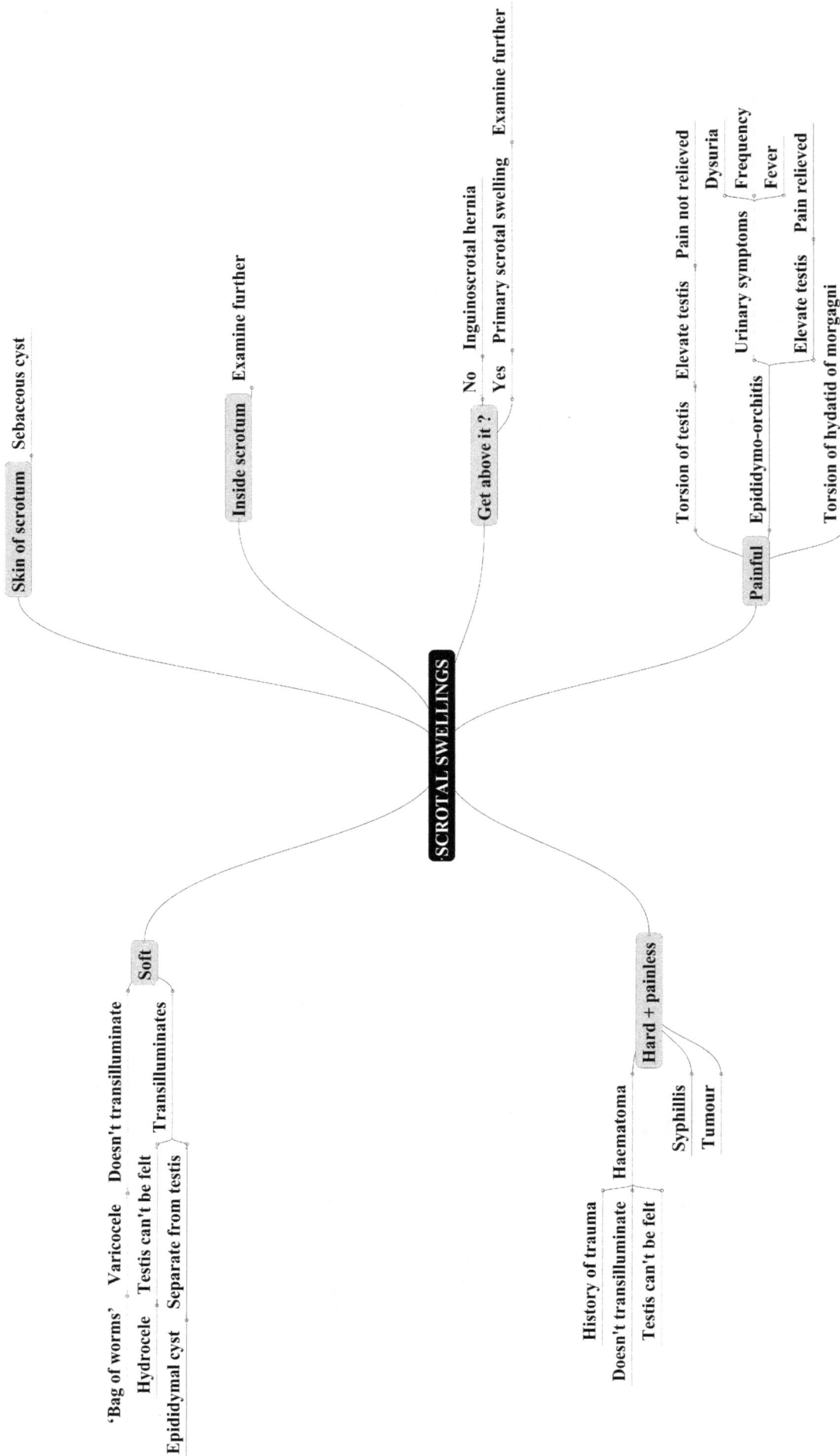

SCROTAL SWELLINGS

Skin of scrotum
- Sebaceous cyst

Inside scrotum — Examine further

Get above it ?
- No — Inguinoscrotal hernia
- Yes — Primary scrotal swelling — Examine further

Painful
- Torsion of testis
- Epididymo-orchitis
  - Elevate testis — Pain not relieved
  - Urinary symptoms
    - Dysuria
    - Frequency
    - Fever
  - Elevate testis — Pain relieved
- Torsion of hydatid of morgagni

Soft
- 'Bag of worms' — Varicocele — Doesn't transilluminate
- Hydrocele — Testis can't be felt — Transilluminates
- Epididymal cyst — Separate from testis

Hard + painless
- History of trauma — Haematoma
- Doesn't transilluminate
- Testis can't be felt
- Syphillis
- Tumour

Chapter 7

THE ACUTELY ILL PATIENT

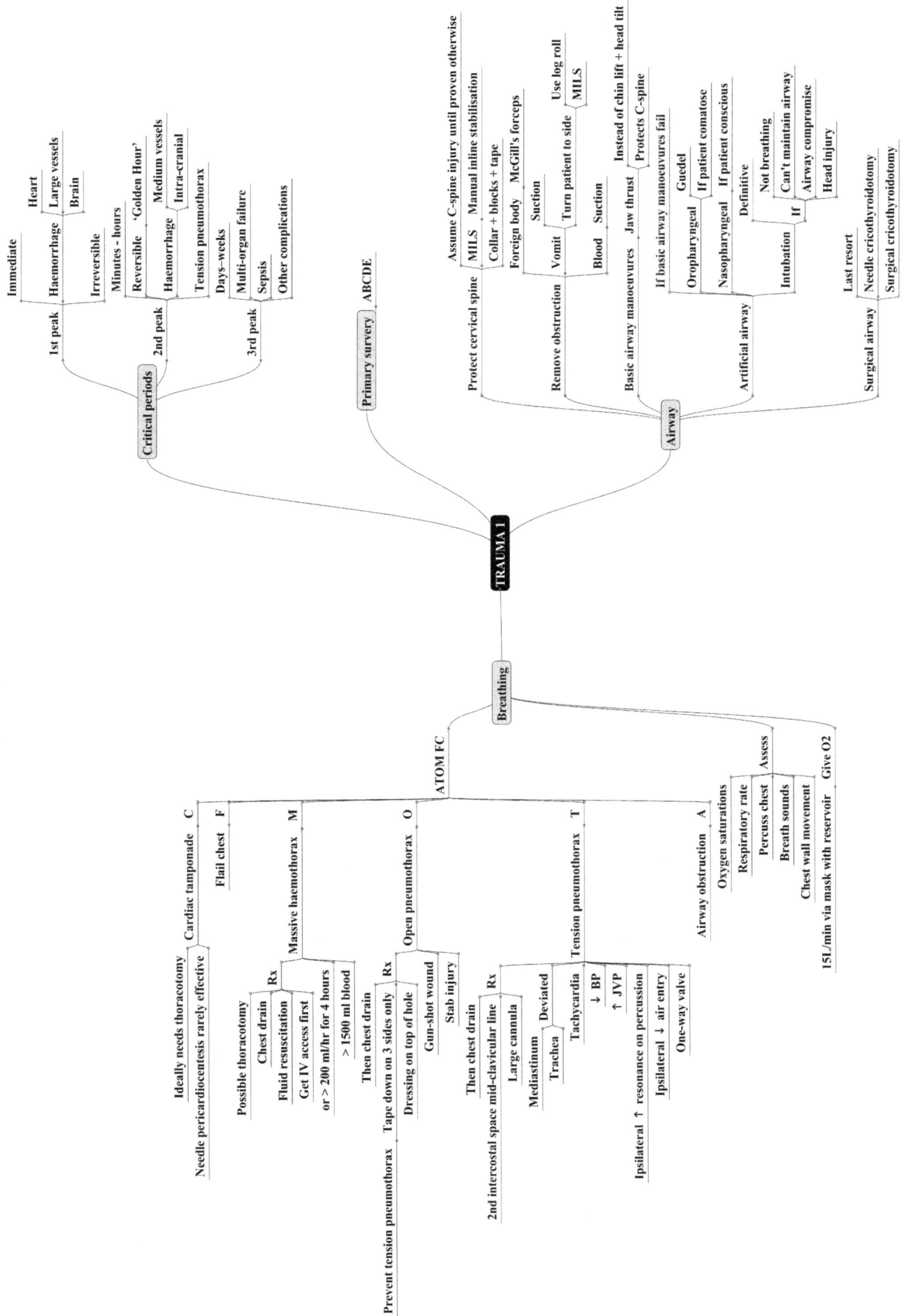

TRAUMA 1

Critical periods

- 1st peak — Immediate
  - Heart
  - Large vessels
  - Brain
- 2nd peak — Irreversible
  - Haemorrhage
  - Minutes – hours
  - Reversible — 'Golden Hour'
    - Haemorrhage
    - Medium vessels
    - Intra-cranial
    - Tension pneumothorax
- 3rd peak — Days–weeks
  - Multi-organ failure
  - Sepsis
  - Other complications

Primary survey — ABCDE

Airway

- Protect cervical spine
  - Assume C-spine injury until proven otherwise
  - Manual inline stabilisation — MILS
  - Collar + blocks + tape
- Remove obstruction
  - Foreign body — McGill's forceps
  - Vomit — Suction
  - Turn patient to side — Use log roll
  - Blood — Suction — MILS
- Basic airway manoeuvres
  - Jaw thrust — Instead of chin lift + head tilt
    - Protects C-spine
- Artificial airway — If basic airway manoeuvres fail
  - Oropharyngeal — Guedel — If patient comatose
  - Nasopharyngeal — If patient conscious
  - Intubation — Definitive
    - If:
      - Not breathing
      - Can't maintain airway
      - Airway compromise
      - Head injury
- Surgical airway — Last resort
  - Needle cricothyroidotomy
  - Surgical cricothyroidotomy

Breathing

ATOM FC

- **A** — Airway obstruction
- **T** — Tension pneumothorax
  - Tachycardia
  - ↓ BP
  - ↑ JVP
  - Mediastinum — Deviated — Trachea
  - Ipsilateral ↑ resonance on percussion
  - Ipsilateral ↓ air entry
  - One-way valve
  - Rx
    - 2nd intercostal space mid-clavicular line
    - Large cannula
    - Then chest drain
- **O** — Open pneumothorax
  - Gun-shot wound
  - Stab injury
  - Rx
    - Dressing on top of hole
    - Tape down on 3 sides only — Prevent tension pneumothorax
    - Then chest drain
- **M** — Massive haemothorax
  - Get IV access first
  - > 200 ml/hr for 4 hours
  - or > 1500 ml blood
  - Rx
    - Possible thoracotomy
    - Chest drain
    - Fluid resuscitation
- **F** — Flail chest
- **C** — Cardiac tamponade
  - Ideally needs thoracotomy
  - Needle pericardiocentesis rarely effective

- Assess
  - Oxygen saturations
  - Respiratory rate
  - Percuss chest
  - Breath sounds
  - Chest wall movement
- Give O2
  - 15l/min via mask with reservoir

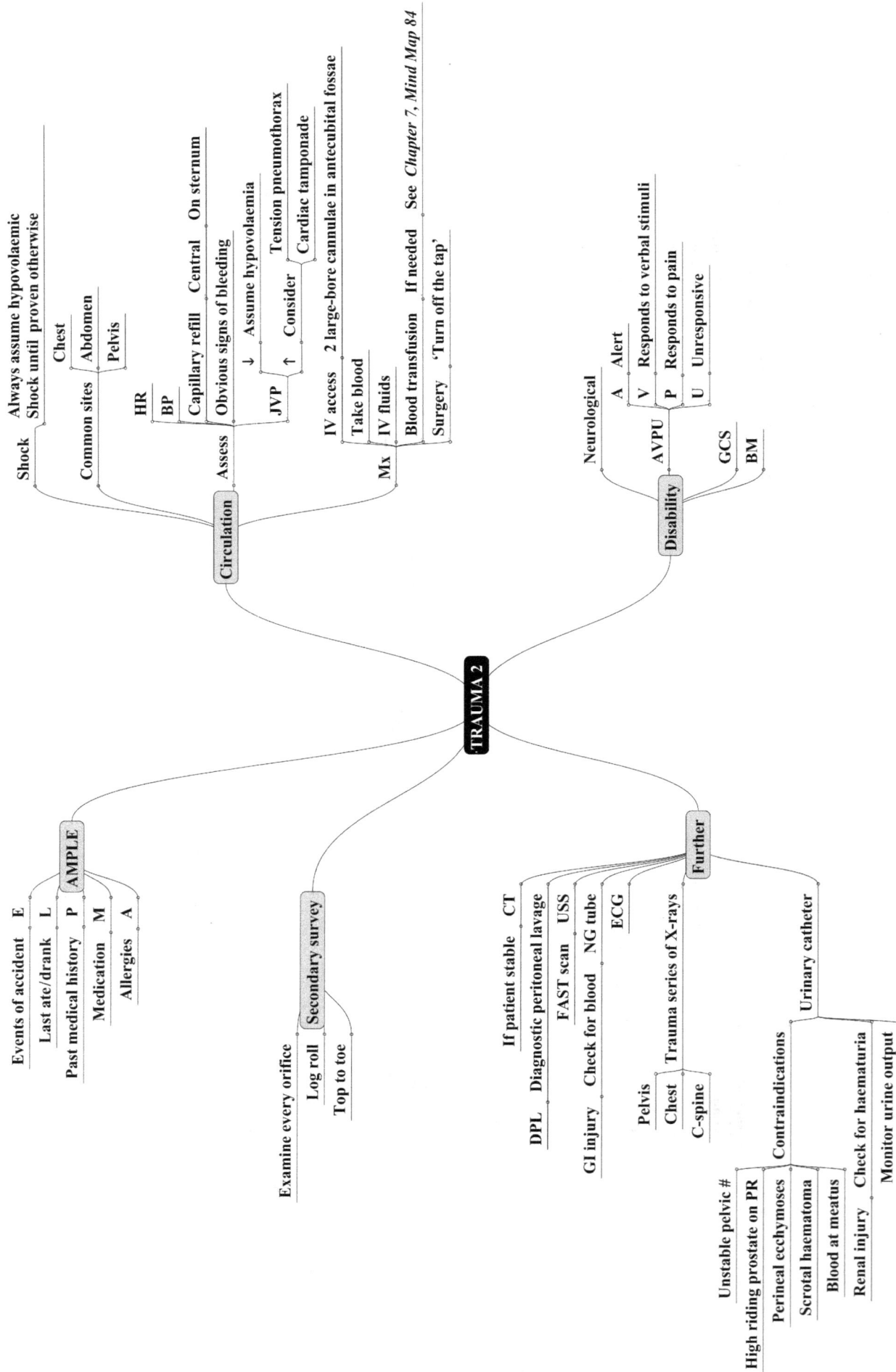

TRAUMA 2

Circulation

Shock
- Always assume hypovolaemic
- Shock until proven otherwise

Common sites
- Chest
- Abdomen
- Pelvis

Assess
- HR
- BP
- Capillary refill — Central — On sternum
- Obvious signs of bleeding
- JVP → Assume hypovolaemia
  - Consider ← Tension pneumothorax / Cardiac tamponade

Mx
- IV access — 2 large-bore cannulae in antecubital fossae
- Take blood
- IV fluids
- Blood transfusion — If needed — See *Chapter 7, Mind Map 84*
- Surgery — 'Turn off the tap'

Disability

Neurological

AVPU
- A — Alert
- V — Responds to verbal stimuli
- P — Responds to pain
- U — Unresponsive

GCS

BM

AMPLE
- Events of accident — E
- Last ate/drank — L
- Past medical history — P
- Medication — M
- Allergies — A

Secondary survey
- Examine every orifice
- Log roll
- Top to toe

Further
- If patient stable — CT
- DPL — Diagnostic peritoneal lavage
- FAST scan — USS
- GI injury — Check for blood — NG tube
- ECG
- Trauma series of X-rays
  - Pelvis
  - Chest
  - C-spine
- Urinary catheter
  - Contraindications
    - Unstable pelvic #
    - High riding prostate on PR
    - Perineal ecchymoses
    - Scrotal haematoma
    - Blood at meatus
  - Renal injury — Check for haematuria
  - Monitor urine output

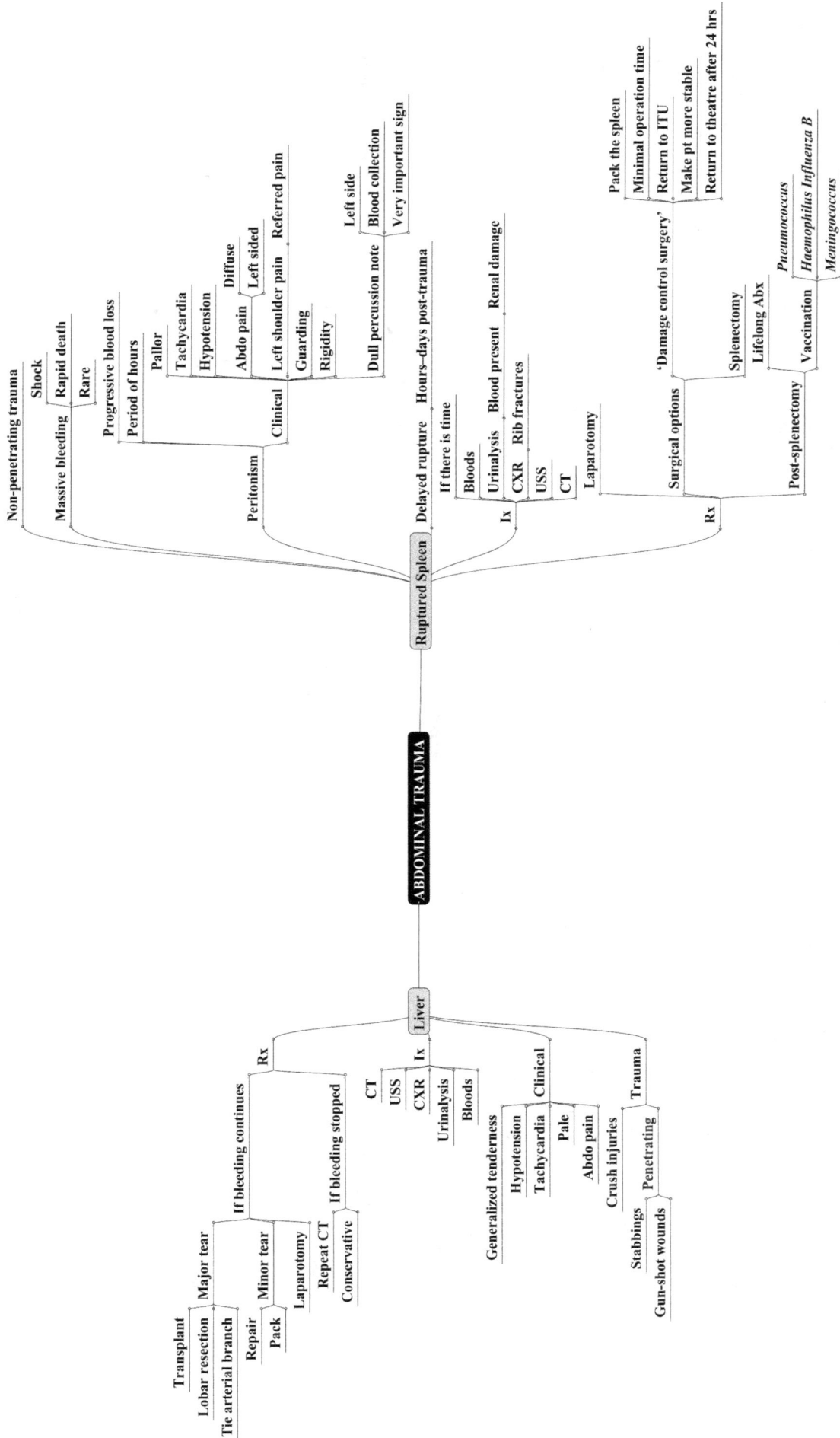

ABDOMINAL TRAUMA

Ruptured Spleen

- Non-penetrating trauma
  - Massive bleeding
    - Shock
      - Rapid death
      - Rare
    - Progressive blood loss
      - Period of hours
- Peritonism
  - Clinical
    - Pallor
    - Tachycardia
    - Hypotension
    - Abdo pain
      - Diffuse
      - Left sided
    - Left shoulder pain — Referred pain
    - Guarding
    - Rigidity
    - Dull percussion note
      - Left side
      - Blood collection
      - Very important sign
- Delayed rupture — Hours–days post-trauma
- Ix
  - If there is time
  - Bloods
  - Urinalysis — Blood present
  - CXR — Rib fractures
  - USS — Renal damage
  - CT
- Rx
  - Laparotomy
  - Surgical options
    - 'Damage control surgery'
      - Pack the spleen
      - Minimal operation time
      - Return to ITU
      - Make pt more stable
      - Return to theatre after 24 hrs
    - Splenectomy
  - Post-splenectomy
    - Lifelong Abx
    - Vaccination
      - *Pneumococcus*
      - *Haemophilus Influenza B*
      - *Meningococcus*

Liver

- Rx
  - If bleeding continues
    - Major tear
      - Transplant
      - Lobar resection
      - Tie arterial branch
    - Minor tear
      - Repair
      - Pack
    - Laparotomy
  - If bleeding stopped
    - Repeat CT
    - Conservative
- Ix
  - CT
  - USS
  - CXR
  - Urinalysis
  - Bloods
- Clinical
  - Generalized tenderness
  - Hypotension
  - Tachycardia
  - Pale
  - Abdo pain
- Trauma
  - Crush injuries
  - Penetrating
    - Stabbings
    - Gun-shot wounds

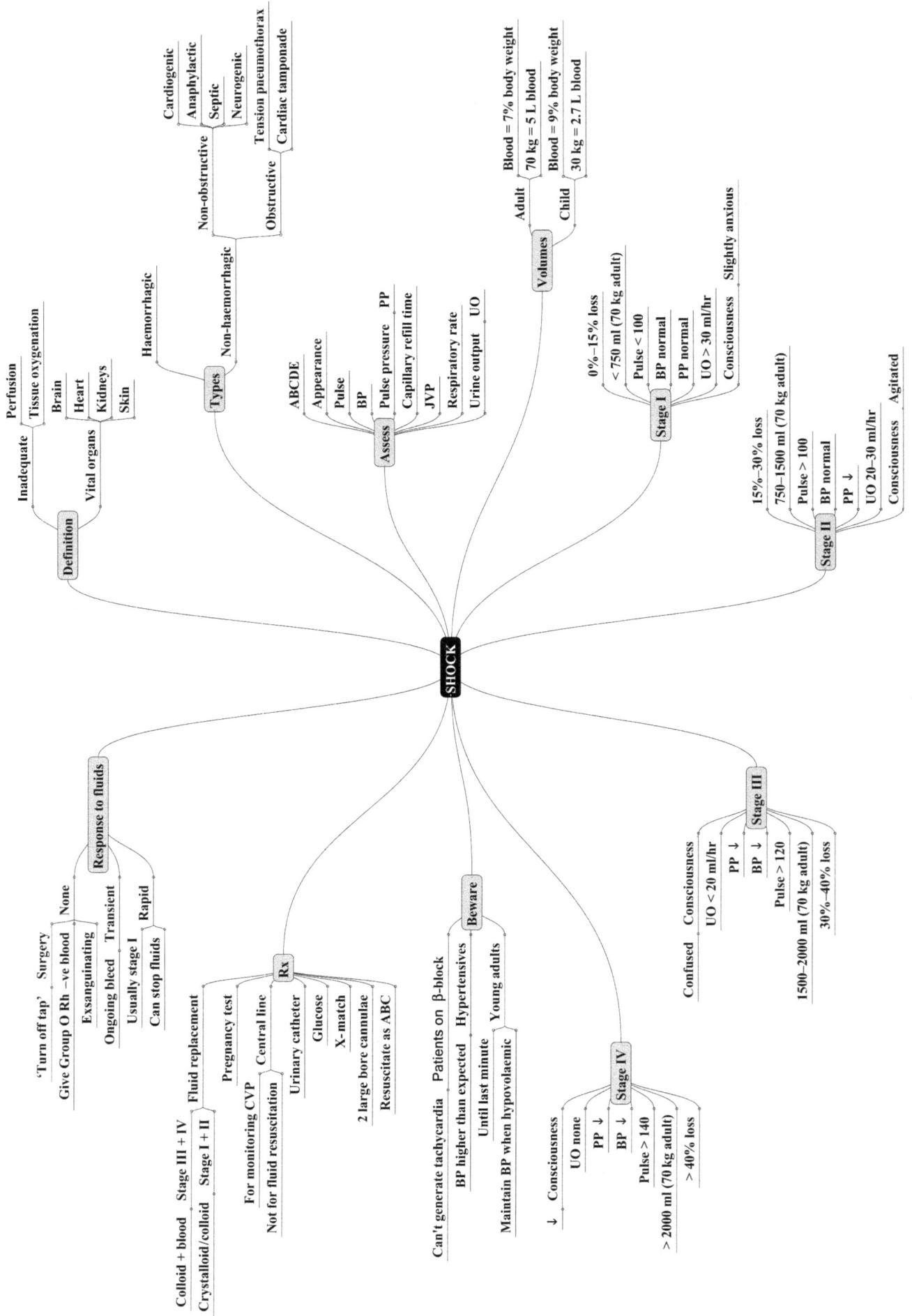

SHOCK

Definition
- Inadequate
  - Perfusion
  - Tissue oxygenation
- Vital organs
  - Brain
  - Heart
  - Kidneys
  - Skin

Types
- Haemorrhagic
- Non-haemorrhagic
  - Non-obstructive
    - Cardiogenic
    - Anaphylactic
    - Septic
    - Neurogenic
  - Obstructive
    - Tension pneumothorax
    - Cardiac tamponade

Assess
- ABCDE
- Appearance
- Pulse
- BP
- Pulse pressure   PP
- Capillary refill time
- JVP
- Respiratory rate
- Urine output   UO

Volumes
- Adult
  - Blood = 7% body weight
  - 70 kg = 5 L blood
- Child
  - Blood = 9% body weight
  - 30 kg = 2.7 L blood

Stage I
- 0%–15% loss
- <750 ml (70 kg adult)
- Pulse < 100
- BP normal
- PP normal
- UO > 30 ml/hr
- Consciousness   Slightly anxious

Stage II
- 15%–30% loss
- 750–1500 ml (70 kg adult)
- Pulse > 100
- BP normal
- PP ↓
- UO 20–30 ml/hr
- Consciousness   Agitated

Stage III
- 30%–40% loss
- 1500–2000 ml (70 kg adult)
- Pulse > 120
- BP ↓
- PP ↓
- UO < 20 ml/hr
- Consciousness   Confused

Stage IV
- >40% loss
- > 2000 ml (70 kg adult)
- Pulse > 140
- BP ↓
- PP ↓
- UO none
- ↓ Consciousness

Beware
- Can't generate tachycardia
  - Patients on β-block
- BP higher than expected
  - Hypertensives
- Maintain BP when hypovolaemic
  - Until last minute
  - Young adults

Rx
- 2 large bore cannulae
  - Resuscitate as ABC
- X-match
- Glucose
- Urinary catheter
- Central line
  - For monitoring CVP
  - Not for fluid resuscitation
- Pregnancy test
- Fluid replacement
  - Crystalloid/colloid
    - Stage I + II
  - Colloid + blood
    - Stage III + IV

Response to fluids
- None
  - 'Turn off tap'
  - Surgery
  - Give Group O Rh −ve blood
  - Exsanguinating
- Transient
  - Ongoing bleed
- Rapid
  - Usually stage I
  - Can stop fluids

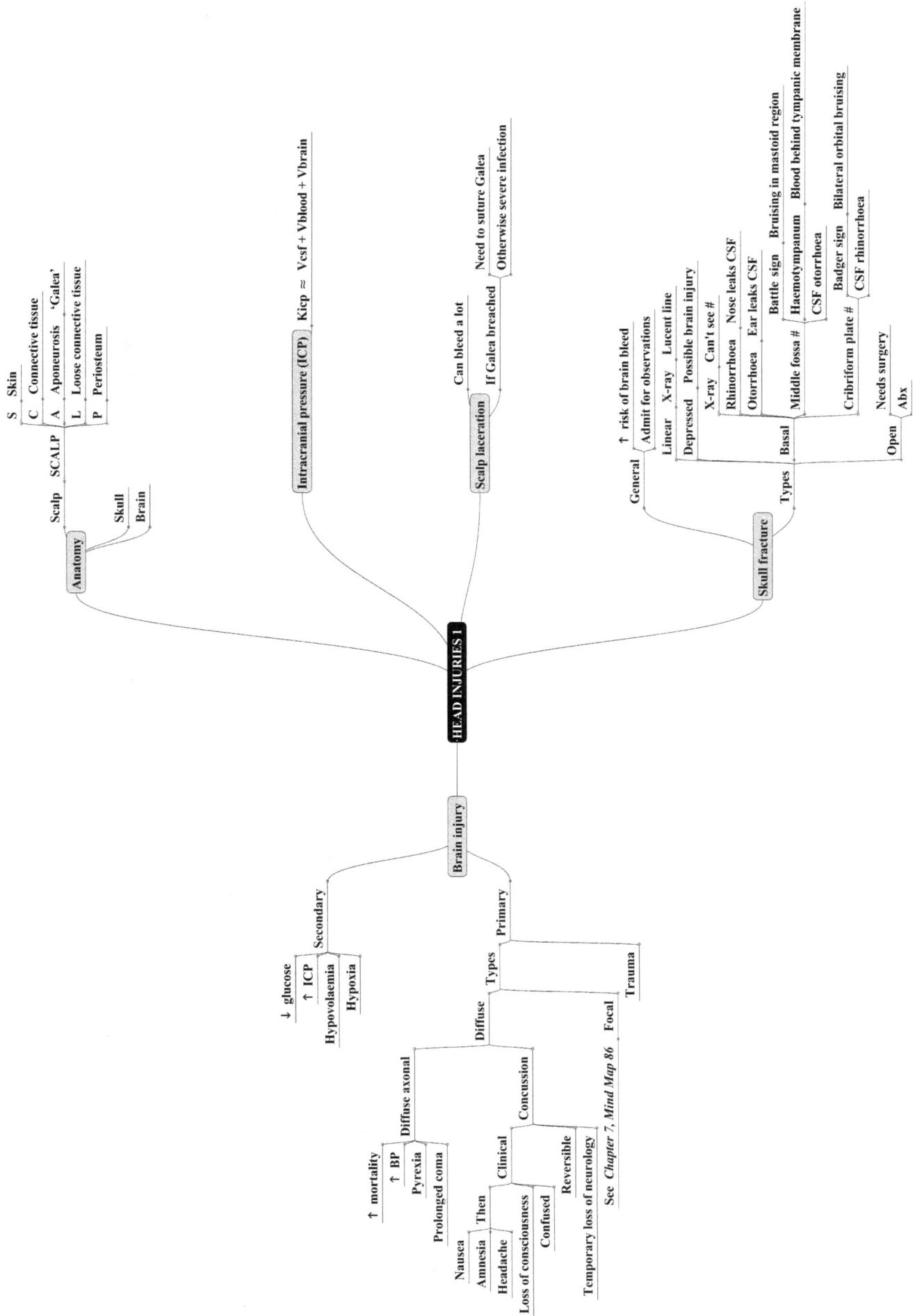

HEAD INJURIES 1

Anatomy

- Scalp — SCALP
  - S — Skin
  - C — Connective tissue
  - A — Aponeurosis 'Galea'
  - L — Loose connective tissue
  - P — Periosteum
- Skull
- Brain

Intracranial pressure (ICP)

$Kicp \approx Vcsf + Vblood + Vbrain$

Scalp laceration

- Can bleed a lot
- If Galea breached
  - Need to suture Galea
  - Otherwise severe infection

Skull fracture

- General
  - ↑ risk of brain bleed
  - Admit for observations
- Types
  - Linear
    - X-ray — Lucent line
  - Depressed
    - Possible brain injury
    - X-ray — Can't see #
  - Basal
    - Rhinorrhoea — Nose leaks CSF
    - Otorrhoea — Ear leaks CSF
    - Middle fossa #
      - Battle sign — Bruising in mastoid region
      - Haemotympanum — Blood behind tympanic membrane
      - CSF otorrhoea
    - Cribriform plate #
      - Badger sign — Bilateral orbital bruising
      - CSF rhinorrhoea
  - Open
    - Needs surgery
    - Abx

Brain injury

- Secondary
  - ↓ glucose
  - ↑ ICP
  - Hypovolaemia
  - Hypoxia
- Primary
  - Types
    - Diffuse
      - Diffuse axonal
        - ↑ mortality
        - ↑ BP
        - Pyrexia
        - Prolonged coma
      - Concussion
        - Clinical
          - Nausea
          - Then
            - Amnesia
            - Headache
            - Loss of consciousness
            - Confused
          - Reversible
          - Temporary loss of neurology
    - Focal
      - See *Chapter 7, Mind Map 86*
  - Trauma

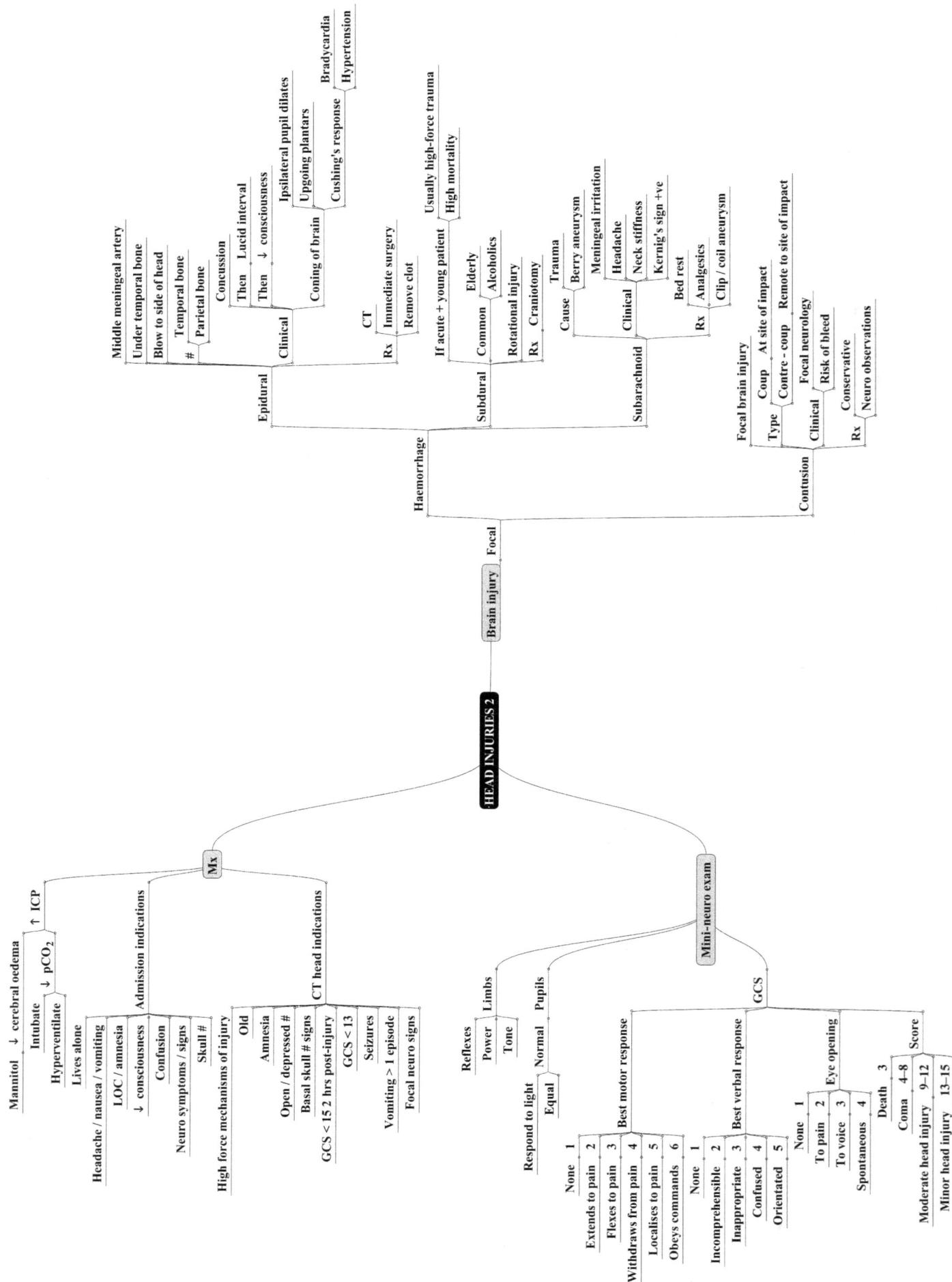

HEAD INJURIES 2

Brain injury

Focal

Haemorrhage

Epidural
- # — Middle meningeal artery
  - Under temporal bone
  - Blow to side of head
  - Temporal bone
  - Parietal bone
- Clinical
  - Concussion
  - Then — Lucid interval
  - Then — ↓ consciousness
    - Ipsilateral pupil dilates
    - Upgoing plantars
    - Coning of brain
  - Cushing's response
    - Bradycardia
    - Hypertension
- Rx — CT
  - Immediate surgery
  - Remove clot

Subdural
- Usually high-force trauma
  - High mortality
- If acute + young patient
- Common
  - Elderly
  - Alcoholics
  - Rotational injury
- Rx — Craniotomy

Subarachnoid
- Cause
  - Trauma
  - Berry aneurysm
- Clinical
  - Meningeal irritation
  - Headache
  - Neck stiffness
  - Kernig's sign +ve
- Rx
  - Bed rest
  - Analgesics
  - Clip / coil aneurysm

Contusion
- Focal brain injury
- Type
  - Coup — At site of impact
  - Contre - coup — Remote to site of impact
- Clinical
  - Focal neurology
  - Risk of bleed
- Rx
  - Conservative
  - Neuro observations

Mx

↑ ICP
- Mannitol — ↓ cerebral oedema
- Intubate — ↓ pCO₂
- Hyperventilate
- Lives alone

Admission indications
- Headache / nausea / vomiting
- LOC / amnesia
- ↓ consciousness
- Confusion
- Neuro symptoms / signs
- Skull #
- High force mechanisms of injury
- Old
- Amnesia
- Open / depressed #
- Basal skull # signs

CT head indications
- GCS <15 2 hrs post-injury
- GCS <13
- Seizures
- Vomiting > 1 episode
- Focal neuro signs

Mini-neuro exam

Limbs
- Reflexes
- Power
- Tone

Pupils
- Normal
- Respond to light
- Equal

GCS

Best motor response
- None — 1
- Extends to pain — 2
- Flexes to pain — 3
- Withdraws from pain — 4
- Localises to pain — 5
- Obeys commands — 6

Best verbal response
- None — 1
- Incomprehensible — 2
- Inappropriate — 3
- Confused — 4
- Orientated — 5

Eye opening
- None — 1
- To pain — 2
- To voice — 3
- Spontaneous — 4

Score
- Death — 3
- Coma — 4–8
- Moderate head injury — 9–12
- Minor head injury — 13–15

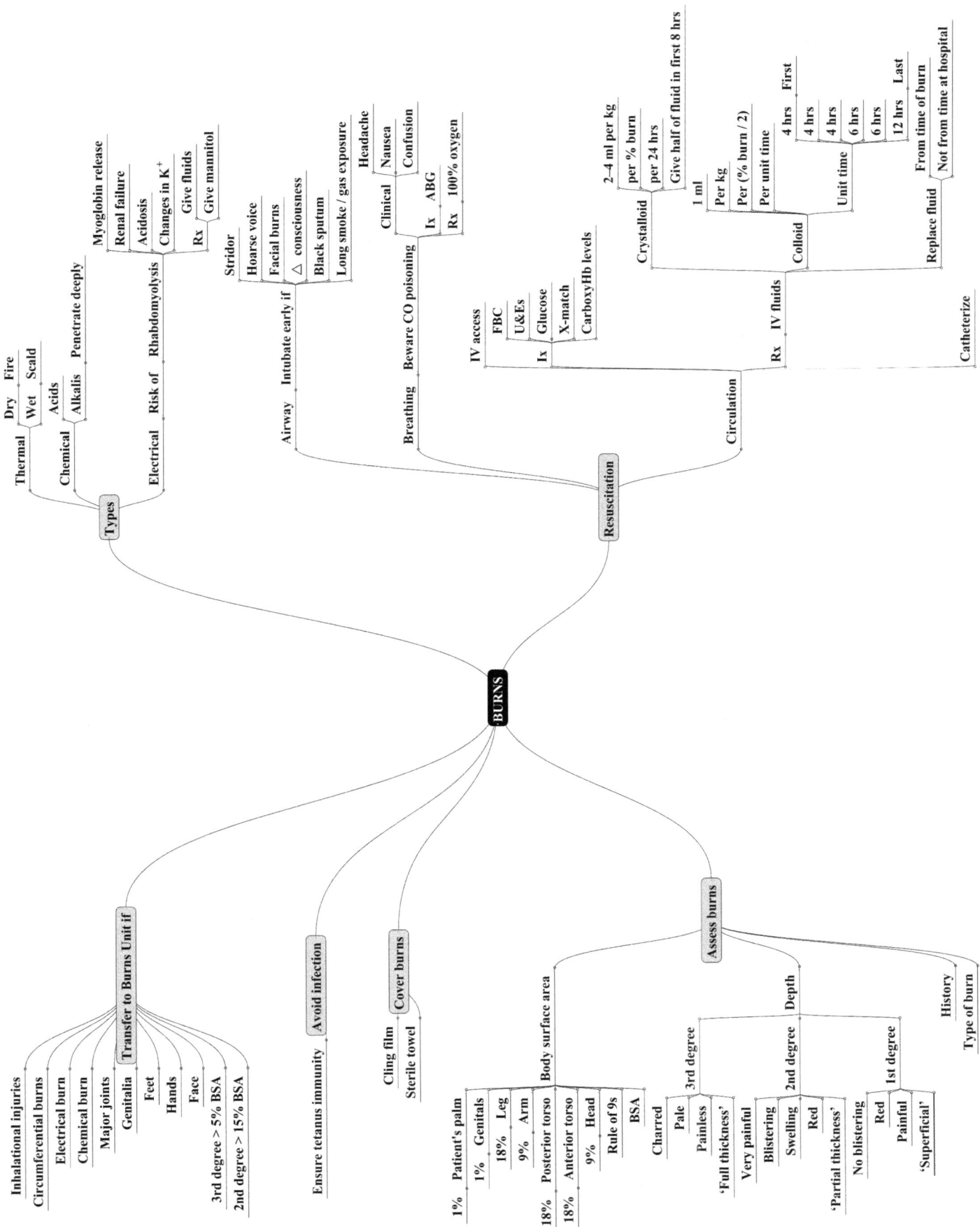

BURNS

Types

- Thermal
  - Dry — Fire
  - Wet — Scald
- Chemical
  - Acids
  - Alkalis — Penetrate deeply
- Electrical
  - Risk of — Rhabdomyolysis
    - Myoglobin release
    - Renal failure
    - Acidosis
    - Changes in K^+
    - Rx
      - Give fluids
      - Give mannitol

Resuscitation

- Airway — Intubate early if
  - Stridor
  - Hoarse voice
  - Facial burns
  - $\triangle$ consciousness
  - Black sputum
  - Long smoke / gas exposure
- Breathing — Beware CO poisoning
  - Clinical
    - Headache
    - Nausea
    - Confusion
  - Ix — ABG — CarboxyHb levels
  - Rx — 100% oxygen
- Circulation
  - IV access
  - Ix
    - FBC
    - U&Es
    - Glucose
    - X-match
    - CarboxyHb levels
  - Rx IV fluids
    - Crystalloid
      - 2–4 ml per kg
      - per % burn
      - per 24 hrs
      - Give half of fluid in first 8 hrs
        - 4 hrs — First
        - 4 hrs
        - 4 hrs
        - 6 hrs — Unit time
        - 6 hrs
        - 12 hrs — Last
    - Colloid
      - 1 ml
      - Per kg
      - Per (% burn / 2)
      - Per unit time
    - Replace fluid
      - From time of burn
      - Not from time at hospital
  - Catheterize

Transfer to Burns Unit if

- Inhalational injuries
- Circumferential burns
- Electrical burn
- Chemical burn
- Major joints
- Genitalia
- Feet
- Hands
- Face
- 3rd degree > 5% BSA
- 2nd degree > 15% BSA

Avoid infection

- Ensure tetanus immunity

Cover burns

- Cling film
- Sterile towel

Assess burns

- Body surface area
  - Patient's palm — 1%
  - Rule of 9s — BSA
    - Genitals — 1%
    - Leg — 18%
    - Arm — 9%
    - Posterior torso — 18%
    - Anterior torso — 18%
    - Head — 9%
- Depth
  - 3rd degree
    - Charred
    - Pale
    - Painless
    - 'Full thickness'
  - 2nd degree
    - Very painful
    - Blistering
    - Swelling
    - Red
    - 'Partial thickness'
  - 1st degree
    - No blistering
    - Red
    - Painful
    - 'Superficial'
- History
- Type of burn

Chapter 8

THE SURGICAL PATIENT

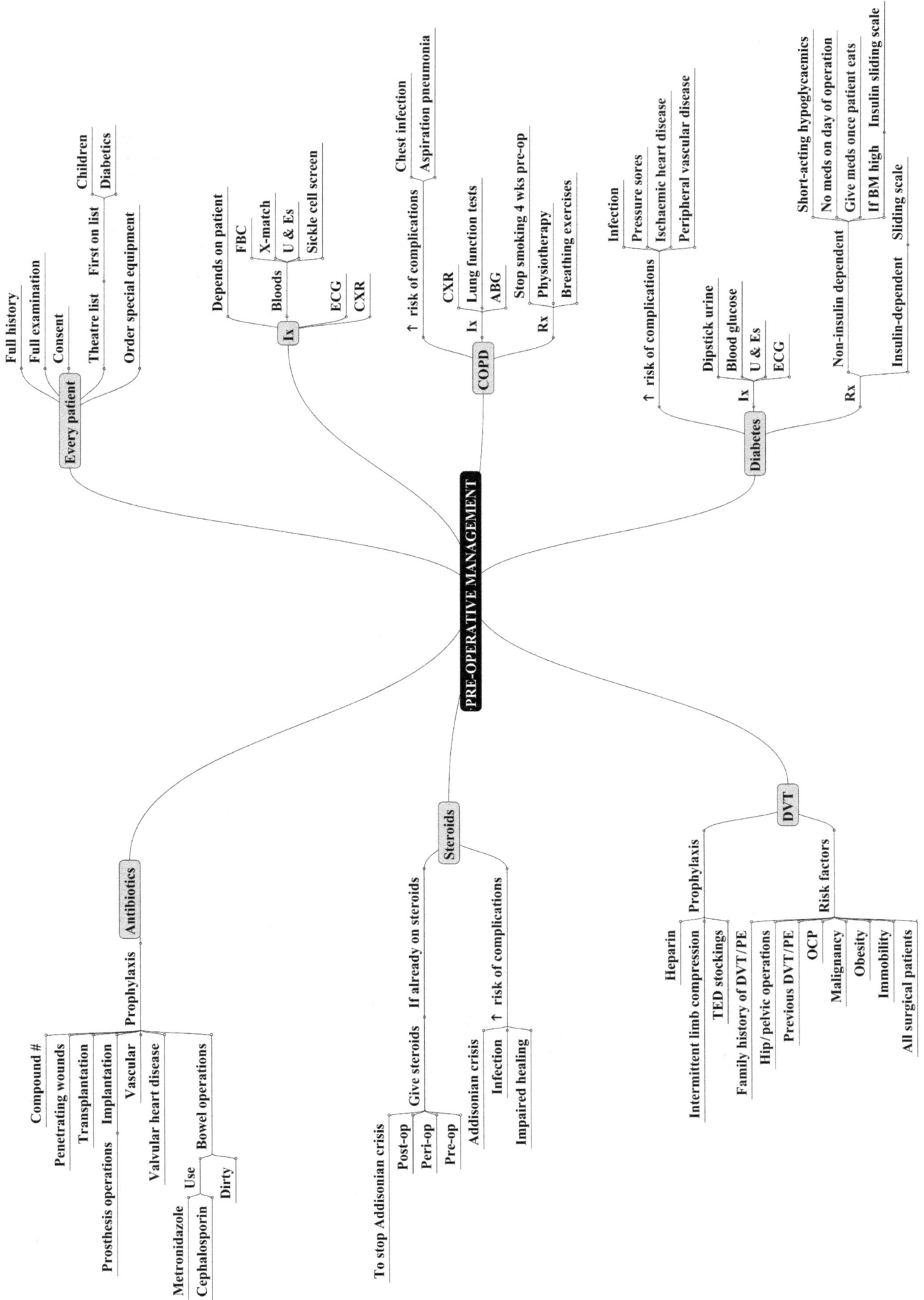

PRE-OPERATIVE MANAGEMENT

Every patient
- Full history
- Full examination
- Consent
- Theatre list
  - First on list
    - Children
    - Diabetics
- Order special equipment

Ix
- Bloods
  - Depends on patient
  - FBC
  - X-match
  - U & Es
  - Sickle cell screen
- ECG
- CXR

COPD
- Ix
  - ↑ risk of complications
    - Chest infection
    - Aspiration pneumonia
  - CXR
  - Lung function tests
  - ABG
- Rx
  - Stop smoking 4 wks pre-op
  - Physiotherapy
  - Breathing exercises

Diabetes
- Ix
  - ↑ risk of complications
    - Infection
    - Pressure sores
    - Ischaemic heart disease
    - Peripheral vascular disease
  - Dipstick urine
  - Blood glucose
  - U & Es
  - ECG
- Rx
  - Non-insulin dependent
    - Short-acting hypoglycaemics
    - No meds on day of operation
    - Give meds once patient eats
    - If BM high
      - Insulin sliding scale
  - Insulin-dependent
    - Sliding scale

Antibiotics
- Prophylaxis
  - Compound #
  - Penetrating wounds
  - Transplantation
  - Implantation
  - Prosthesis operations
  - Vascular
  - Valvular heart disease
  - Bowel operations
- Use
  - Metronidazole
  - Cephalosporin
  - Dirty

Steroids
- If already on steroids
  - To stop Addisonian crisis
  - Give steroids
    - Post-op
    - Peri-op
    - Pre-op
- ↑ risk of complications
  - Addisonian crisis
  - Infection
  - Impaired healing

DVT
- Prophylaxis
  - Heparin
  - Intermittent limb compression
  - TED stockings
- Risk factors
  - Family history of DVT/PE
  - Hip/pelvic operations
  - Previous DVT/PE
  - OCP
  - Malignancy
  - Obesity
  - Immobility
  - All surgical patients

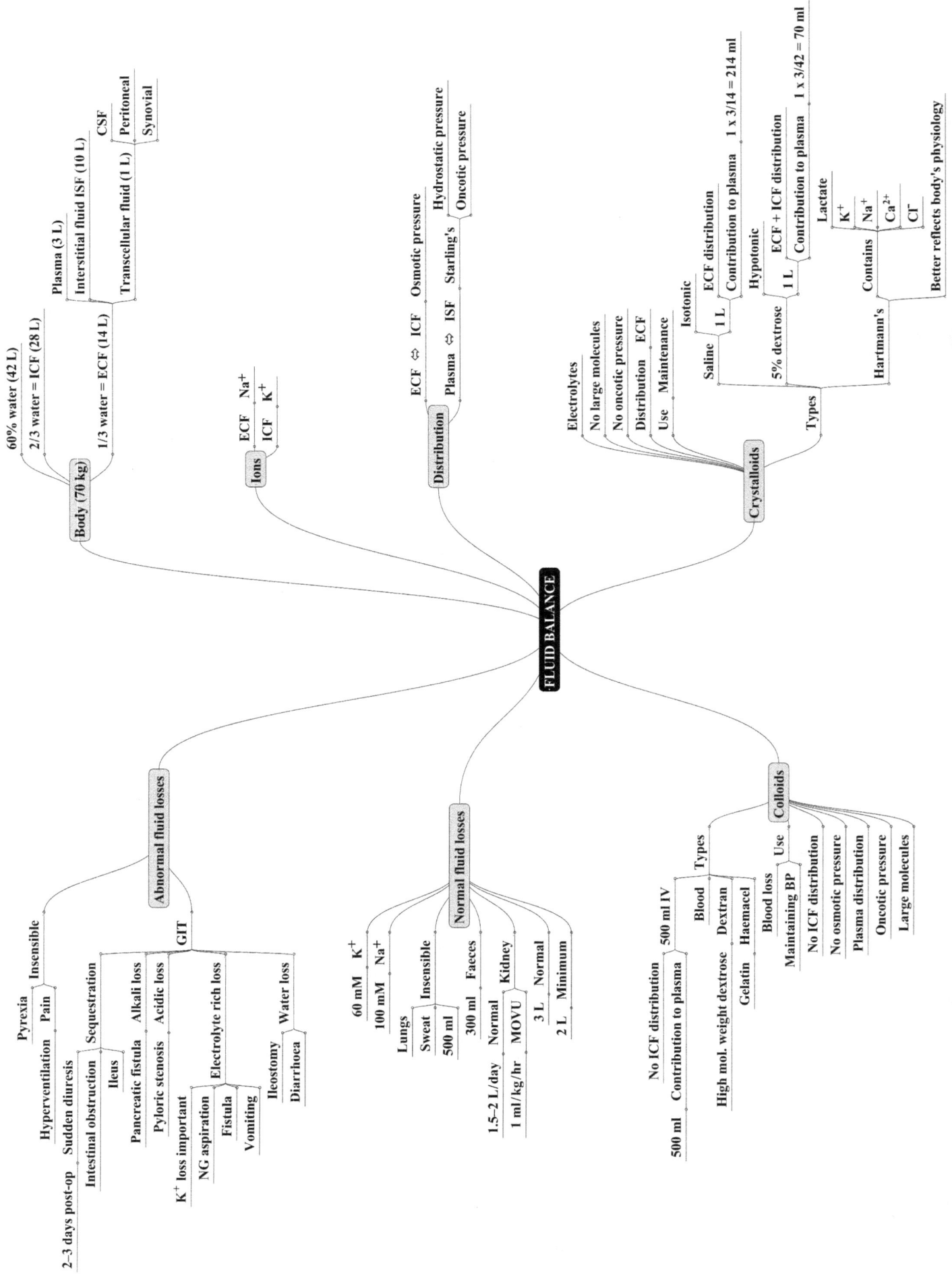

FLUID BALANCE

Body (70 kg)
- 60% water (42 L)
  - 2/3 water = ICF (28 L)
  - 1/3 water = ECF (14 L)
    - Plasma (3 L)
    - Interstitial fluid ISF (10 L)
    - Transcellular fluid (1 L)
      - CSF
      - Peritoneal
      - Synovial

Ions
- ECF — Na^+
- ICF — K^+

Distribution
- $ECF \Leftrightarrow ICF$ — Osmotic pressure
- $Plasma \Leftrightarrow ISF$ — Starling's
  - Hydrostatic pressure
  - Oncotic pressure

Crystalloids
- Electrolytes
- No large molecules
- No oncotic pressure
- Distribution — ECF
- Use — Maintenance
- Types
  - Saline
    - Isotonic
    - 1 L — ECF distribution
    - Contribution to plasma $1 \times 3/14 = 214$ ml
  - 5% dextrose
    - Hypotonic
    - 1 L — ECF + ICF distribution
    - Contribution to plasma $1 \times 3/42 = 70$ ml
  - Hartmann's
    - Contains — Lactate, K^+, Na^+, Ca^{2+}, Cl^-
    - Better reflects body's physiology

Abnormal fluid losses
- Insensible
  - Pyrexia
    - 2–3 days post-op
  - Pain
  - Hyperventilation
  - Sudden diuresis
- GIT
  - Sequestration
    - Intestinal obstruction
    - Ileus
  - Alkali loss
    - Pancreatic fistula
  - Acidic loss
    - Pyloric stenosis
  - Electrolyte rich loss
    - K^+ loss important
    - NG aspiration
    - Fistula
    - Vomiting
  - Water loss
    - Ileostomy
    - Diarrhoea

Normal fluid losses
- K^+ — 60 mM
- Na^+ — 100 mM
- Insensible
  - Lungs
  - Sweat — 500 ml
- Faeces — 300 ml
- Kidney
  - Normal — 1.5–2 L/day
  - MOVU — 1 ml/kg/hr
  - Normal — 3 L
  - Minimum — 2 L

Colloids
- Types
  - Blood — 500 ml IV
    - No ICF distribution
    - Contribution to plasma — 500 ml
  - Dextran — High mol. weight dextrose
  - Gelatin — Haemacel
- Use
  - Blood loss
  - Maintaining BP
- No ICF distribution
- No osmotic pressure
- Plasma distribution
- Oncotic pressure
- Large molecules

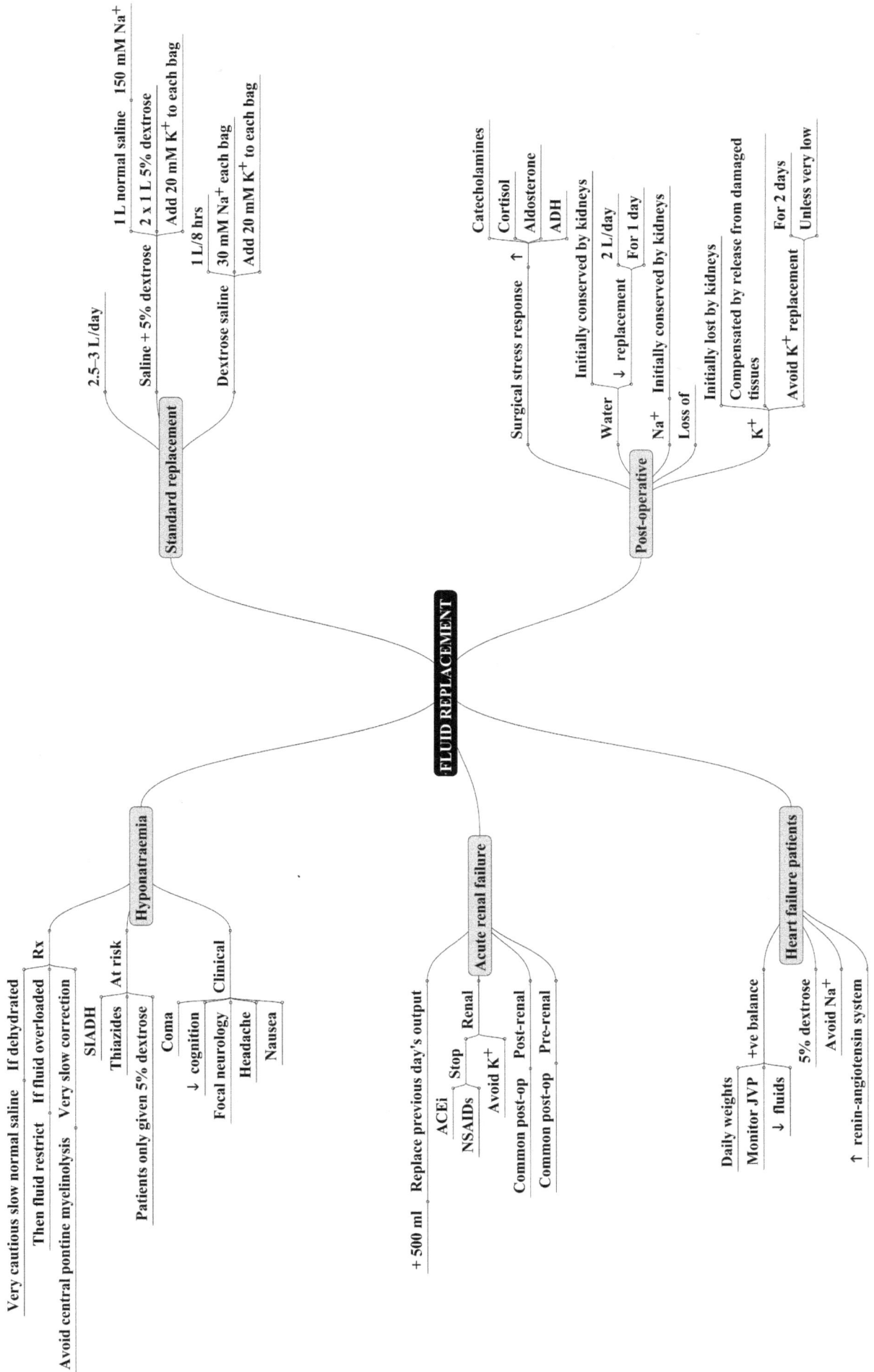

FLUID REPLACEMENT

Standard replacement

- 2.5–3 L/day
- Saline + 5% dextrose
  - 1 L normal saline — 150 mM Na$^+$
  - 2 x 1 L 5% dextrose
    - Add 20 mM K$^+$ to each bag
- Dextrose saline
  - 1 L/8 hrs
  - 30 mM Na$^+$ each bag
    - Add 20 mM K$^+$ to each bag

Post-operative

- Surgical stress response ↑
  - Catecholamines
  - Cortisol
  - Aldosterone
  - ADH
- Water
  - Initially conserved by kidneys
  - ↓ replacement — 2 L/day — For 1 day
- Na$^+$ — Initially conserved by kidneys
- Loss of
- K$^+$
  - Initially lost by kidneys
  - Compensated by release from damaged tissues
  - Avoid K$^+$ replacement — For 2 days — Unless very low

Hyponatraemia

- Rx
  - If dehydrated — Very cautious slow normal saline
  - If fluid overloaded — Then fluid restrict
  - Very slow correction — Avoid central pontine myelinolysis
- At risk
  - SIADH
  - Thiazides
  - Patients only given 5% dextrose
- Clinical
  - Coma
  - ↓ cognition
  - Focal neurology
  - Headache
  - Nausea

Acute renal failure

- Replace previous day's output + 500 ml
- Stop
  - ACEi
  - NSAIDs
- Renal — Avoid K$^+$
- Post-renal — Common post-op
- Pre-renal — Common post-op

Heart failure patients

- Daily weights
- Monitor JVP
  - +ve balance
  - ↓ fluids
    - 5% dextrose
    - Avoid Na$^+$
    - ↑ renin-angiotensin system

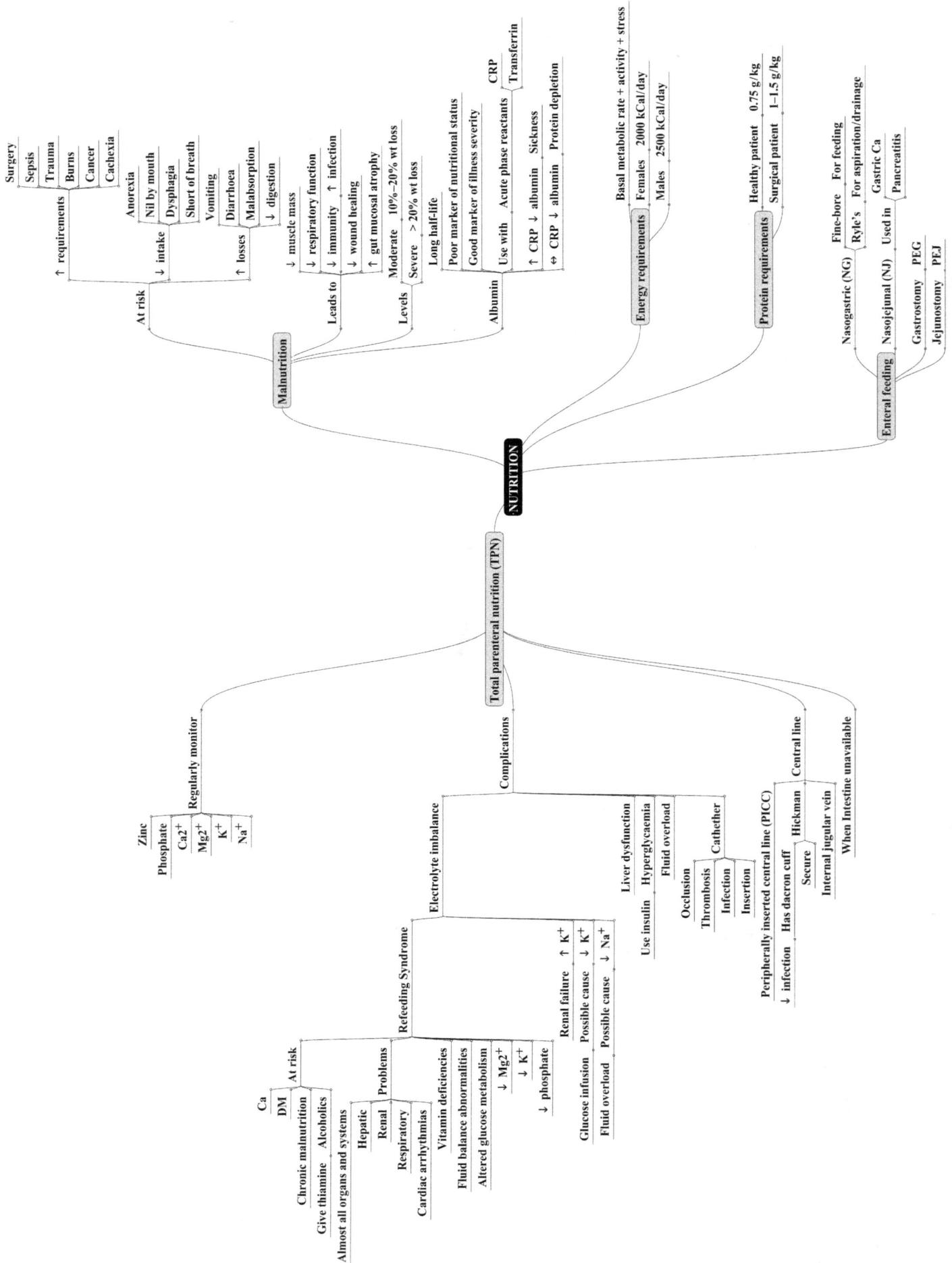

NUTRITION

Malnutrition

At risk
- ↑ requirements
  - Surgery
  - Sepsis
  - Trauma
  - Burns
  - Cancer
  - Cachexia
- ↓ intake
  - Anorexia
  - Nil by mouth
  - Dysphagia
  - Short of breath
- ↑ losses
  - Vomiting
  - Diarrhoea
  - Malabsorption
  - ↓ digestion

Leads to
- ↓ muscle mass
- ↓ respiratory function
- ↓ immunity   ↑ infection
- ↓ wound healing
- ↓ gut mucosal atrophy

Levels
- Moderate   10%–20% wt loss
- Severe   > 20% wt loss

Albumin
- Long half-life
- Poor marker of nutritional status
- Good marker of illness severity
- Use with   Acute phase reactants
  - CRP
  - Transferrin
  - ↑ CRP   ↓ albumin   Sickness
  - ⇔ CRP   ↓ albumin   Protein depletion

Energy requirements
- Basal metabolic rate + activity + stress
- Females   2000 kCal/day
- Males   2500 kCal/day

Protein requirements
- Healthy patient   0.75 g/kg
- Surgical patient   1–1.5 g/kg

Enteral feeding
- Nasogastric (NG)
  - Fine-bore   For feeding
  - Ryle's   For aspiration/drainage
- Nasojejunal (NJ)   Used in
  - Gastric Ca
  - Pancreatitis
- Gastrostomy   PEG
- Jejunostomy   PEJ

Total parenteral nutrition (TPN)

Regularly monitor
- Zinc
- Phosphate
- Ca2+
- Mg2+
- K+
- Na+

Complications
- Electrolyte imbalance
  - Refeeding Syndrome
    - At risk
      - Ca
      - DM
      - Chronic malnutrition   Alcoholics
      - Give thiamine
      - Almost all organs and systems
    - Problems
      - Hepatic
      - Renal
      - Respiratory
      - Cardiac arrhythmias
      - Vitamin deficiencies
      - Fluid balance abnormalities
      - Altered glucose metabolism
        - ↓ Mg2+
        - ↓ K+
        - ↓ phosphate
  - Renal failure   ↑ K+
    - Possible cause   ↓ K+
      - Glucose infusion
    - Possible cause   ↓ Na+
      - Fluid overload
- Liver dysfunction
- Hyperglycaemia   Use insulin
- Fluid overload
- Catheter
  - Occlusion
  - Thrombosis
  - Infection
  - Insertion
- Peripherally inserted central line (PICC)   ↓ infection
- Central line
  - Has dacron cuff   Secure
  - Hickman
  - Internal jugular vein
  - When Intestine unavailable

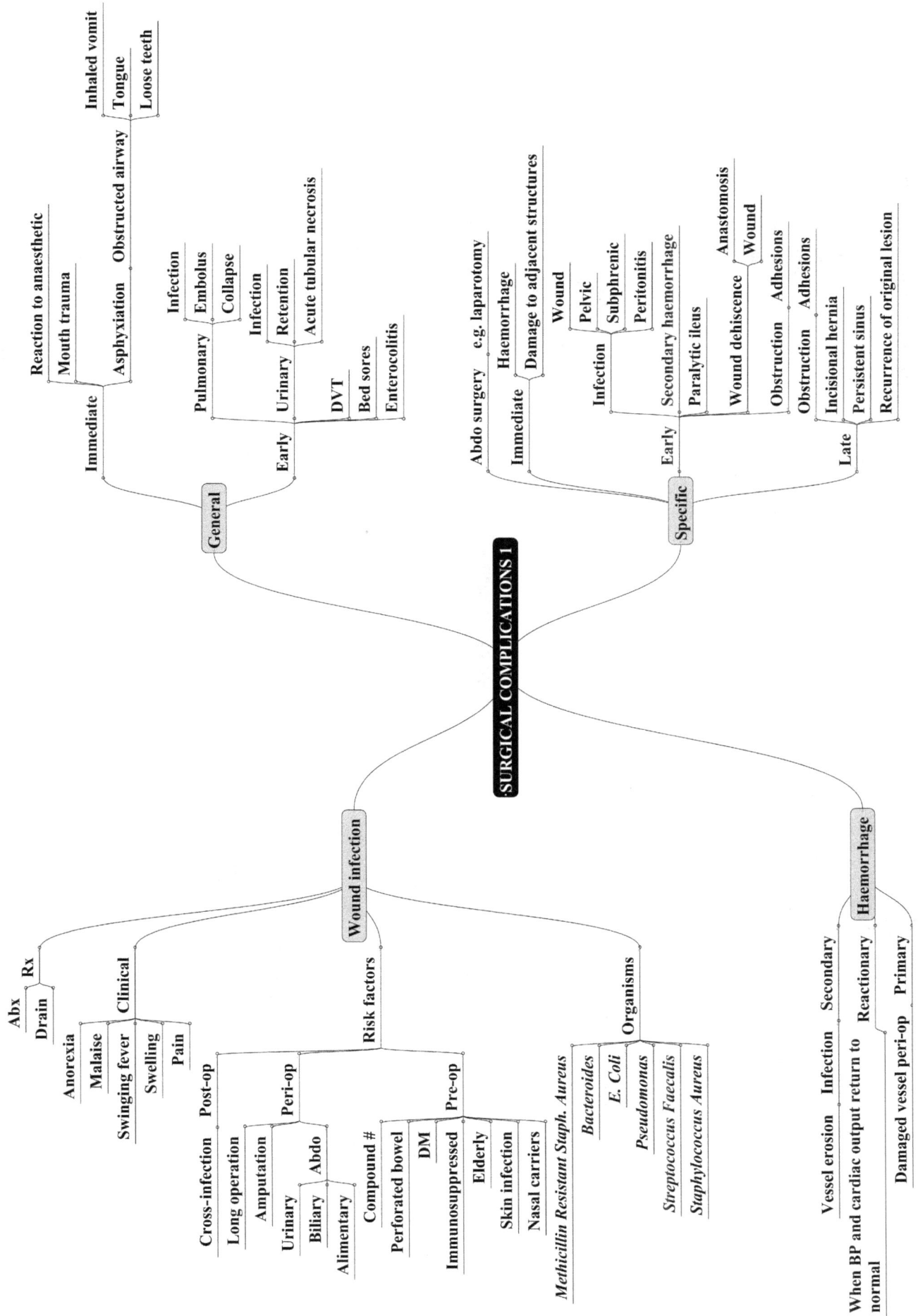

SURGICAL COMPLICATIONS 1

General

Immediate
- Reaction to anaesthetic
- Mouth trauma
- Asphyxiation
  - Obstructed airway
    - Inhaled vomit
    - Tongue
    - Loose teeth

Early
- Pulmonary
  - Infection
  - Embolus
  - Collapse
- Urinary
  - Infection
  - Retention
  - Acute tubular necrosis
- DVT
- Bed sores
- Enterocolitis

Specific

Immediate
- Abdo surgery e.g. laparotomy
- Haemorrhage
- Damage to adjacent structures

Early
- Wound
  - Pelvic
  - Subphrenic
  - Peritonitis
- Infection
- Secondary haemorrhage
- Paralytic ileus
- Wound dehiscence
  - Anastomosis
  - Wound
- Obstruction — Adhesions

Late
- Obstruction — Adhesions
- Incisional hernia
- Persistent sinus
- Recurrence of original lesion

Wound infection

Rx
- Abx
- Drain

Clinical
- Anorexia
- Malaise
- Swinging fever
- Swelling
- Pain

Risk factors
- Post-op
  - Cross-infection
- Peri-op
  - Long operation
  - Amputation
  - Urinary
  - Biliary
  - Abdo
  - Alimentary
- Pre-op
  - Compound #
  - Perforated bowel
  - DM
  - Immunosuppressed
  - Elderly
  - Skin infection
  - Nasal carriers

Organisms
- *Methicillin Resistant Staph. Aureus*
- *Bacteroides*
- *E. Coli*
- *Pseudomonas*
- *Streptococcus Faecalis*
- *Staphylococcus Aureus*

Haemorrhage

- Secondary
  - Vessel erosion
  - Infection
- Reactionary
  - When BP and cardiac output return to normal
- Primary
  - Damaged vessel peri-op

SURGICAL COMPLICATIONS 2

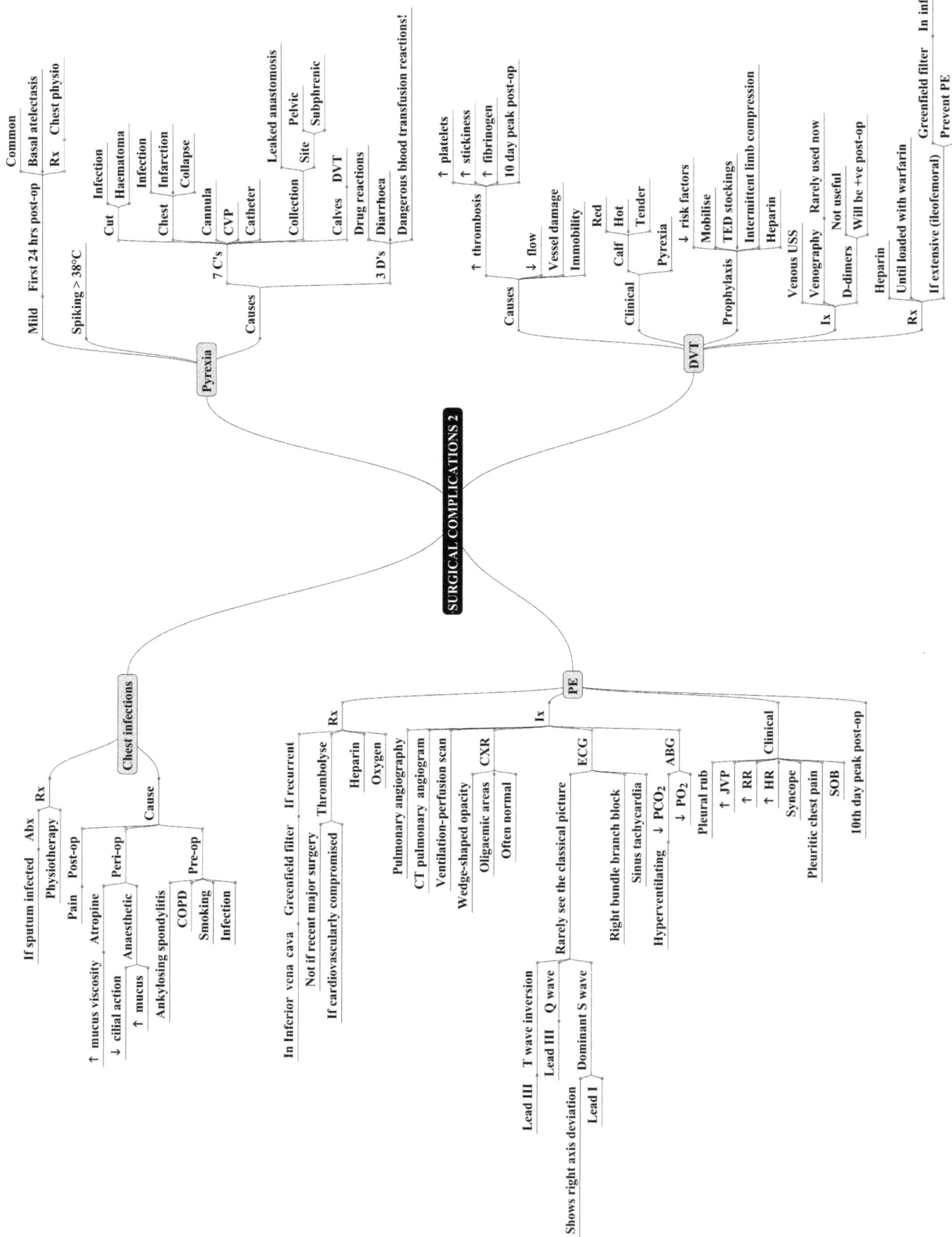

Pyrexia

- **Mild** First 24 hrs post-op
- Spiking > 38°C
- **Common** — Basal atelectasis — **Rx** Chest physio
- **Causes**
  - **7 C's**
    - Cut — Infection
    - Haematoma
    - Chest — Infection
      - Infarction
      - Collapse
    - Cannula
    - CVP
    - Catheter
  - Leaked anastomosis — **Site** — Pelvic
    - Subphrenic
  - Collection
  - DVT — Calves
  - **3 D's**
    - Drug reactions
    - Diarrhoea
    - Dangerous blood transfusion reactions!

DVT

- **Causes**
  - ↑ thrombosis
    - ↑ platelets
    - ↑ stickiness
    - ↑ fibrinogen
    - 10 day peak post-op
  - ↓ flow
  - Vessel damage
  - Immobility
- **Clinical**
  - Calf — Red
    - Hot
    - Tender
  - Pyrexia
- **Prophylaxis**
  - ↓ risk factors
  - Mobilise
  - TED stockings
  - Intermittent limb compression
  - Heparin
- **Ix**
  - Venous USS
  - Venography — Rarely used now
  - D-dimers — Not useful — Will be +ve post-op
- **Rx**
  - Heparin
  - Until loaded with warfarin
  - If extensive (ileofemoral) — Greenfield filter — In inferior vena cava — Prevent PE

Chest infections

- **Rx**
  - If sputum infected — Abx
  - Physiotherapy
  - Pain
- **Cause**
  - Post-op
  - Peri-op — Atropine — ↑ mucus viscosity
    - ↓ cilial action
  - Anaesthetic — ↑ mucus
  - Ankylosing spondylitis
  - Pre-op — COPD
    - Smoking
    - Infection

PE

- **Rx**
  - In Inferior vena cava — Greenfield filter — If recurrent
    - Not if recent major surgery
  - Thrombolyse — If cardiovascularly compromised
  - Heparin
  - Oxygen
- **Ix**
  - Pulmonary angiography
  - CT pulmonary angiogram
  - Ventilation-perfusion scan
  - CXR — Wedge-shaped opacity
    - Oligaemic areas
    - Often normal
  - ECG — Rarely see the classical picture
    - Right bundle branch block
    - Sinus tachycardia
    - Lead III — T wave inversion
      - Q wave
    - Lead I — Dominant S wave
    - Shows right axis deviation
  - ABG — Hyperventilating — ↓ PCO_2
    - ↓ PO_2
- **Clinical**
  - Pleural rub
  - ↑ JVP
  - ↑ RR
  - ↑ HR
  - Syncope
  - Pleuritic chest pain
  - SOB
  - 10th day peak post-op

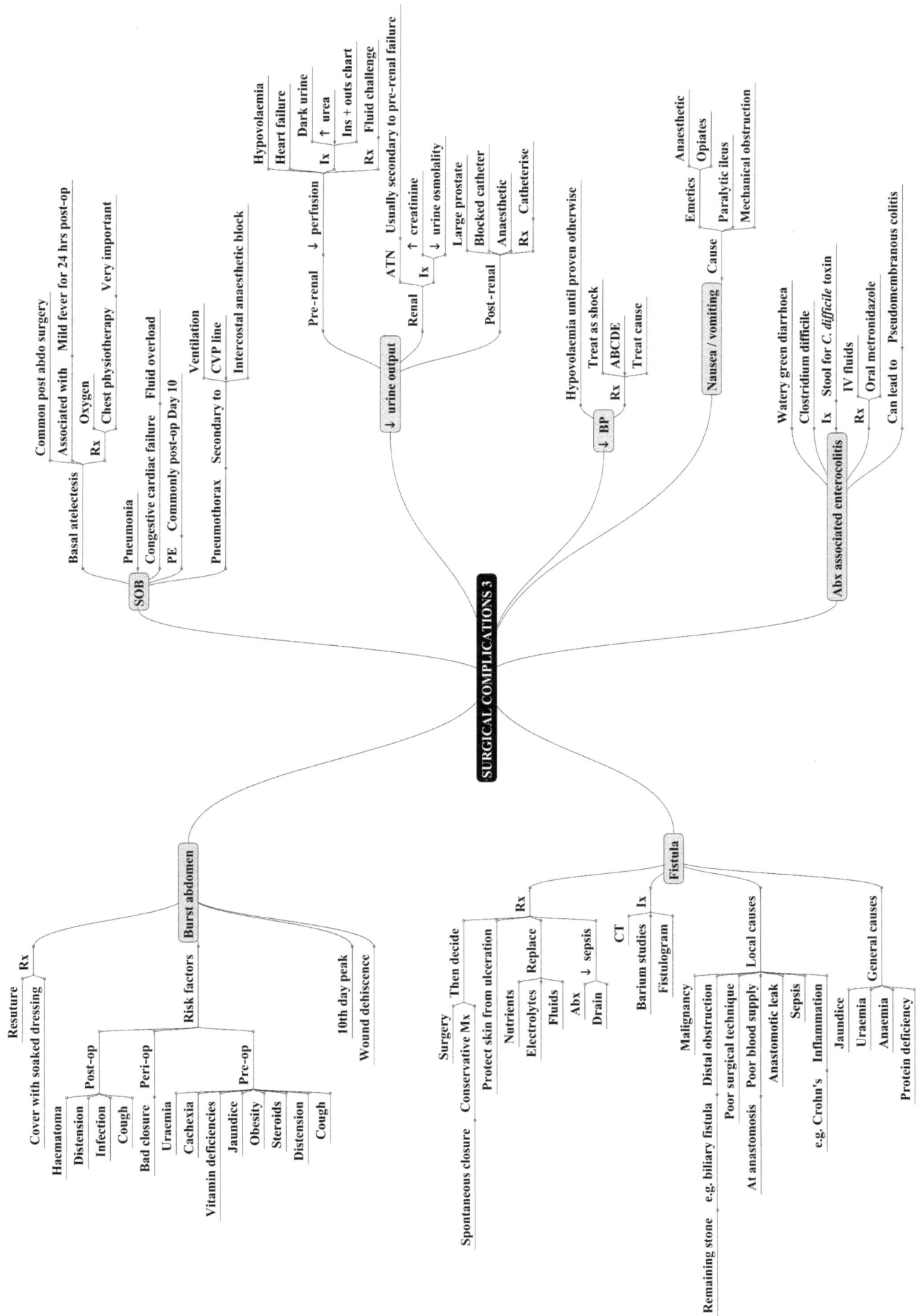

SURGICAL COMPLICATIONS 3

SOB
- Basal atelectesis
  - Common post abdo surgery
  - Associated with — Mild fever for 24 hrs post-op
  - Rx
    - Oxygen
    - Chest physiotherapy — Very important
- Pneumonia
- Congestive cardiac failure — Fluid overload
- PE — Commonly post-op Day 10
- Pneumothorax — Secondary to
  - Ventilation
  - CVP line
  - Intercostal anaesthetic block

↓ urine output
- Pre-renal — ↓ perfusion
  - Hypovolaemia
  - Heart failure
  - Ix
    - Dark urine
    - ↑ urea
    - Ins + outs chart
  - Rx — Fluid challenge
- Renal
  - ATN — Usually secondary to pre-renal failure
  - Ix
    - ↑ creatinine
    - ↓ urine osmolality
- Post-renal
  - Large prostate
  - Blocked catheter
  - Anaesthetic
  - Rx — Catheterise

↓ BP
- Hypovolaemia until proven otherwise
- Treat as shock
- Rx
  - ABCDE
  - Treat cause

Nausea / vomiting
- Cause
  - Emetics
  - Anaesthetic
  - Opiates
  - Paralytic ileus
  - Mechanical obstruction

Abx associated enterocolitis
- Watery green diarrhoea
- Clostridium difficile
- Ix — Stool for *C. difficile* toxin
- Rx
  - IV fluids
  - Oral metronidazole
- Can lead to — Pseudomembranous colitis

Burst abdomen
- Rx
  - Resuture
  - Cover with soaked dressing
- Risk factors
  - Post-op
    - Haematoma
    - Distension
    - Infection
    - Cough
  - Peri-op
    - Bad closure
  - Pre-op
    - Uraemia
    - Cachexia
    - Vitamin deficiencies
    - Jaundice
    - Obesity
    - Steroids
    - Distension
    - Cough
- 10th day peak
- Wound dehiscence

Fistula
- Rx
  - Surgery — Then decide
  - Conservative Mx
    - Spontaneous closure
    - Protect skin from ulceration
    - Replace
      - Nutrients
      - Electrolytes
      - Fluids
    - Abx — ↓ sepsis
    - Drain
- Ix
  - CT
  - Barium studies
  - Fistulogram
- Local causes
  - Malignancy
  - Distal obstruction
  - Poor surgical technique
  - Poor blood supply
  - Anastomotic leak — At anastomosis
  - Sepsis
  - Inflammation — e.g. Crohn's
  - e.g. biliary fistula — Remaining stone
- General causes
  - Jaundice
  - Uraemia
  - Anaemia
  - Protein deficiency

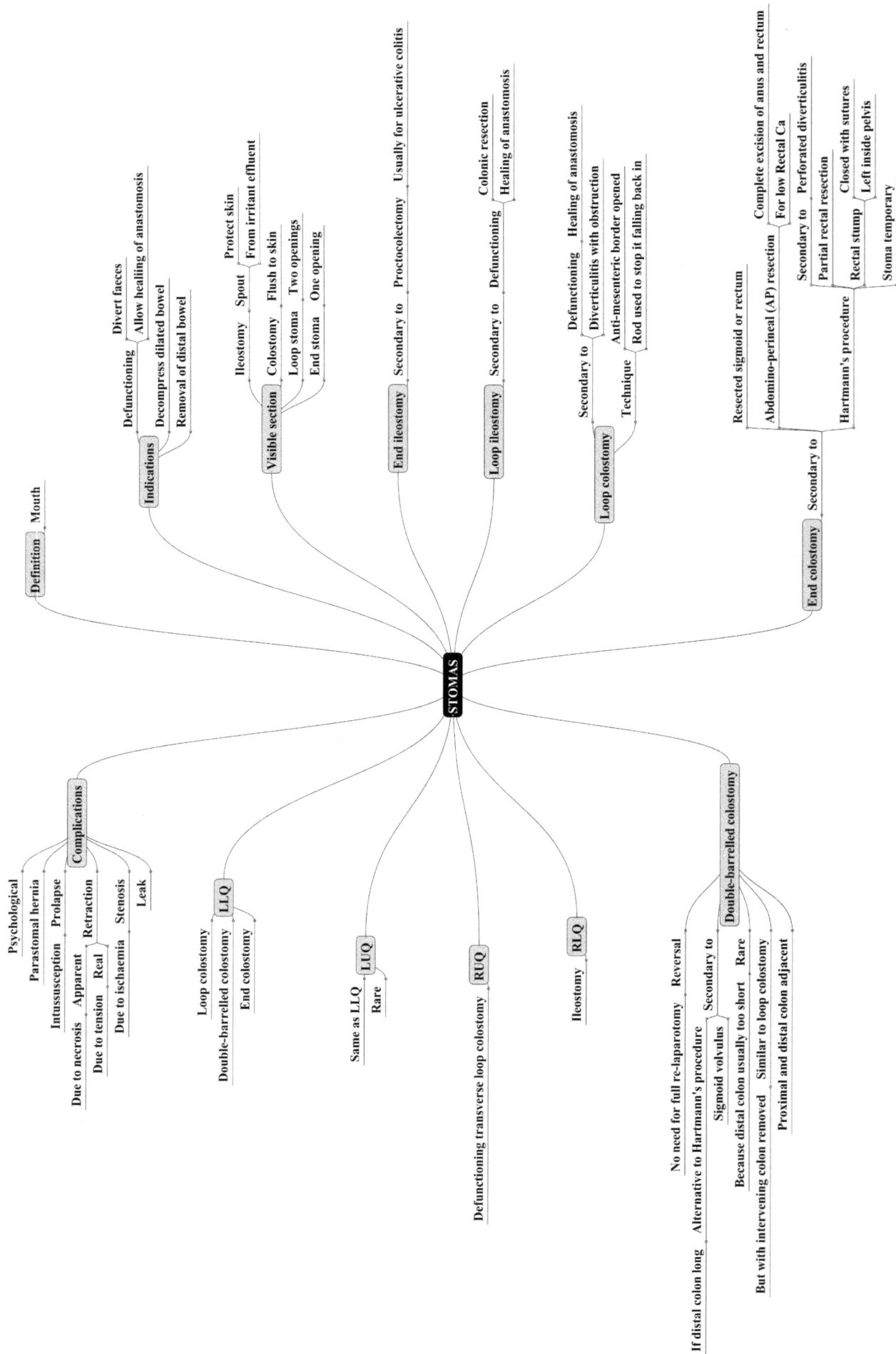

STOMAS

Definition — Mouth

Indications
- Defunctioning
  - Divert faeces
  - Allow healing of anastomosis
- Decompress dilated bowel
- Removal of distal bowel

Visible section
- Ileostomy — Spout — Flush to skin
  - Protect skin
  - From irritant effluent
- Colostomy
  - Loop stoma — Two openings
  - End stoma — One opening

End ileostomy
- Secondary to — Proctocolectomy — Usually for ulcerative colitis

Loop ileostomy
- Secondary to — Defunctioning
  - Colonic resection
  - Healing of anastomosis

Loop colostomy
- Secondary to
  - Defunctioning — Healing of anastomosis
  - Diverticulitis with obstruction
- Technique
  - Anti-mesenteric border opened
  - Rod used to stop it falling back in

End colostomy
- Secondary to
  - Resected sigmoid or rectum
  - Abdomino-perineal (AP) resection
    - Complete excision of anus and rectum
    - For low Rectal Ca
  - Hartmann's procedure
    - Secondary to — Perforated diverticulitis
    - Partial rectal resection
    - Rectal stump
      - Closed with sutures
      - Left inside pelvis
    - Stoma temporary

Complications
- Psychological
- Parastomal hernia
- Prolapse
- Intussusception
- Retraction
  - Apparent — Due to tension
  - Real — Due to ischaemia
- Stenosis — Due to necrosis
- Leak

LLQ
- Loop colostomy
- Double-barrelled colostomy
- End colostomy

LUQ
- Same as LLQ
- Rare

RUQ
- Defunctioning transverse loop colostomy

RLQ
- Ileostomy

Double-barrelled colostomy
- No need for full re-laparotomy — Reversal
- Alternative to Hartmann's procedure
- Secondary to — Sigmoid volvulus
- Because distal colon usually too short — Rare
- Similar to loop colostomy
- If distal colon long
- But with intervening colon removed
- Proximal and distal colon adjacent

Chapter 9

SPECIFIC EXAMINATIONS

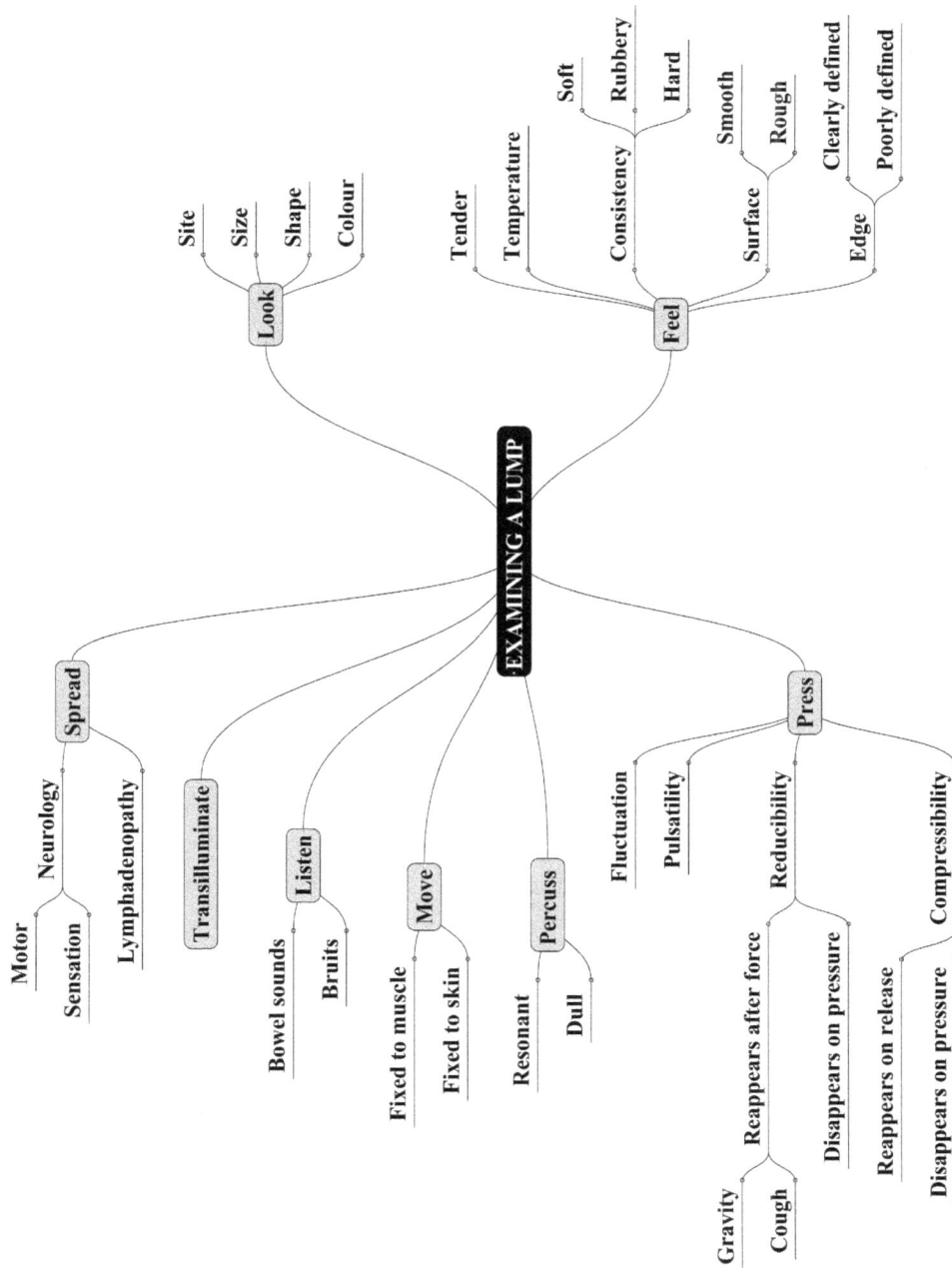

EXAMINING A LUMP

Look
- Site
- Size
- Shape
- Colour

Feel
- Tender
- Temperature
- Consistency
  - Soft
  - Rubbery
  - Hard
- Surface
  - Smooth
  - Rough
- Edge
  - Clearly defined
  - Poorly defined

Spread
- Neurology
  - Motor
  - Sensation
- Lymphadenopathy

Transilluminate

Listen
- Bowel sounds
- Bruits

Move
- Fixed to muscle
- Fixed to skin

Percuss
- Resonant
- Dull

Press
- Fluctuation
- Pulsatility
- Reducibility
  - Gravity
  - Cough
  - Reappears after force
  - Disappears on pressure
- Compressibility
  - Reappears on release
  - Disappears on pressure

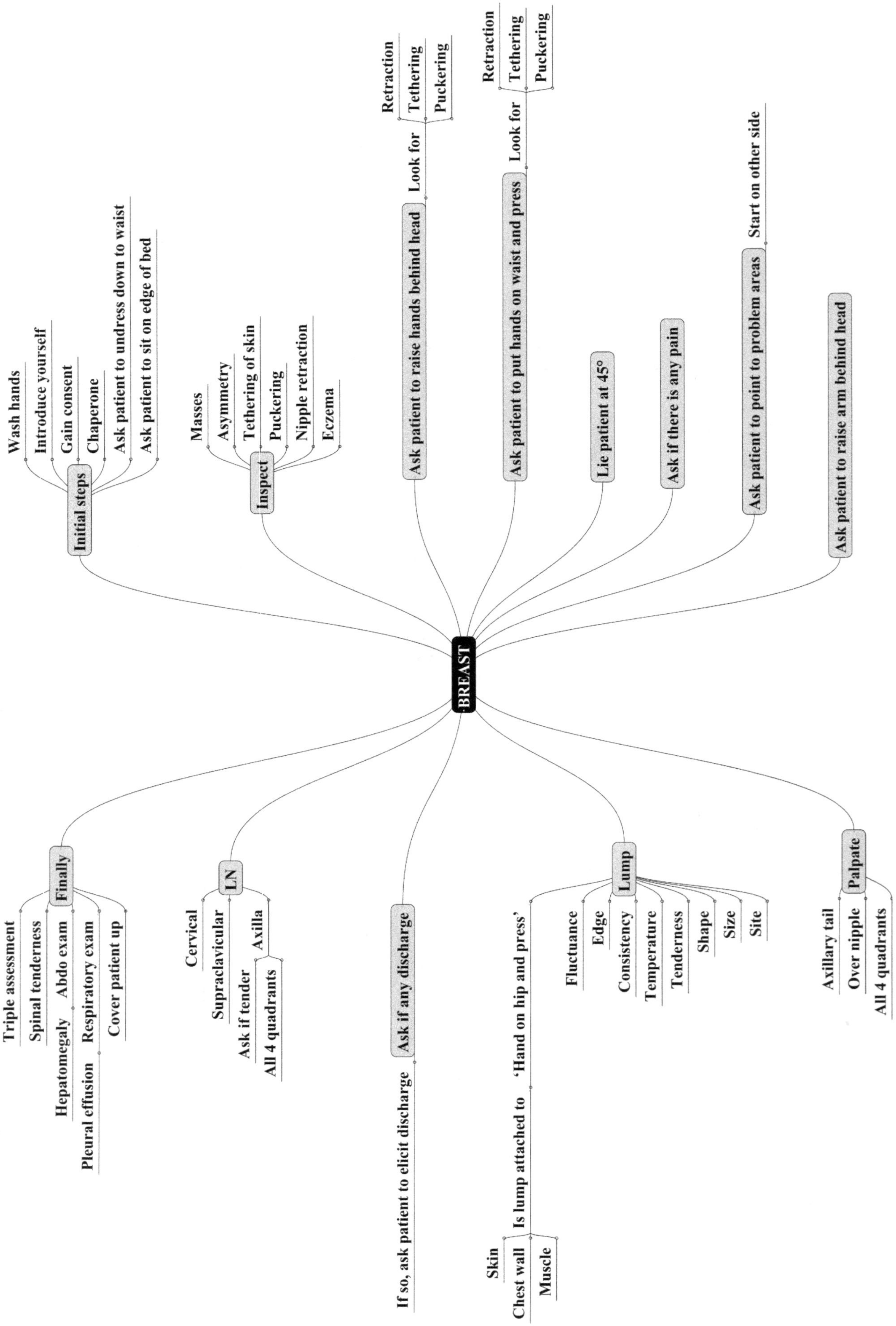

BREAST

Initial steps
- Wash hands
- Introduce yourself
- Gain consent
- Chaperone
- Ask patient to undress down to waist
- Ask patient to sit on edge of bed

Inspect
- Masses
- Asymmetry
- Tethering of skin
- Puckering
- Nipple retraction
- Eczema

Ask patient to raise hands behind head — Look for
- Retraction
  - Tethering
  - Puckering

Ask patient to put hands on waist and press — Look for
- Retraction
  - Tethering
  - Puckering

Lie patient at 45°

Ask if there is any pain

Ask patient to point to problem areas — Start on other side

Ask patient to raise arm behind head

Palpate
- Axillary tail
- Over nipple
- All 4 quadrants

Lump
- Fluctuance
- Edge
- Consistency
- Temperature
- Tenderness
- Shape
- Size
- Site
- Is lump attached to 'Hand on hip and press'
  - Skin
  - Chest wall
  - Muscle

Ask if any discharge
- If so, ask patient to elicit discharge

LN
- Cervical
- Supraclavicular
- Axilla
  - Ask if tender
  - All 4 quadrants

Finally
- Triple assessment
- Spinal tenderness
- Abdo exam
- Hepatomegaly
- Respiratory exam
- Pleural effusion
- Cover patient up

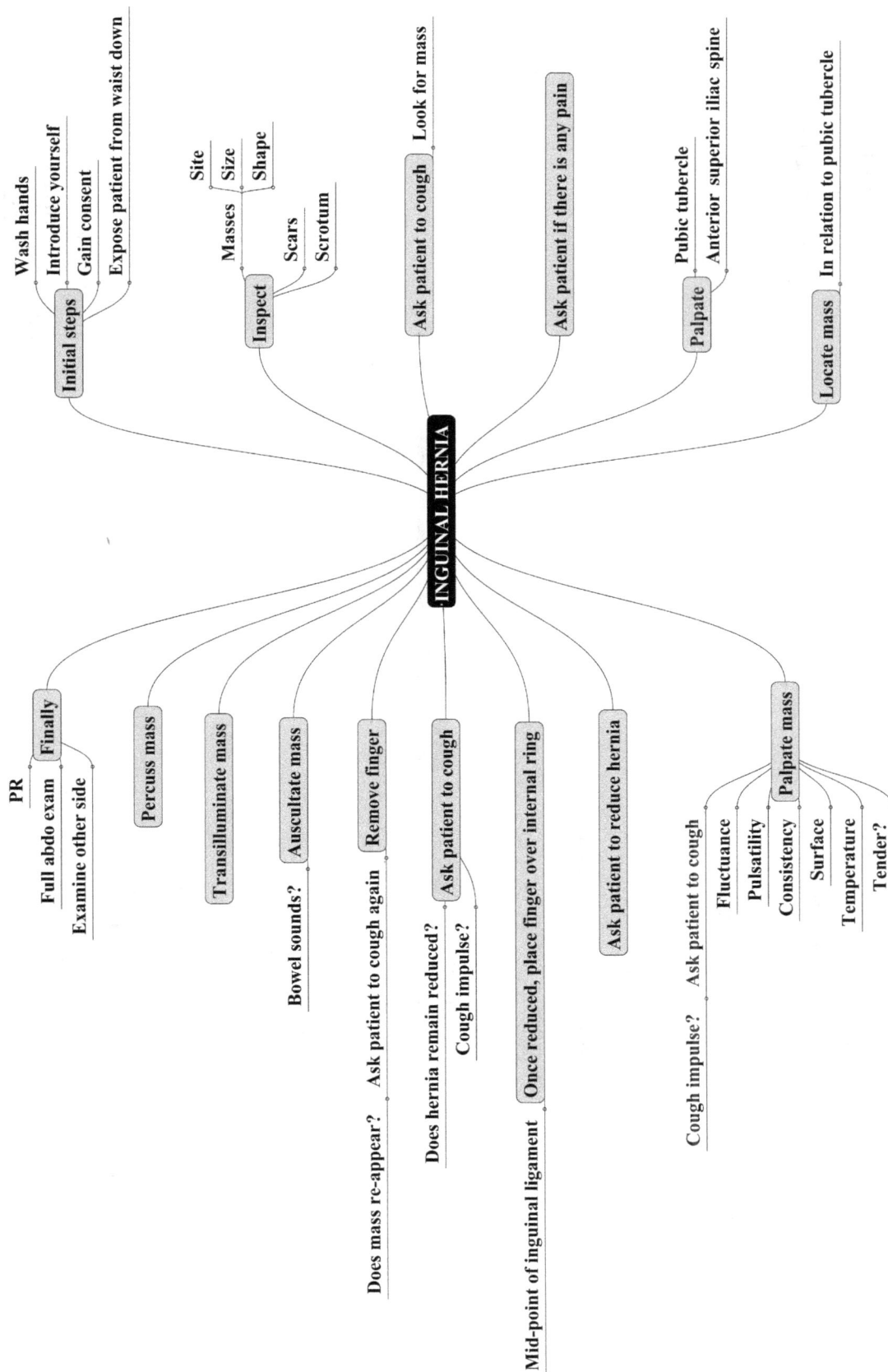

INGUINAL HERNIA

Initial steps
- Wash hands
- Introduce yourself
- Gain consent
- Expose patient from waist down

Inspect
- Masses
  - Site
  - Size
  - Shape
- Scars
- Scrotum

Ask patient to cough
- Look for mass

Ask patient if there is any pain

Palpate
- Pubic tubercle
- Anterior superior iliac spine

Locate mass
- In relation to pubic tubercle

Palpate mass
- Ask patient to cough
  - Cough impulse?
- Fluctuance
- Pulsatility
- Consistency
- Surface
- Temperature
- Tender?

Ask patient to reduce hernia

Once reduced, place finger over internal ring
- Mid-point of inguinal ligament

Ask patient to cough
- Cough impulse?
- Does hernia remain reduced?

Remove finger
- Ask patient to cough again
  - Does mass re-appear?

Auscultate mass
- Bowel sounds?

Transilluminate mass

Percuss mass

Finally
- PR
- Full abdo exam
- Examine other side

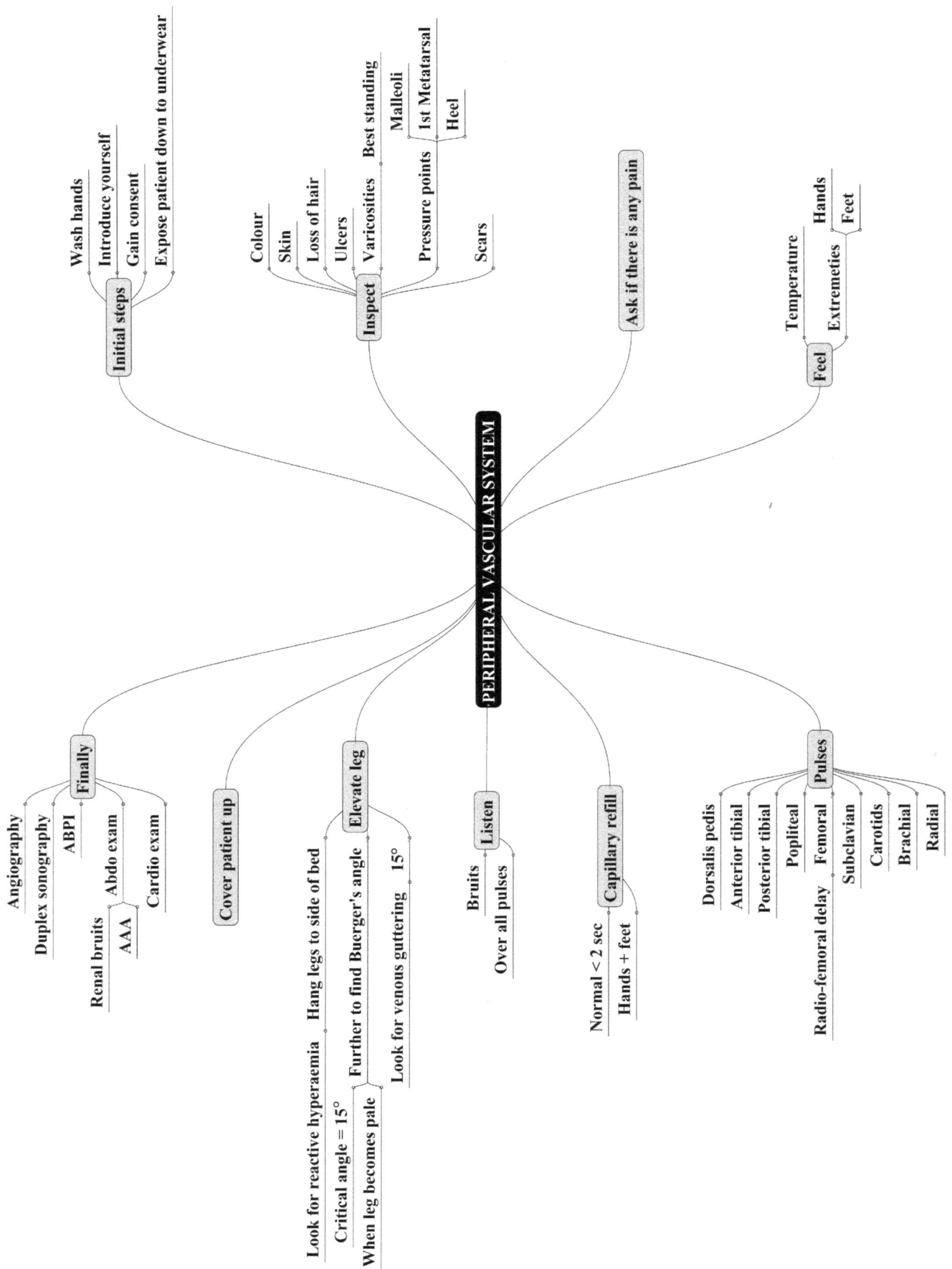

PERIPHERAL VASCULAR SYSTEM

Initial steps
- Wash hands
- Introduce yourself
- Gain consent
- Expose patient down to underwear

Inspect
- Colour
- Skin
  - Loss of hair
- Ulcers
- Varicosities
  - Best standing
- Pressure points
  - Malleoli
  - 1st Metatarsal
  - Heel
- Scars

Ask if there is any pain

Feel
- Temperature
- Extremeties
  - Hands
  - Feet

Finally
- Angiography
- Duplex sonography
- ABPI
- Renal bruits
  - AAA
- Abdo exam
- Cardio exam

Cover patient up

Elevate leg
- Look for reactive hyperaemia
- Hang legs to side of bed
- Further to find Buerger's angle
  - Critical angle = 15°
  - When leg becomes pale
- Look for venous guttering 15°

Listen
- Bruits
- Over all pulses

Capillary refill
- Normal < 2 sec
- Hands + feet

Pulses
- Dorsalis pedis
- Anterior tibial
- Posterior tibial
- Popliteal
- Femoral
  - Radio-femoral delay
- Subclavian
- Carotids
- Brachial
- Radial

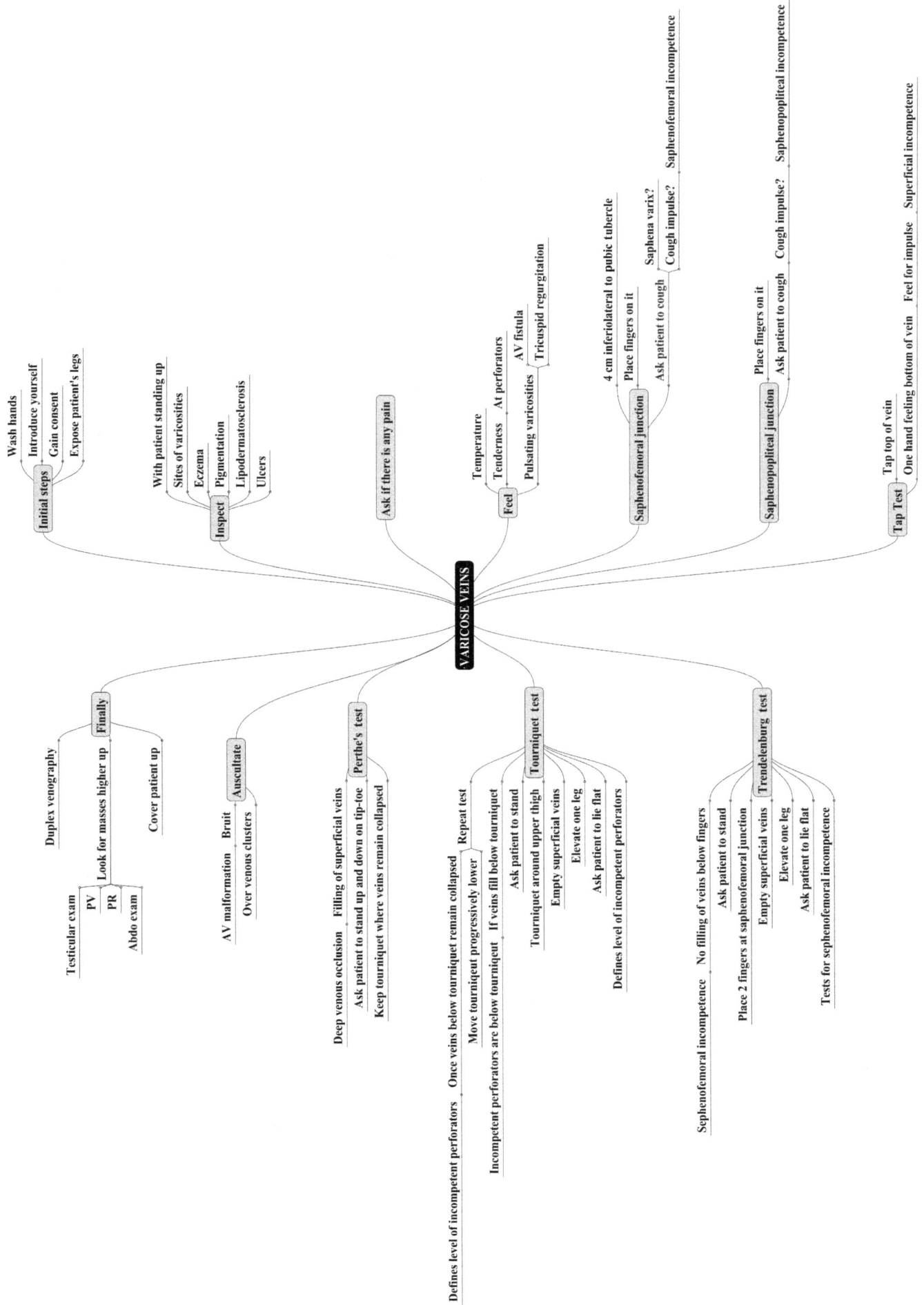

VARICOSE VEINS

Initial steps
- Wash hands
- Introduce yourself
- Gain consent
- Expose patient's legs

Inspect
- With patient standing up
- Sites of varicosities
- Eczema
- Pigmentation
- Lipodermatosclerosis
- Ulcers

Ask if there is any pain

Feel
- Temperature
- Tenderness — At perforators
- Pulsating varicosities
  - AV fistula
  - Tricuspid regurgitation

Saphenofemoral junction
- 4 cm inferiolateral to pubic tubercle
- Place fingers on it
- Ask patient to cough
  - Saphena varix?
  - Cough impulse? — Saphenofemoral incompetence

Saphenopopliteal junction
- Place fingers on it
- Ask patient to cough
  - Cough impulse? — Saphenopopliteal incompetence

Tap Test
- Tap top of vein
- One hand feeling bottom of vein
- Feel for impulse — Superficial incompetence

Finally
- Duplex venography
- Look for masses higher up
  - Testicular exam
  - PV
  - PR
  - Abdo exam
- Cover patient up

Auscultate
- AV malformation — Bruit
- Over venous clusters

Perthe's test
- Deep venous occlusion — Filling of superficial veins
- Ask patient to stand up and down on tip-toe
- Keep tourniquet where veins remain collapsed

Tourniquet test
- Defines level of incompetent perforators — Once veins below tourniquet remain collapsed — Repeat test
- Move tourniquet progressively lower
- Incompetent perforators are below tourniquet — If veins fill below tourniquet
- Ask patient to stand
- Tourniquet around upper thigh
- Empty superficial veins
- Elevate one leg
- Ask patient to lie flat
- Defines level of incompetent perforators

Trendelenburg test
- Saphenofemoral incompetence — No filling of veins below fingers
- Ask patient to stand
- Place 2 fingers at saphenofemoral junction
- Empty superficial veins
- Elevate one leg
- Ask patient to lie flat
- Tests for saphenofemoral incompetence

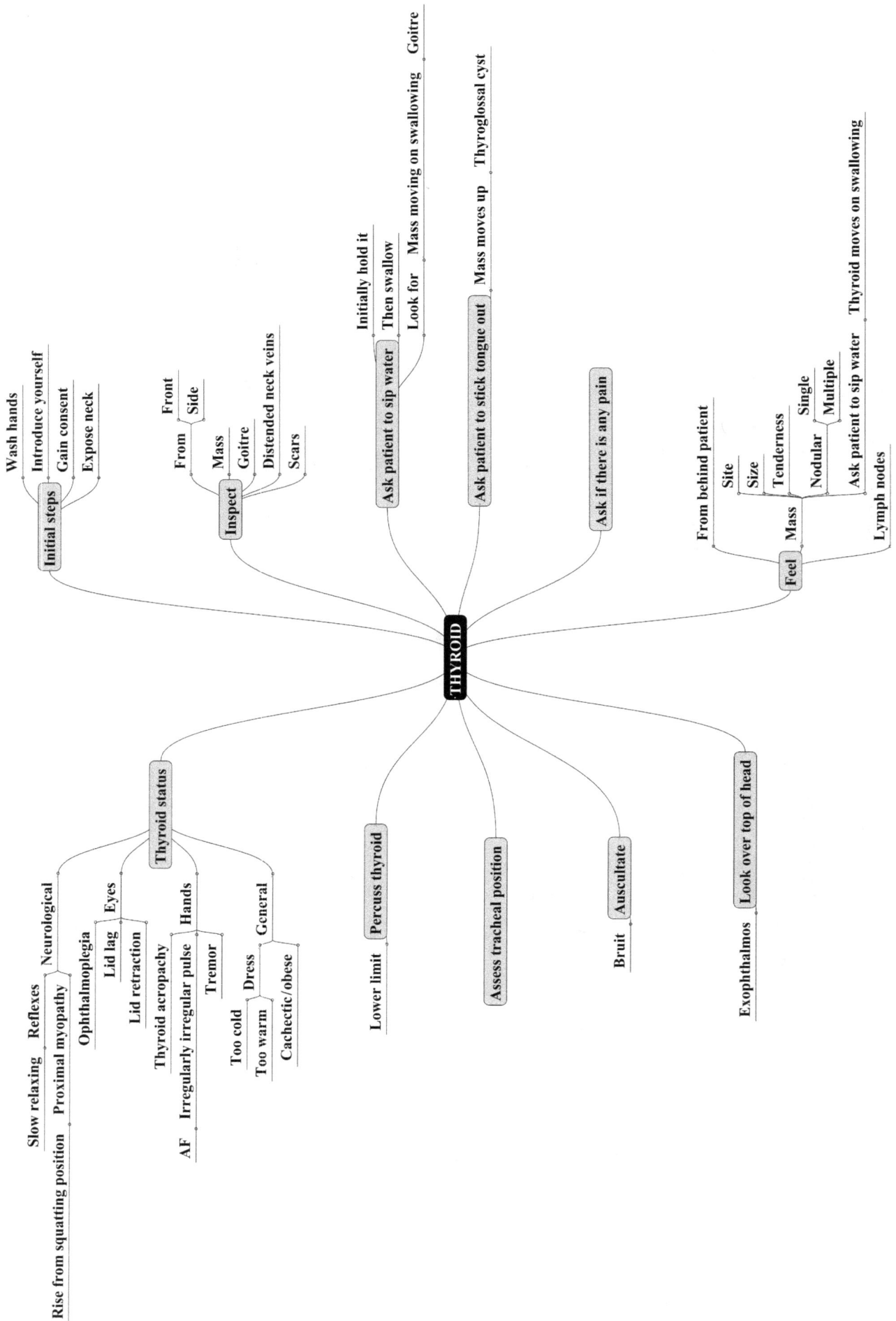

THYROID

Initial steps
- Wash hands
- Introduce yourself
- Gain consent
- Expose neck

Inspect
- From
  - Front
  - Side
- Mass
- Goitre
- Distended neck veins
- Scars

Ask patient to sip water
- Initially hold it
- Then swallow
- Look for Mass moving on swallowing   Goitre

Ask patient to stick tongue out
- Mass moves up   Thyroglossal cyst

Ask if there is any pain

Feel
- From behind patient
- Mass
  - Site
  - Size
  - Tenderness
  - Nodular
    - Single
    - Multiple
  - Ask patient to sip water   Thyroid moves on swallowing
- Lymph nodes

Thyroid status
- Neurological
  - Reflexes
    - Slow relaxing
  - Proximal myopathy
    - Rise from squatting position
- Eyes
  - Ophthalmoplegia
  - Lid lag
  - Lid retraction
- Hands
  - Thyroid acropachy
  - Irregularly irregular pulse   AF
  - Tremor
- General
  - Dress
    - Too cold
    - Too warm
  - Cachectic/obese

Percuss thyroid
- Lower limit

Assess tracheal position

Auscultate
- Bruit

Look over top of head
- Exophthalmos

INDEX*

---

* The corresponding page mumbers of the mind maps can be found on the Contents page.

www.ingramcontent.com/pod-product-compliance
Lightning Source LLC
Chambersburg PA
CBHW081108220326
41598CB00038B/7280